Strabismus
Simplified

Second Edition

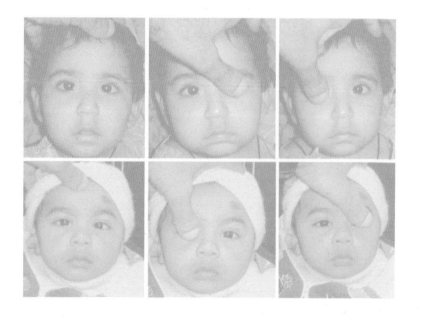

Strabismus
Simplified

Second Edition

Pradeep Insan Sharma MD FAMS
Professor and Head
Pediatric Ophthalmology, Strabismus and Oculoplasty
Officer Incharge, Orthoptics
Dr Rajendra Prasad Centre for Ophthalmic Sciences
All India Institute of Medical Sciences
New Delhi, India

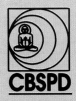

CBSPD

CBS Publishers & Distributors Pvt Ltd

New Delhi • Bengaluru • Chennai • Kochi • Kolkata • Lucknow • Mumbai
Hyderabad • Jharkhand • Nagpur • Patna • Pune • Uttarakhand

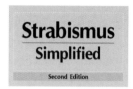

ISBN: 978-81-239-2303-1

Copyright © Author

Second Edition 2013
 Reprint: 2015, 2016, 2019, 2020, 2021, 2022
First Edition 1999
 Reprint: 2000, 2001, 2008, 2011, 2012

Published by Satish Kumar Jain and produced by Varun Jain for

CBS Publishers & Distributors Pvt Ltd
4819/XI Prahlad Street, 24 Ansari Road, Daryaganj, New Delhi 110 002, India
Ph: 011-23289259, 23266861, 23266867   Website: www.cbspd.com
Fax: 011-23243014   e-mail: delhi@cbspd.com; cbspubs@airtelmail.in.

Corporate Office: 204 FIE, Industrial Area, Patparganj, Delhi 110 092, India
Ph: 011-4934 4934   Fax: 011-4934 4935   e-mail: publishing@cbspd.com;
                        publicity@cbspd.com

Branches

• **Bengaluru:** Seema House 2975, 17th Cross, KR Road, Banasankari 2nd Stage, Bengaluru 560 070, Karnataka, India
  Ph: +91-80-26771678/79   Fax: +91-80-26771680   e-mail: bangalore@cbspd.com
• **Chennai:** 7, Subbaraya Street, Shenoy Nagar, Chennai 600 030, Tamil Nadu, India
  Ph: +91-44-26680620, 26681266   Fax: +91-44-42032115   e-mail: chennai@cbspd.com
• **Kochi:** 42/1325, 1326, Power House Road, Opp KSEB, Power House, Ernakulum Kochi 682 018, Kerala, India
  Ph: +91-484-4059061-65,67   Fax: +91-484-4059065   e-mail: kochi@cbspd.com
• **Kolkata:** 147, Hind Ceramics Compound, 1st Floor, Nilgunj Road, Belghoria, Kolkata-700056, West Bengal, India
  Ph: +033-25633055, 033-25633056   e-mail: kolkata@cbspd.com
• **Lucknow:** Basement, Khushnuma Complex, 7 Meerabai Marg (Behind Jawahar Bhawan),Lucknow-226001, UP, India
  Ph: +0522-4000032   e-mail: tiwari.lucknow@cbspd.com
• **Mumbai:** PWD Shed, Gala no 25/26, Ramchandra Bhatt Marg, Next to JJ Hospital Gate no. 2, Opp. Union Bank of India, Noorbaug, Mumbai-400009, Maharashtra, India
  Ph: 022-66661880/89   e-mail: mumbai@cbspd.com

Representatives

• Hyderabad	0-9885175004	• Jharkhand	0-9811541605	• Nagpur	0-9421945513
• Patna	0-9334159340	• Pune	0-9623451994	• Uttarakhand	0-9716462459

Printed at HT Media Ltd., Greater Noida, UP, India

to
my patients
my teachers
my parents, Mahavir–Shanti
my wife, Dr Anuradha and
my daughter, Dr Anudeepa
for their contributions in making me a better:
human being, ophthalmologist, teacher, and author

Foreword

Strabismus exists in two worlds. There is the world of the physical. In this world, after learning the patient's history, the practitioner analyzes ocular alignment and rotations, near versus distant measurements, and movement limitations. He/she then relates these findings to the patient's age, refractive error, systemic or syndromal findings, and finally reaches a diagnosis and treatment plan.

Strabismus Simplified will be of great value to anyone practising strabismus. It is concise, yet marked by extreme clarity. The superb illustrations and text bring almost every point to life; encouraging the reader to carry on and learn more about the topic. It is particularly a useful and practical work, to the point of teaching the reader about the various surgical instruments and orthoptic devices to permit a "hands on" approach to treatment.

The second world is more esoteric; almost reaching the mystical and spiritual. In this world, the practitioner analyzes the impact of strabismus on the brain by evaluating diplopia, retinal correspondence, suppression patterns, binocularity, stereopsis, and other modalities. The ophthalmologist leaves the mechanical sphere and enters the mysterious world of trying to understand how the brain functions — an almost impossible challenge. Yet *Strabismus Simplified* concisely and clearly explains these cerebral adaptations to the satisfaction of the reader which will ultimately improve patient care.

This consideration of these two worlds of strabismus is a reflection of the author. Dr. Pradeep Sharma is a man who also exists in two worlds. He is a careful and exact diagnostician employing all modalities to reach the correct diagnosis. His treatment plans are based on his long experience, his wisdom, and the latest in the medical literature. In fact, he has been a great contributor to the latest in clinical strabismus research, benefiting strabismus practitioners worldwide with his innovative and well considered publications.

Dr. Sharma's second world is that of the spiritual. He is a deeply religious and philosophical man who seeks more from life than the physical. It is perhaps this spiritual perception that allows him to have a better perspective on the physical world than most physicians.

Strabismus Simplified is a work to be cherished. If I allow my residents and fellows to pry it out of my hands, I will insist that they read it "cover to cover", refer to it often, and thus straddle both worlds of strabismus.

Dr Sherwin Isenberg MD
Ex Emeritus Editor, J AAPOS,
Gerber Professor of Pediatric Ophthalmology
Vice-Chairman, Department of Ophthalmology, and
Jules Stein Eye Institute
David Geffen School of Medicine at UCLA
Los Angeles, California, USA

Preface to the Second Edition

Twelve long years have passed since the first edition and there has been a sea-change in the interest of the ophthalmologists. The awe and fear of strabismus has evaporated and part of this could be attributed to the *Strabismus Simplified* of which there have been several reprints and a continuing demand for a new edition. This was also overdue because of a gradual change in the techniques. Moreover, the author after having an advanced fellowship in strabismus in different centres in the US has had the opportunity to work with some of the best strabismologists of the world such as Drs Robert Reinecke, Arthur Rosenbaum, Sherwin Isenberg, Joseph Calhoun, Joseph Demer, Leonard Nelson, Federico Velez, Keith McNeer and interact with Drs Marilyn Miller, Burton Kushner, David Guyton, Stephen Kraft, Richard Hertle, David Stager, Lionel Kowal, Ken Nischal and so many others from whom the author has imbibed so much. The advances in publishing technology have facilitated four-colour printing for better images to transmit the clinical material with clarity. Moreover, the stress is now in managing strabismus early in childhood and the role of testing stereopsis as also the newer surgical techniques has mandated this new edition. An accompanying CD carries some of the surgical procedures as well as common clinical tests for the beginners.

I would like to thank once again all those,whom I have thanked in the first edition, as well as all those, whom I have enumerated above and also all my strabismology colleagues in India. My gratitude is also due to Dr RC Deka, Director of All India Institute of Medical Sciences, Dr RV Azad, Chief of Dr RP Centre for Ophthalmic Sciences, AIIMS, for permitting me to venture in this task. I want to specially thank Dr Shailesh and Lt Col Dr Anirudh for helping me in proofreading and Dr Digvijay for the help in editing the CD. I also thank Mr SK Jain, Managing Director, Mr YN Arjuna, Senior Director — Publishing, Editorial and Publicity, of CBS Publishers & Distributors and their team especially Mrs Ritu Chawla, Mrs Jyoti Kaur, Mr Neeraj, Mr Kshirod and all others whom I have not been able to name due to lack of word-space. I hope the readers will find this edition more useful than ever before. If there are some errors, I would like to apologize and expect the readers to communicate to me. I remain:

still Strabismologically yours
Pradeep Insan Sharma

Preface to the First Edition

An old story comes to my mind of a boy who found learning Sanskrit grammar too tough and being repeatedly reprimanded by his Guru decided to run away. So many of us have contemplated the same while coming to terms with strabismology or mathematics. And things we find difficult, we develop an aversion and convince ourselves that it is not important. But this school-drop-out Varadraj, that I was talking about, was different. He sat beside a well and was surprised to see the dents cast in the stone by the earthen pots and pulley rope. He decided to return to his school with determined perseverance. He not only mastered the Sanskrit grammar of Panini, but brought out a simplified version called "Laghu siddhant kaumidi", which made the job of other pursuants much easier.

Strabismus has generally been confounded and many of us have avoided, despised or denied its importance for the lack of our comprehension. But in ophthalmic practice, the most common problems are related with problems of binocular vision or ocular motility. Next to cataract surgery, squint surgery is the most common surgery performed by ophthalmic practitioners. We cannot evade it. In fact, we would love it, for it is the least demanding except for a little understanding. There are far fewer facts to memorise by rote compared to other specialities. It is more or less like mathematics, which serves all out life, once we comprehend it.

The attempt of this book is to simplify strabismus, demystify the myths surrounding it. That's why the title *Strabismus Simplified*. I had the great fortune to learn the tricks of the trade from Dr. Prem Prakash, one of pioneers of strabismology in this country. The sweet fruits of this 16 years of association I offer for you all to share. Over the years I have also had the opportunity to interact with strabismologists like Drs. Hanumantha Reddy, S.K. Narang, B.S. Goel, D.K. Sen, Vimala Menon, T.S. Surendran, P.Vijaylakhsmi, Ravi Thomas, Kamini Audich, K. Mc Neer, Dr. RD Reinecke, MT Miller, AO Ciancia, S Isenberg and many others. In addition I have liberally acquired information from standard textbooks: *Binocular Vision and Ocular Motility* by GK Von Noorden, *Atlas of Strabismology* by EH Helveston, *Practical Orthoptics* by T Keith Lyle and KC Wybar, *Adler's Physiology* by W Hart and several important monographs from various journals. This book is a crystallization of thoughts instilled from so many quarters. I thank them all from the core of my heart.

My gratitude is also due to Prof PK Dave, Director and Prof MC Maheshwari, Dean of All India Institute of Medical Sciences, Prof VK Dada, Chief, Dr RP Centre for Ophthalmic Sciences, AIIMS, for permitting me to venture in this task. The idea of writing a book actually came in from Prof VK Dada. I thank all my faculty colleagues and residents.

Special thanks are due to Dr Ravindranath, Mrs Kulwant and Mr MM Sachdeva, Mr Harminder Singh, of Dr RP Centre for Ophthalmic Sciences. The artist Mr. Sunil Dutt deserves tribute for beautifying the sketches that were drafted by me. And above all Mr Malhotra, Mr Naresh Malik, Dr Ramesh Kumar, Dr Anil Sharga and Maya Kandpal of Modern Publishers deserve my gratitude for taking pains to publish this book.

Strabismologically yours
Pradeep Insan Sharma

Contents

1. An Overview of Strabismology   1

Introduction to binocular vision, basic terms, types of strabismus, consequences of strabismus and their adaptations, role of a strabismologist.

2. Applied Anatomy and Physiology of Extraocular Muscles   9

Anatomy of extraocular muscles, their origins, insertions and other characteristics, nerves supplying them, action of extraocular muscles, agonists–synergists, antagonists. Hering's law, Sherrington's law, Donder's and Listing's law, the physiology of eye movements: pulse step and ramp innervations, torsional eye movements, physiological basis of strabismus surgery, length-tension curves, Muscle pulleys.

3. Related Aspects   23

Histopathology of extraocular muscles, embryology. accommodation—convergence relationship, types of eye movements, relevant neuroanatomy.

4. The Physiology of Binocular Vision, Amblyopia and Anomalous Retinal Correspondence   34

Understanding sensory aspects, localization in space, horopter, Panum's area, stereopsis, monocular cues, binocular vision and squint, adaptations to squint: motor and sensory. amblyopia—its types, clinical features and pathophysiology, anomalous retinal correspondence: pre-requisites, diagnosis by various tests.

5. The Preliminary Examination and Assessment of Visual Acuity   52

History taking, refraction, cycloplegia, examination of anterior and posterior segment, fundus examination for torsion. Visual acuity, types of visual acuity, methods of assessment in children, hyperacuity, vernier acuity, stereoacuity, screening methods in children.

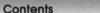

Brown's superior oblique sheath syndrome, strabismus fixus, congenital muscle fibrosis, dysthyroid orbitomyopathy, other restrictive conditions.

CD Contents

A. Clinical Skills Videos
1. Covertest to confirm manifest squint
2. Detection of latent deviation by uncover test
3. Alternate cover-uncover
4. Alternate PBCT
5. Simultaneous PBCT
6. Mod horizontal Lang test for stereopsis

B. Surgical Videos
1. Recession resection horizontal recti
2. Adjustable important steps
3. Inf oblique Mod E&N
4. Inf oblique compilation of different techniques
5. Posterior tenectomy of Sup oblique
6. Sup oblique tucking
7. Adjustable Harada-Ito
8. Faden with recession
9. Periosteal anchoring of LR
10. Partial vert rectus transpositioning

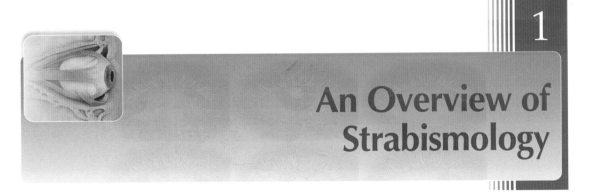

An Overview of Strabismology

Binocular single vision (BSV) is one of the hallmarks of the human race that has bestowed on it the supremacy in the hierarchy of the animal kingdom. It is not without reason that about 60% of the brain tissue and more than half of the twelve cranial nerves subserve the eyes. BSV is accomplished by a perfect sensorimotor coordination of the two eyes both at rest and during movement. The two two-dimensional images of an object of interest formed at the fovea of each eye, transmitted to the respective visual cortex are processed and perceived as one three-dimensional (3-D) percept (Fig. 1.1). This requires constant and controlled activity of the appropriate eye muscles to maintain fixation of the two eye-cameras on the concerned object, irrespective of the movement between it and the observer. It also requires the accommodational mechanism to maintain clear view even as the object moves closer or farther.

EXTRAOCULAR MUSCLES

Each eye is equipped with six extraocular muscles (EOM) for this purpose (Figs 1.2 and 1.3).

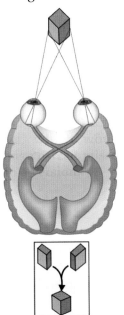

Fig. 1.1: A schematic diagram showing how we see the three-dimensional world. Inset shows two two-dimensional figures seen by each eye, having some disparity are fused together to become one three-dimensional percept.

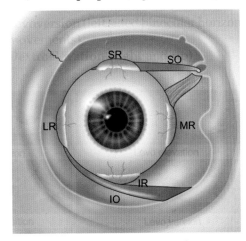

Fig. 1.2: Front view of right eye in orbit. Superior rectus: SR, Inferior rectus: IR, lateral rectus: LR, Medial rectus: MR, Superior oblique: SO and Inferior oblique: IO.

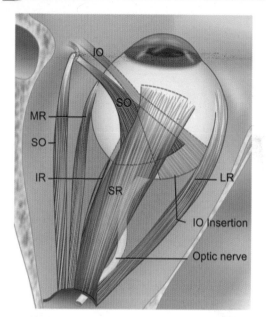

Fig. 1.3: An overview of right eye from top.

- Two horizontal recti: **Medial** and **lateral recti**.
- Two vertical recti: **Superior** and **inferior recti**.
- Two obliques: **Superior** and **inferior obliques**.

PLANES AND AXES

These six EOM together allow each eye free motility in all the three dimensions in innumerable planes and axes. For convenience we take three planes of eye movement, **(Listing's planes)** and their three respective axes **(Fick's axes)** perpendicular to the planes: Listing's plane is vertical plane that includes 'X', 'Z' and oblique axes that pass through center of eye (Fig. 1.4).

- **Horizontal plane:** Horizontal eye movements around Z-axis
- **Vertical plane:** Vertical eye movements around X-axis (in three vertical planes: eyes in primary position, eyes in adduction and eyes in abduction)
- **Torsional:** Torsional eye movements around Y-axis, which is anteroposterior.

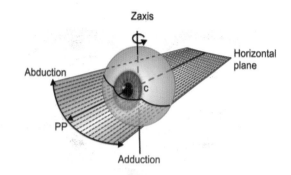

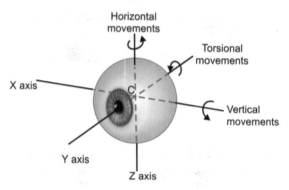

Fig. 1.4: Planes and axes for different eye movements.

DUCTIONS AND VERSIONS

The eye movements when tested uniocularly are called **ductions** and when tested binocularly are called **versions**.

Ductions

Ductions in the three planes mentioned above are (Fig. 1.5):

- **Adduction** (nasally directed horizontal movement)
- **Abduction** (temporally directed horizontal movement)
- **Sursumduction** or **elevation** (upward movement): It can be in primary position, in adduction, or in abduction.
- **Deorsumduction** or **depression** (downward movement): Like sursumduction it can also be in primary position, in adduction, or in abduction.
- **Incycloduction** or **intorsion** (nasally directed tilting of 12 o'clock meridian)

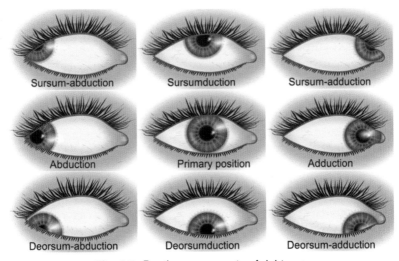

Fig. 1.5: Duction movements of right eye.

- **Excycloduction** or **extorsion** (temporally directed tilting of 12 o'clock meridian)

Ductions give a good idea of the ability of excursion of eyes in different directions, but have a disadvantage in case of paresis (partial loss of power of eye muscles), when normal ductions may be observed. This is due to extra innervation called in to compensate for the paresis. In case of versions, however, this extra innervation also goes to the yoke muscle of the other eye, which would show an overaction. **Thus a paresis missed on duction is picked up in a version.**

Versions

Versions are binocular eye movements that are in the same direction (conjugate eye movements). Binocular eye movements in the opposite directions (**disjugate** eye movements) are called **vergences**.

Versions are labelled in the three diagnostic planes (Fig. 1.6) as.
- **Dextroversion** (right sided binocular horizontal movements)
- **Levoversion** (left sided binocular horizontal movements)
- **Dextroelevation** (right and up)

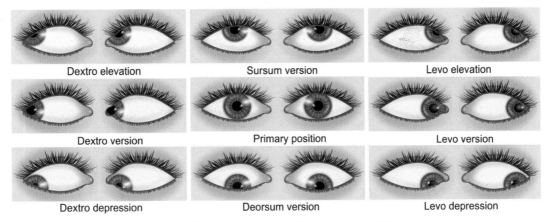

Fig. 1.6: Version movements in nine gaze positions.

- **Levoelevation** (left and up)
- **Dextro-depression** (right and down)
- **Levo-depression** (left and down).

Other positions also used are: Sursum-version (straight up), deorsum-version (straight down), and for torsional movements:

- **Dextrocycloversion** (right eye extorts, left eye intorts),
- **Levocycloversion** (right eye intorts, left eye extorts).

Vergences

Vergences are **convergence** (both eye move nasally) and **divergence** (both eye move temporally) in the horizontal plane (Fig. 1.7).

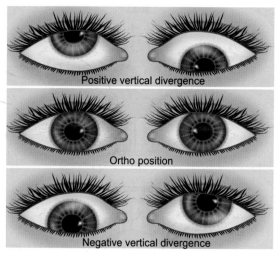

Fig. 1.8: Vertical divergence.

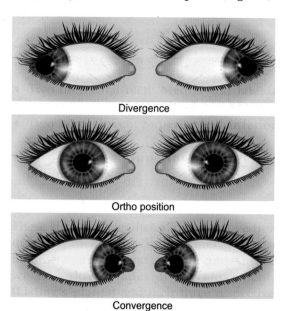

Fig. 1.7: Horizontal vergences.

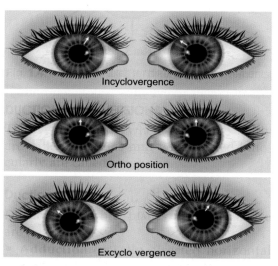

Fig. 1.9: Cyclovergence.

Positive vertical divergence (right eye up, left eye down) and **negative vertical divergence** (right eye down, left eye up) are the vergences in the vertical plane (Fig. 1.8).

Incyclovergence (both eyes intort) and **excyclovergence** (both eyes extort) are the torsional vergences (Fig. 1.9).

Vergences are very important as they can be helpful in keeping a tendency of squint under control **(fusional vergences)**.

AGONISTS AND ANTAGONISTS

It is obvious that the two eyes work in unison as one unit. The respective extraocular muscles which are working in pairs, said to be "yoked" are called **synergists** or **agonists** which may be of the same eye **(ipsilateral)** or of the other eye **(contralateral)**. The opposing muscle is called the **antagonist**. For example, due to a dextroversion, right lateral rectus has left medial rectus as its contralateral synergist and right medial rectus as its ipsilateral antagonist. However, for a convergence the right and left medial recti become the synergists and the two lateral recti become the antagonists.

It would be desired that for the two eyes to look at the same object, the synergists should move equally in the desired direction. Indeed this happens so, and this is governed by the **Hering's law of equal innervation which states that for any movement the synergists receive equal and simultaneous innervation. In addition the respective antagonists are inhibited to facilitate a smooth and unobstructed movement, inhibition not innervation the Sherrington's law of reciprocal inhibition.**

CORRESPONDENCE

Having two eyes would necessitate a normal sensory system to collect the two visual images at the corresponding visual cortices and further to co-ordinate the two informations to make a single percept. Each fovea has a primary visual direction (the direction of its straight-ahead gaze), and the two fovea share a **common visual direction**. Any object imaged on the visual direction of either of the fovea would be superimposed and seen in the common visual direction, which is of neither eyes but of an imaginary **cyclopean eye** (Fig. 1.10).

The two foveas are said to have a **normal retinal correspondence (bifoveal correspondence)**. The other areas of the retina have a relationship with their fovea, and also correspond with a specific retinal area of the other eye **(corresponding point or area)**. Objects imaged on the corresponding areas are seen binocularly single (Fig. 1.11).

An imaginary plane on which the corresponding points are projected is called the **horopter**. A little area on either sides of the horopter, which allows the sensory fusion despite the disparity is called the **Panum's area of fusion**. This fusion despite disparity,

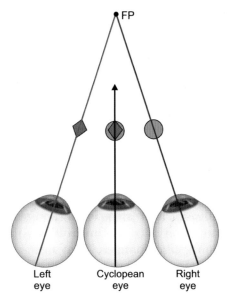

Fig. 1.10: Bifoveal correspondence with normal alignment while fixating on a fixation point. FP two objects located separately in space but on the visual directions appear in one line of common visual direction of cyclopean eye.

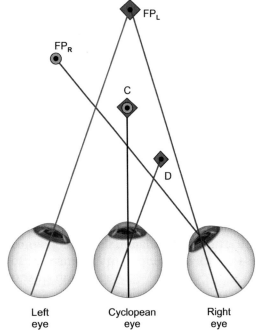

Fig. 1.11: Bifoveal correspondence with convergent strabismus of right eye. Confusion (C) due to two fixation points of each eye, FP$_L$ & FP$_R$. Diplopia (D) due to projection of the FP$_L$ in right eye.

however, produces a three-dimensional vision **(stereopsis)**.

All the other areas are said to be disparate points and objects imaged on the disparate points are seen as double **(diplopia)**. This diplopia is binocular and is not perceived under monocular conditions.

STRABISMUS

Normally the two visual axes meet at the point of regard or the object of attention. The eyes are said to be in alignment (**orthophoria** or **orthotropia**). Due to some unfortunate reason the two visual axes may not be aligned to the point of regard, that is one eye fixates at the point but the other eye does not. A **strabismus or squint or heterotropia** results. When this tendency is overcome by the fusional vergences the subject does not manifest squint. This **latent squint** is called **heterophoria**. When the squint is present at times and controlled at other times, it is called **intermittent** as against a **constant** squint.

Classification of Strabismus

The strabismus may be **concomitant** (also called **comitant)** when the deviations are equal in all the different gazes, and **incomitant** when the deviations are more in one gaze than the other. The concomitant strabismus is classified as: **horizontal, vertical, or torsional**. The horizontal strabismus may be **convergent: esotropia (ET), or divergent: exotropia (XT)**. The corresponding latent strabismus or heterophorias are called: **esophoria(E) and exophoria(X),** and the intermittent heterotropias are called: **intermittent esotropia E(T)** and **intermittent exotropia X(T)**.

Esotropias are further divided into **accommodative, nonaccommodative** and **partially accommodative** depending on the role of accommodative element in its causation. A more detailed classification will be described in the relevant chapters.

Vertical concomitant strabismus is described as **hypertropia** (upward deviation) and **hypotropia** (downward deviation). But since whenever one eye is hypertropic, the other eye would be hypotropic, by convention vertical strabismus is designated by the hypertropic eye, that is we would talk of right hypertropia–RHT (right eye up) and left hypertropia–LHT (left eye up). In short we may also describe the squint as R/L or L/R.

Torsional squints or **cyclotropia** or **cyclodeviations** are described as: **incyclotropia** (12 o'clock meridian intorted or turned in) or **excyclotropia** (12 o'clock meridian extorted or turned out) of the respective eye.

The **incomitant strabismus** can be subdivided into **paralytic, restrictive** and **spastic,** depending on the cause of underaction in the first two conditions and overaction in the third type. The paralytic type can be **neurogenic (supranuclear, infranuclear** or **nuclear)** or myogenic. Specific nerve lesions are designated as the nerve supplying it like: **third nerve (oculomotor), fourth nerve (trochlear),** or **sixth nerve (abducens)** paralysis.

A **paralysis** implies a total involvement and **paresis** implies a partial involvement.

Consequences of Strabismus

Whenever a strabismus occurs, only one eye can fix at the object of regard, the other gets fixated elsewhere so that the two fovea receive two different images, each producing rival cortical perceptions, this is called **confusion**. Fortunately the cortex has strong foveal rivalry which immediately decides for one perception and suppresses the other image, so that this "confusion" actually causes no confusion. Because of the misalignment of the eyes the same object is imaged on some other retinal area of the other eye, which has a different projection value in space, so that an object gets projected at two different positions in space, this is called **diplopia** or double vision. Diplopia is a troublesome thing, the asset of binocular vision of the two eyes for once becomes a liability.

The **motor system** tries to overcome the consequences of strabismus by **fusion,** converting a tropia into phoria, if that is possible, as in intermittent exotropia. When the fusion mechanism is overwhelmed, and if there is incomitance, that is the deviation is less in a particular gaze position, a **head posture** is assumed to once again regain the paradise lost. Head posture may at times be assumed such that the deviation is aggravated so much so that the other image falls in the retinal periphery, which can be easily ignored. Unusually the other image may fall (or made to fall in an incomitant esotropia) on the **blind spot** of the retina alleviating the double image. These are called the **motor adaptations of strabismus**. In adult onset strabismus these are the usual "remedial" steps.

The **sensory system** also gears up to face the challenge of a strabismus by the **sensory adaptations**. These are mainly two: **suppression** and **anomalous retinal correspondence**. In suppression the cortex disregards the other image from cognition. Thus under binocular conditions the other eye does not actively participate in perception, though each eye may retain its full potential under monocular conditions. Suppression is generally possible easily when the other image is weak, that is imaged in the retinal periphery. But when the deviation is small angle, the other image being strong cannot be easily set aside by suppression, so the sensory system tries to have a readjustment, so that the fovea of one eye can now have a correspondence with the extra-foveal area which shares the same image due to the strabismus. This is called **harmonious anomalous retinal correspondence**. This is like recalibrating the interocular relationship (*resetting the scale to adjust for the zero error*). An analogy may be simple to understand: if you have a difference of opinion with some one, you ignore him if he is ignorable, but otherwise you try to readjust your relationship with him. The sensory adaptations are possible only during the stage of plasticity of the neurodevelopment, that is early childhood, up to 6–7 years of age. In adults though suppression does not occur a **visual ignorance** is usually possible to avoid the troublesome double image.

The suppression in childhood can be **facultative** or **obligatory,** the former is only under the binocular conditions, with no residual effect under monocular conditions. The obligatory suppression carries on under monocular conditions also, like an undesirable hangover. The effect of the obligatory suppression is **amblyopia,** which results in a functional diminution of vision of the suppressed eye. Thus amblyopia would be most likely to occur in the sensitive age group of plasticity of the neural development.

THE ROLE OF A STRABISMOLOGIST

Let us now understand the role of a strabismologist in dealing with his patients which may be in any age group but more so in the pediatric age group. This is a desirable thing from the view of maximal effectivity as binocular vision can be ensured only in the younger age group, the younger the better. A strabismologist's role is:

1. Assessment of **vision of each eye** and proper correction of refractive error, if any, by suitable optical means in order to achieve good, equal and maintainable visual acuity in each eye. This is to restore and maintain a normal balance between the two eyes so that a normal binocular vision with good stereopsis is maintained.

2. Assessment of the **accommodation** and **convergence relationship**, and correction of the same if any required, with glasses, prisms or exercises.

3. Defect of vision in the form of **suppression** or **amblyopia** with or without eccentric fixation may require occlusion and other measures to correct amblyopia in order to restore and maintain equal vision in both eyes.

4. When the motor fusional reserves are low, orthoptic treatment in the form of fusional exercises, with anti-suppression measures when required. This is to overcome the heterotropia and maintain heterophoria, so that the two eyes can function together asymptomatically.

5. And finally the assessment and correction of significant ocular deviations by prisms, chemical denervation or surgery on one or more of extraocular muscles as may be required to re-establish the normal ocular motor co-ordination.

6. Many cases of squint may have systemic problems like thyroid disorder, or may have an underlying neurological disturbance, over-looking of which can be fatal for the patient, and a gross negligence on the part of the doctor. A high index of suspicion, attention to details and a thorough but relevant investigation is desired.

Thus the **practice of strabismology** shall entail the clinician taking up the role of a pediatrician, a refractionist, an orthoptist, a neuro-ophthalmologist and last but not the least an eye-surgeon with the ability to investigate, interpret and integrate all the ocular and systemic findings for re-establishing the three-dimensional world of the patient, *to regain the paradise lost.*

Suggested Reading

1. Noorden GK von. Binocular Vision and Ocular Motility. Theory and Management of Strabismus, Fifth Edition. The CV Mosby Company, St. Louis 1996.

2. Lyle TK and Wybar KC Lyle and Jackson's Practical Orthoptics in the Treatment of Squint (and other anomalies a binocular vision) 15th Edition. HK Lewis & Co. Ltd., London, 1970.

3. Helveston EH. Surgical Management of Strabismus. An Atlas of Strabismus Surgery ed. 4. St. Louis, 1978.

4. Duke Elder S and Wybar K System of Ophthalmology, vol. 6, Ocular Motility and Strabismus, St. Louis. 1973, Mosby—Year Book Inc.

5. Lancaster WB "Terminology" with extended comments on the position of rest and fixation. In Allen JH editor. Strabismus Ophthalmic Symposium St. Louis. 1950. The CV Mosby Co.

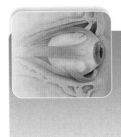

Applied Anatomy and Physiology of Extraocular Muscles

An appraisal of relevant applied anatomy and physiology of the extraocular muscles is pertinent before we undertake the examination.

ANATOMY

There are six extraocular muscles: Four recti and two obliques on either sides. They are named based on their location, thus: **medial, lateral, superior** and **inferior recti;** and **superior** and **inferior, obliques** (Figs 2.1 and 2.2).

The distance between the adjacent recti varies between different sets of the recti muscles. It is about 7–8 mm (this limits the

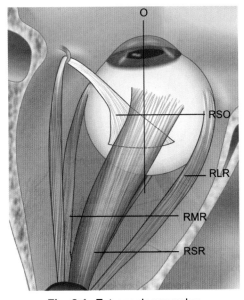

Fig. 2.1: Extraocular muscles.

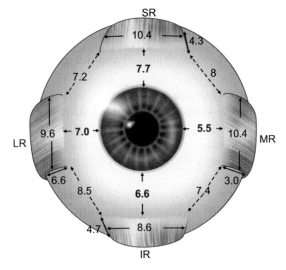

Fig. 2.2: Facts and figures of the four recti muscles of EOM insertions in relation to limbus, and to each other, as also tendon length and tendon width.

transposition horizontally or vertically). The table summarizes the anatomic features of the four recti (Table 2.1).

The Recti

All the recti take origin from the annulus of Zinn, which surrounds the optic canal and in part the superior orbital fissure. While the medial rectus runs almost straight, parallel to the sagittal plane, the lateral rectus runs anterolaterally. It makes an angle of about 40°–45° with the sagittal plane. The two vertical recti make an angle of about 23° with

Table 2.1: Anatomic features of the four recti

Muscles	Medial rectus	Lateral rectus	Superior rectus	Inferior rectus
Length of muscle	37.7 (32.0–44.5)	36.3 (27.0–42.0)	37.3 (31.0–45.0)	37.0 (33.0–42.5)
Length of tendon	3.0 (1.0–7.0)	7.2 (4.0–11.0)	4.3 (2.0–6.0)	4.7 (3.0–7.0)
Width of insertion	10.4 (8.0–13.0)	9.6 (8.0–13.0)	10.4 (7.0–12.0)	8.6 (7.0–12.0)
Distance of limbus from mid-insertion	5.3 (3.6–7.0)	6.9 (5.4–8.5)	7.9 (6.2–9.2)	6.8 (4.8–8.5)

Note: All figures in mm, mean and ranges in parentheses
Courtesy: Length of muscle and tendon from Lang and co-workers and Distance from limbus from Apt as cited in von Noorden's Binocular Vision and Ocular Motility,1996

the sagittal plane. The recti then curve around the globe strapping it, the lateral rectus the most, and the medial rectus the least. They finally get inserted anterior to the equator, at a varying distance from the limbus (Table 2.1). These insertions form the **spiral of Tillaux.**

The Obliques

The two oblique muscles differ from the recti in taking their functional origin from the anteronasal part of the orbit. They run posterolaterally at an angle of 100° to 105° to the vertical recti. On contraction, they would pull the globe nasally and outwards. This is an important fact that on slippage, they are not lost retro-orbitally, like the recti. When taut, they do not retract the globe. And to test their tautness during forced duction test (FDT) the globe needs to be pushed backwards!

The **superior oblique** actually arises from the superomedial part of the optic foramen, runs parallel close to the upper part of the medial wall up to the trochlea, where it turns around and runs posterolaterally making an angle of 54° with the sagittal plane. For practical purposes, the **trochlea** acts like its functional origin, and is formed medially by the trochlear fossa of frontal bone and laterally by a cartilaginous tissue. A bursa like structure between the saddle and the superior oblique tendon is postulated. Anomalies of this structure result in Brown's superior oblique sheath syndrome. About 10 mm of the distal **pre-trochlear** part, the **trochlear** part (4–6 mm),

and the **post-trochlear** part is tendinous. The post-trochlear part becomes fan-shaped, passes beneath the superior rectus and gets attached posterior to the equator. The anterior and lateral end is about 4 mm posterior to the lateral end of superior rectus. The posterior and medial end is about 14 mm posterior to the medial end of superior rectus. The width of the insertion is about 11 mm (range 7–18 mm). **The posterior fibres of the fan are primarily responsible for depression and the anterior fibres are responsible for intorsion.** The total length is 60 mm, 40 mm being pre-trochlear and 20 mm post-trochlear. It is the longest extraocular muscle (Fig. 2.3).

The **inferior oblique** muscle is the shortest of all, just 37 mm with virtually no tendon or just about 1–2 mm. Its origin is in the

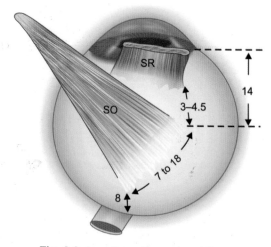

Fig. 2.3: Insertion of superior oblique.

anteroinferior angle of the bony orbit in a shallow depression in the orbital plate of the maxilla. From here it runs posterolaterally 51° to the sagittal plane, passing below the inferior rectus, inserting in a fan shaped manner. The insertion is about 9 mm wide (range: 5–14 mm). Its anterior end is located about 9.5 mm behind and 1–2 mm lateral to the macula. Some of its fibres merge with the fascia surrounding the optic nerve, responsible for pain on elevation in optic neuritis. **Its posterior fibres are primarily responsible for elevation and the anterior fibres for extorsion** (Fig. 2.4).

The fascia of the inferior oblique and inferior rectus get meshed to form the suspensory ligament of Lockwood (Fig. 2.5).

Some of the fibres of the lower lid are also attached to this and a large recession of IR without separating these fibres causes drooping of the lower lid. Similarly with a large resection there is a narrowing of the palpebral fissure. A similar effect, though less pronounced is seen in the position of the upper lid on large recession and resections of the superior rectus, without separating the

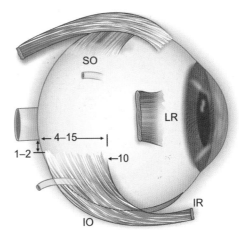

Fig. 2.4: Insertion of inferior oblique.

fibrous attachment between the upper lid and the superior rectus. A recession causing a retraction and a resection causing a ptosis.

Tenon's Capsule (Fig. 2.6). If the globe is enucleated the anterior orifice of Tenon's capsule is seen, attached to the sclera 2 mm from limbus. The posterior orifice is fused with the optic nerve sheaths. The muscles enter through slits and vortex veins make small openings.

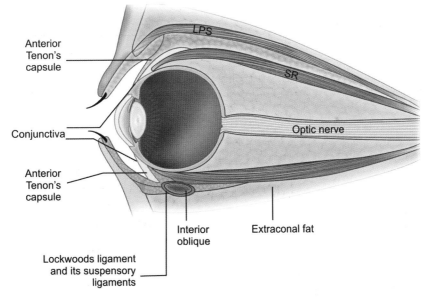

Fig. 2.5: A longitudinal section of the eye showing the fascial connections.

2

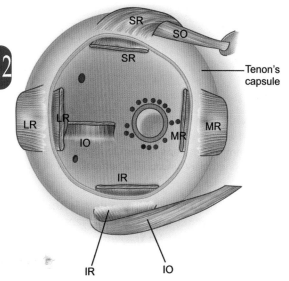

Fig. 2.6: Anterior and posterior orifice of Tenon's capsule (Charpy, 1912).

Each extraocular muscle has an extracapsular (outside Tenon's) and intracapsular portions. In the extracapsular portion it is encased in a muscle sheath: a reflection of Tenon's capsule running backwards for a distance of 10–12 mm. The muscle sheaths of the four recti are connected by a fascial formation called the intermuscular septum. The intracapsular portion has no muscle sheath.

Blood Supply

All the recti and superior oblique get their vascular supply and innervation on its inner aspect at the junction of the middle and distal third. The inferior oblique gets its innervation and blood supply as it crosses the nasal border of the inferior rectus. The obliques do not contribute to the anterior ciliary circulation Each of the recti, except the lateral rectus, contributes two anterior ciliary arteries (Fig. 2.7).

The lateral rectus gives only one. In addition there is a significant contribution by the medial long ciliary artery on the medial

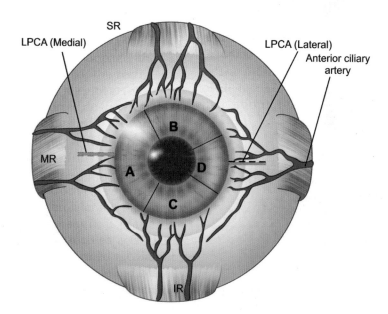

Fig. 2.7: Anterior segment circulation. The anterior ciliary arteries, two per recti except lateral rectus. The long posterior ciliary arteries medial and lateral also contribute. The perfusion of sectors of iris are (A): medial LPCA and anterior ciliary (AC) of MR, (B): AC of SR, (C): AC of IR, (D): AC of LR and AC of SR and IR overlap with very little contribution by lateral LPCA.

aspect, sparing the burden from the medial rectus to some extent. But the supply of the lateral rectus anterior ciliary artery is crucial, **thus a surgery on the two vertical recti along with the lateral rectus can cause anterior segment ischemia.**

Nerve Supply

The **oculomotor nerve** (third cranial) supplies to superior rectus, medial rectus, inferior rectus, inferior oblique and also the levator palpebrae superioris and the intraocular muscles: sphincter pupillae, dilator pupillae and ciliary muscles. The **abducens nerve** (sixth cranial) supplies the lateral rectus. And the **trochlear nerve** (fourth cranial) supplies the superior oblique (Fig. 2.8).

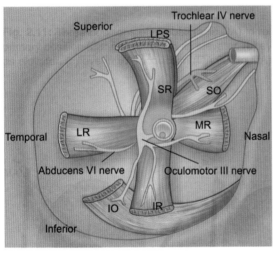

Fig. 2.8: Nerve supply to extraocular muscles, Oculomotor (IIIN) superior division (LPS, SR), inferior division (MR, IR, IO, ciliary ganglion); Abducens (VI N) LR, and Trochlear (IV N) (SO).

THE PHYSIOLOGY OF EYE MOVEMENTS

If one keeps in mind the anatomy of the extraocular muscles, the understanding of their actions appears simple. The primary action of the **horizontal recti** is to perform abduction (lateral rectus) and adduction (medial rectus) in the primary position. But

in the extreme upgaze, they would have a vector acting downwards also causing depression as a secondary action. Similarly in extreme downgaze they would also cause elevation as a secondary action (Figs 2.9 and 2.10).

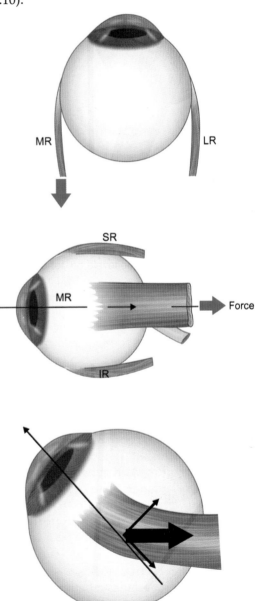

Fig. 2.9: Horizontal muscles act in horizontal plane. If eyeball elevated the horizontal force has significant vertical vector component.

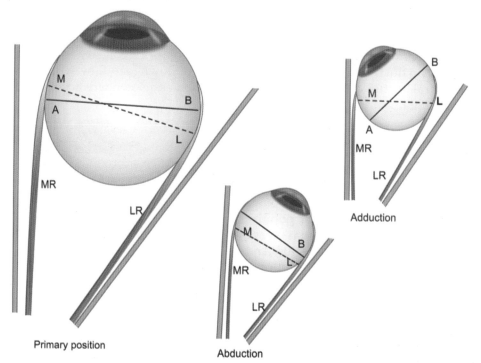

Fig. 2.10: Anatomical and functional equators. Anatomical equator, AB is the widest horizontal diameter, about 13–14 mm from limbus. Functional equator, ML, varies in different gaze positions depending on the arc of contacts. M is the tangential point for MR and L, that of LR. In the primary position M is 2 mm anterior to A and L is 2–4 mm posterior to B, the functional equator ML is obliquely placed. In adduction the arc of contact for MR decreases and increases for LR. In abduction reverse occurs.

The **vertical recti** and the **obliques** have overlapping functions and can be termed as **cyclo-vertical muscles**.

The **superior rectus** primarily acts as an elevator in the **primary position**, its secondary action being intorsion. When **abducted 23°** it is a pure elevator. And when adducted it becomes more and more an intorter, especially if the eyeball were to be **adducted 67°** it would be a pure intorter (this is a hypothetical situation as the eyeball cannot be adducted as much) (Fig. 2.11).

The inferior rectus, a depressor in the primary position becomes a better depressor in abduction and on adduction it becomes a better extorter.

The superior oblique (Fig. 2.12) is primarily an intorter in the primary position, if adducted it becomes more and more a depressor. When **adducted 54°**, it becomes a pure depressor, remember superior oblique is a depressor because of its insertion being posterior to the equator. When abducted progressively it becomes an intorter, and it is a **pure intorter at 36° abduction**. Similarly the **inferior oblique**, primarily an elevator and extorter becomes a pure elevator at 51° adduction, and a pure extorter in 39° abduction.

In the **primary position** the elevation is done by both the superior rectus and the inferior oblique in a 60–40 ratio. And depression by the inferior rectus and the superior oblique in a 60–40 ratio. Both the recti act as adductors in the primary position and **adduction**, but act as abductors when abducted more than 23°.

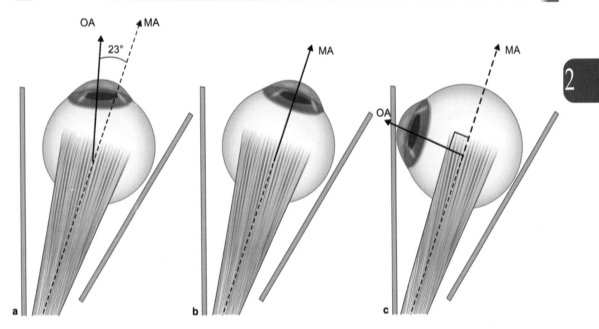

Fig. 2.11: Three positions of eyeball (axis OA) in relation to muscle axis (MA) of superior rectus. (a) eye in primary position (23° nasal). SR main elevator, (b) eye in 23° abduction (aligned with MA) SR 100% effective as elevator, (c) eye in 67° adduction (OA 90° to MA) SR pure intorter, no elevation.

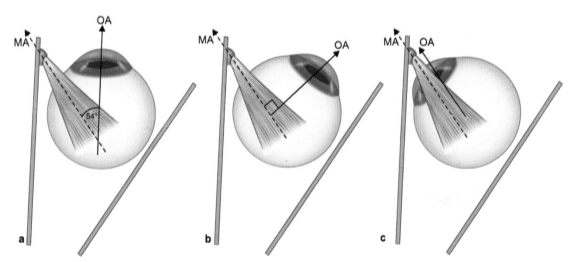

Fig. 2.12: Three positions of eyeball (axis OA) in relation to the muscle axis (MA) of superior oblique; (a) eye in primary position (OA 23° temporal to MA) so acts as an intorter mainly, also has depression, (b) eye in 36° abduction (OA 90° to MA) so acts as a pure intorter, no depressor effect, (c) eye in 54° adduction (OA parallel to MA) so acts as a pure depressor, no intorsion.

2

Actions of cyclovertical muscles			
Muscle/eye position	Primary position	Adduction	Abduction
Superior rectus	Elevator primarily also intorter and adductor	Weaker elevator better intorter	Better elevator weaker intorter
Inferior rectus	Depressor primarily also extorter and adductor	Weaker depressor better extorter	Better depression weaker extorter
Superior oblique	Intorter primarily also depressor and abductor	Mainly depressor weaker intorter	Better intorter
Inferior oblique	Extorter primarily also elevator and abductor	Mainly elevator weaker extorter	Better extorter

Both the obliques act as abductors in the primary position, in abduction as well as in most part of adduction. They would become adductors if the eyeball was adducted more than 60°!

Yoke Muscles

To co-ordinate the movements of the two eyes one muscle of each eye acts together for any eye movement, these two muscles are said to be **yoke muscles** or **synergists** or **agonists** (**Table 2.2**). For example, the right medial rectus and left lateral rectus are yoke muscles for a levoversion. And the right superior rectus and left inferior oblique are yoke muscles for a dextro-elevation. And for a convergence the two medial recti become the yoke muscles.

Hering's Law of Motor Correspondence

The Hering's law states that for an binocular movement the corresponding (yoke) muscles receive equal and simultaneous innervation. It is obvious that in any binocular movement in order to maintain alignment, equal and simultaneous movement of each eye would be desirable. If this were not to happen a squint would result! So the Hering's law ensures the **motor correspondence**. This is true not only for versions but also for vergences. In a **symmetric convergence** the two medial recti receive equal and simul-taneous innervation. In an **asymmetric convergence**, though apparently only one eye appears to converge, while the other eye appears to be steady, as an object approaches in the line of vision of one (let's say right) eye,

Table 2.2: Synergists and antagonists		
Action	Agonist or synergist	Antagonists
1. Dextro-version	RLR, LMR	RMR, LLR
2. Dextro elevation	RSR, LIO	RIR, LSO
3. Dextro depression	RIR, LSO	RSR, LIO
4. Sursum version	RSR, LSR (RIO, LIO)*	RIR, LIR (RSO, LSO)*
5. Deorsum version	RIR, LIR (RSO, LSO)*	RSR, LSR (RIO, LIO)*
6. Levo version	RMR, LLR	RLR, LMR
7. Levo elevation	RIO, LSR	RSO, LIR
8. Levo depression	RSO, LIR	RIO, LSR

Note: *The vertical recti are the main elevators but the obliques also contribute to some extent.
RSR: Right superior rectus, RLR: Right lateral rectus, RIR: Right inferior rectus, RIO: Right infra\oblique, RMR: Right medial rectus, RSO: Right superior oblique, LSR: Left superior rectus, LLR: Left lateral rectus, LIR: Left inferior rectus, LIO: Left inferior oblique, LMR: Left medial rectus, LSO: Left superior oblique.

the reality is different. Actually it is a combination of a symmetric convergence (both medial recti act) and a lateral version (right lateral rectus + left medial rectus act). While the action of right medial and lateral recti cancel out each other, the left medial rectus acts double-strong to have that extra adduction (Figs 2.13a and b).

Whereas in normal circumstances the Hering's law ensures maintenance of alignment of the two eyes in different gazes, in a concomitant squint it ensures that the deviations are the same in different gazes. Concomitant actually means "moving together". The deviations with each eye fixing are also the same in a concomitant squint, as against the incomitant squint, where the primary and secondary deviations differ, (*see* paralytic squint).

Sherrington's Law of Reciprocal Inhibition

The Sherrington's law states that for any binocular movement the direct antagonist receives an equal and simultaneous inhibition of its innervation. The eye muscles have a constant tonic innervation even as the eye is still, unlike the skeletal muscles. For a smooth movement to occur the antagonist needs to relax, as the agonist muscle acts. This is called **reciprocal inhibition of innervation**. A failure of observance of this law would result in a simultaneous contraction of the agonist and the antagonist, a **co-contraction** allowing no movement and resulting in a retraction of the globe. This is actually seen in a clinical condition, the Duane's retraction syndrome, and is called **paradoxic innervation**. Similarly in aberrant regenerations the abnormal innervations flout the above law.

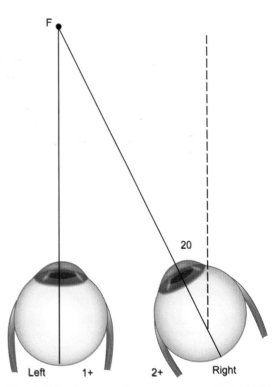

Fig. 2.13a: Symmetric convergence RMR, LMR both receive equal innervation (1+) for convergence.

Fig. 2.13b: Asymmetric convergence RMR, LMR receive 1+ innervation, and LLR and RMR also receive 1+ innervation (symmetric convergence + levoversion).

Donder's and Listing's Laws

The **Donder's law** states that to each position of the line of sight belongs a definite orientation of the horizontal and vertical meridians relative to the co-ordinates of space. That means in a tertiary position the orientation of the meridians of the eye will be the same no matter through which route it has come to that position. This orientation of meridians is perceived as a **torsion**, but since it is not a true torsion occurring around the anteroposterior axis it is called **pseudotorsion** (Fig. 2.14).

The **Listing's law** also states the same thing: that there is **no real torsion or cyclorotation** of the eye around the anteroposterior axis, when it comes to a tertiary position from the primary position.

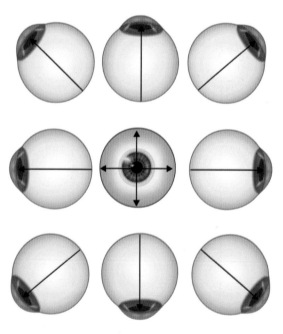

Fig. 2.14: Pseudotorsion. Donder's and Listing's laws. Eye in tertiary positions undergoes a pseudotorsion by virtue of its globular structure.

NEUROPHYSIOLOGY OF EYE MOVEMENTS

To understand the eye movements and the differential action of each extraocular muscle for different movements, the work of Boeder and Robinson cannot be forgotten. They have applied the laws of mechanics and kinematics to explain the eye movements. A **simple resume** is given here:

In the primary position, all the six extra-ocular muscles are innervated and a balance of tone between the antagonist pairs is responsible for the position of globe in that position. Now for an abduction, say of 30°, suddenly the tone for lateral rectus is increased (a **pulse** of + 3), and that of medial rectus is decreased (–3), while the superior and inferior recti and superior and inferior obliques maintain their resting tone. This allows a net tone of +6 for abduction, the tone of vertical and oblique muscles serves to steady the globe in this movement. The viscoelastic forces of the orbit are the dampeners. The lateral rectus continues to have extra innervation, more than what it had in primary position, but much less than the sudde pulse, it may be + 0.5 or + 1. This is called **step**. This **pulse-step innervation** is responsible for a fast eye movement or **saccade**, first a pulse and then a step to maintain the eye in the net position (30° abduction in our example) (Fig. 2.15).

For a slow, steady pursuit or tracking eye movement, the innervation is slowly and steadily increased in the agonist **(ramp)** (Fig. 2.16). At the same time the antagonist receives a reciprocal inhibition.

For the **vertical eye movements**, it should be understood that both the vertical recti and obliques work together. The vertical recti are the primary elevators and depressors especially in the abduction, primary position and up to 10° adduction (Fig. 2.17). The superior rectus contributes about 60% in elevation with inferior oblique chipping in 30%, the rest 10% by the medical and lateral recti. For depression the inferior rectus contributes 80% with superior oblique adding just 10% and the horizontal recti adding the rest. In adduction of beyond 10° to 30°, the

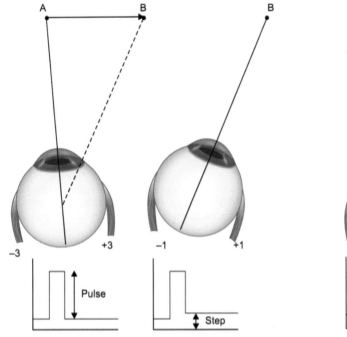

Fig. 2.15: Refixation saccade.

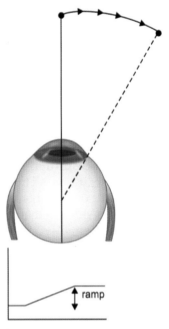

Fig. 2.16: Following pursuit.

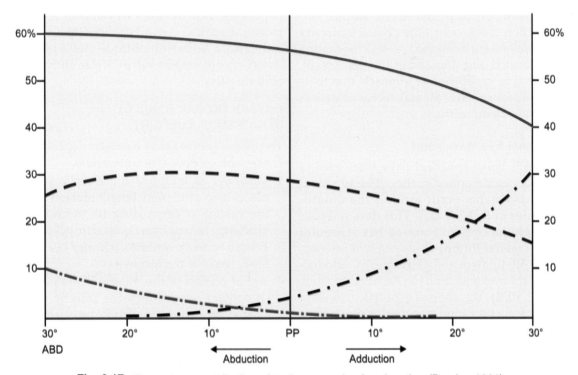

Fig. 2.17: Percentage contribution of various muscles for elevation (Boeder, 1961).

share of superior rectus in elevation is 40% while inferior oblique may have 25–5%. A significant effect coming from lateral recti (about 30–5%). For depression again the inferior rectus gives 50% and superior oblique about 20%, lateral rectus adding 30% (Boeder P. Am. J. Ophthalmol 5, 469, 1961).

Thus it must be noted that **the vertical recti are the primary elevators or depressors. The oblique muscles are the primary torsional muscles, even in the adduction position** (their diagnostic positions). Though their contribution for vertical movement increases, in these positions it is still less than that of the vertical recti. Theoretically speaking the obliques would be the prime elevators or depressors in the 55° adduction position. But practically this never happens, even in the 30° adduction positions their contribution does not increase dramatically because of their fan-shaped insertions.

Another point should be noted that though lateral recti significantly contribute to either elevation or depression in about 30° adduction, this is only if the eyeball is already in an elevated or depressed position (elevating the elevated and depressing the depressed). This is due to slippage of a muscle due to its long arc of contact. Medial rectus slips less than the lateral rectus.

Torsional Eye Movements

Eye balls being spherical have three axes of rotation, as described earlier. **The torsional eye movements occur around the antero-posterior or Fick's Y axis. This does not pass through the centre of cornea but at a point on the lateral limbus** as shown by Linwong, (Fig. 2.18) (Linwong M. Herman SJ; Cycloduc-tion of the eyes with head tilt, Arch Ophthalmol. 85.570, 1971). The applied aspect is in looking for an intorsion (due to superior oblique) in the presence of oculomotor nerve palsy, on attempted depression, one should focus the attention on superonasal limbal vessels, the lateral vessels move the least.

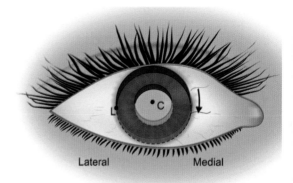

Fig. 2.18: Right eye showing intorsion with axis at lateral limbus (L) not at the centre of cornea (C) (Linwong, 1971).

Compensatory torsional movements on head tilt are at best partial and variable in different individuals. A 30° head tilt causes a mean incycloduction of the ipsilateral eye of 7.00 ± 3.10 degrees and an excycloduction of the contralateral eye of 8.36 ± 2.50 degrees (Linwong, 1971). In addition the ipsilateral eye elevates slightly and the contralateral eye depresses. But in cases of oblique muscle palsies, a marked vertical upshoot (ipsilateral) indicates a superior oblique palsy and a downshoot (contralateral) indicates an inferior oblique palsy.

PHYSIOLOGICAL BASIS OF STRABISMUS SURGERY

The torque generated by a muscle depends on:
1. Strength or power of the muscle.
2. Tautness or laxity of the muscle which places it on a different, **length tension curve** increasing or decreasing its mechanical efficiency (a taut muscle is more efficient).
3. Length of the lever limb, (shorter the lever limb, lesser is the torque).
4. Arc of contact of the muscle. A longer arc of contact necessitates the muscle to be fixated far behind to significantly alter its lever limb (Fig. 2.19). **(Retroequatorial fixation or faden is most efficient on medial rectus and least on the lateral rectus).**

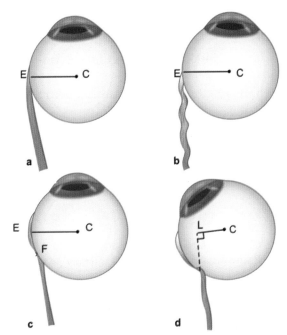

Fig. 2.19: Recession and Faden. Retroequatorial myopexy. (a) Normal muscle with lever arm of EC. (b) Recessed muscle upto equator lever arm same EC (c) Faden operation done at F lever arm with eye in primary position is only slightly shorter, (d) Faden operation eye in the direction of action of muscle lever arm, LC reduced, weakening the muscle in this position.

The above principles are utilised in the different surgical procedures.

Strengthening procedures like resection or advancement, make the muscle more taut, putting it on a higher length tension curve making it more effective. But resection is limited by the size of the fibrous tendon as more resection will reduce the muscle strength by taking away the active muscle fibres (making it a myectomy, a weakening procedure).

A **recession** or a **lengthening** procedure, makes the muscle lax, putting it on a lower length tension curve, reducing its effectivity. But this is limited by the arc of contact of the muscle, recessing it beyond will make the muscle ineffective for that action and merely make it a retractor muscle. Thus we have limits for these procedures, **safe limits** (Fig. 2.20).

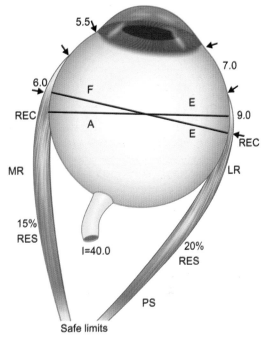

Fig. 2.20: Safe limits.

A **retroequatorial myopexy** or **faden** by fixing the muscle posteriorly shortens the lever limb, reducing the torque.

Length-Tension Curves

A muscle can be stretched upto a length which depends on its tension. Any extra stretch would be passive stretch depending on its elasticity and an excess of stretch may snap the muscle (its sarcoplasmic reticulum) which would cause permanent damage. Length tension curves indicate the muscle characteristics, its elasticity and contractility. Work done by Robinson, Scott, Collins and O'Meara has generated families of length tension curves for the horizontal recti (Fig. 2.21). The minimum force is for 15° in the opposite direction (15° temporal for MR). Beyond 15° T the muscle may receive less innervation, but the passive stretch on it increases the tension in it.

This is an important fact that the antagonist muscle, though relaxes, still starts to have an increasing tone in the extreme opposite direction to its field of action due to passive

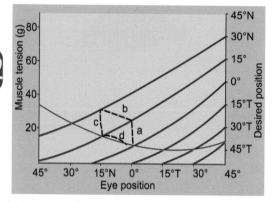

Fig. 2.21: A family of length tension curves for medial rectus showing muscle tension (g) for each desired position at each eye position. The thicker line indicates the resting muscle tension at different eye positions. It is minimum for 15° temporal (not primary position). A15° adduction is shown by dotted lines (a) isometric tension build up, (b) contraction, (c) isometric relaxation, and (d) a return to the old position by return saccade.

stretch. At the same time the agonist which contracts due to active innervation, has a lowering of tension as the eye movement is executed in its direction. The sum total of this effect reestablishes a **dynamic equilibrium in the new eccentric position** and holds the eye in that position, till a new impulse changes that.

During an adduction, the medial rectus first builds up tension due to isometric contraction (a) then has an isotonic shortening (b) (as the eye movement occurs) followed by an **isometric relaxation** (c) (lowering the tone in the new position to match that of the antagonist). During a return abduction saccade, similar changes would occurs in the lateral rectus, the medial rectus then would occur in the lateral rectus, the medial rectus then would have an increase in tension (d).

- A family of length tension curves of MR, determined from indwelling strain-guage measures
- Heavy line is the actual realized force (Resting muscle tension).

- Minimum force is at 15° T
- The loop, showing forces during a saccade
  a. An isometric contraction an isotonic change
  b. In length, followed by an isometric
  c. Relaxation.
- The rise in tension during the return saccade is due to viscosity

Suggested Reading

1. Apt L. An anatomical evaluation of rectus muscle insertions. Trans. Am. Ophthalmol. Soc. 78 365 1980.
2. Charpy A. Muscle et capsule de Tenon. In Poirier, P and Charpy A. editors. Traite de anatomic humaine, new ed., vol 512, Paris, 1912. Masson and Lie Editeurs.
3. Duke Elder S and Wybar, KC: The anatomy of the visual system. System of Ophthalmology. Vol. 2, St. Louis, 1961. The CV Mosby Co.
4. Fink WH: Surgery of the vertical muscles of the eyes ed. 2 Springfield, 111. 1962. Charles C Thomas.
5. Wolff E. Anatomy of the eye and orbit, ed. 6 revised by Last RJ Philadelphia, 1968. HK Lewis and Co.
6. Boeder P. The cooperation of the extra ocular muscles. Am. J. Ophthalmol. 51 469, 1961.
7. Robinson D. Control of eye movements. In Brooks, VB, editor. Handbook of Physiology Vol II. Part 2 The Nervous System, Baltimore, 1981. William and Wilkins.
8. Robinson DA. A quantitative analysis of extraocular muscle cooperation and squint. Invest ophthalmol. 14. 801, 1975.
9. Linwong M and Herman SJ Cycloduction of the eyes with head tilt Arch. Ophthalmol. 85, 570. 1971.
10. Hart WM ed. Adler's Physiology of the Eye: Clinical Applications 9th ed. St. Louis, Mo. CV Mosby 1992.
11. von Noorden G. Binocular Vision and Ocular Motility5th edition Mosby 1997.
12. Collins CC, Scott AB, O' Meara D: Muscle tension during unrestrained human eye movements. J. Physiol (Lond) (1975. 245. 351–69).

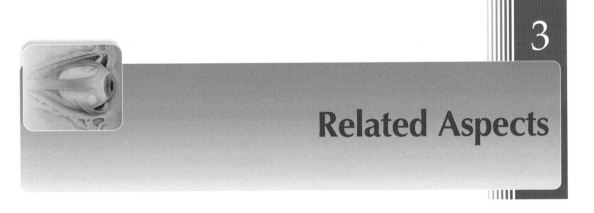

3

Related Aspects

HISTOPATHOLOGY OF EXTRAOCULAR MUSCLES

Extraocular muscles are striated muscle and share several characteristics with the skeletal muscles though differing in some.

Muscle sheath: The muscle is enclosed in a collagenous connective tissue sheath called the **epimysium**. Extensions from the epimysium subdivide the muscle into bundles or fascicles each surrounded by a well defined collagenous layer, the **perimysium**. The individual muscle fibres are separated from each other by a network of connective tissue called the **endomysium**.

Muscle structure: The individual muscle fibres are multinucleated **syncytia** (several fused cells), surrounded by a cell membrane the **sarcolemma**. The nuclei are elliptical and exhibit a prominent nucleolus, which lies just under the sarcolemma. Each muscle fibre is composed of myofibril units which are separated from each other by **sarcoplasmic reticulum**. Tubular invaginations of the sarcolemma form the t-tubule system which brings the latter into the direct contact with the elements of sarcoplasmic reticulum. The myofibril is composed of a bundle of **actin and myosin myofilaments** aligned regularly to form repeating structures called **sarcomeres**. This regular alternation gives the appearance of the typical striations associated with this type of muscle. Each sarcomere is composed of a dark **anisotropic band (A band)** flanked on either side by a light **isotropic band (I band)**. The filaments of I band are attached to a narrow dense z-line demarcating one sarcomere from the other (Fig. 3.1).

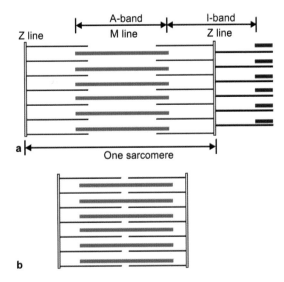

Fig. 3.1: Structure of a sarcomere (a) and changes after contraction (b) (After Huxley).

Contraction of the myofibril occurs by the sliding of actin myofilaments along the myosin filaments towards the centre of A band **(M line)**. This shortens the sarcomere longitudinally causing the muscle contraction. The release of Acetyl choline (Ach neurotransmitter) from the motoneuron triggers this process. Interaction of Ach with the muscle surface receptors results in depolarization and an action potential is propagated along and inside the muscle through the t-tubule system. The opening of sarcoplasmic reticulum causes release of intracellular calcium which acting through a troponin-tropomysin complex, removes barriers to interaction of actin and myosin filaments. The contraction that ensues is an energy dependent process which is provided by aerobic (Mitochondrial oxidative or anaerobic (glycolytic) mechanisms.

The **multiply innervated fibres** may not have propagation of action potential, instead, they undergo slow, graded contractions at each synaptic site instead of twitches, characteristic of singly innervated fibres.

The two properties of **contraction speed** and **fatigue resistance** in different combinations leads to classification of skeletal muscles into four types

a. Slow twitch, fatigue resistant

b. Fast twitch, fatigue resistant

c. Fast twitch, fatiguable

d. Fast twitch intermediate

Characteristics of Extraocular Muscles

The extraocular muscles differ from other striated muscles in their job requirements:

1. Have to maintain a constant tone at all times to keep the eye position steady **(position maintenance).**

2. Have to subserve the different types of eye movements: **Saccades** (fast eye movements for refixation or corrective movements), **pursuit** (slow tracking or follow movements), vergence (slow convergence or divergence movements), **vestibular, optokinetic** and **neck reflex** eye movements.

The job of carrying the globe steady so as not to disturb the critical sense of vision is a very demanding job. Certain special characteristics of the extraocular muscles make this possible.

Classification of Extraocular Muscles

The extraocular muscles are classified on the basis of **location (orbital or global), colour (red, intermediate or pale)** and **innervation pattern (singly or multiply innervated)** (Fig. 3.2). The differentiation into **orbital** (outer, towards the orbit) layer and global (inner,

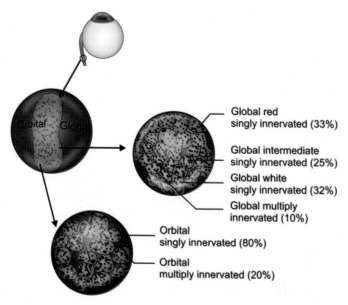

Fig. 3.2: Histopathology of EOM.

towards the eyeball) is unique for the recti and oblique muscles. The levator palpebrae superioris and other accessory muscles lack this differentiation (Table 3.1).

1. **Orbital singly innervated fibre (OSIF):** This type of fibre contains 80% of the orbital muscle fibres belong to this type. They are singly innervated and have numerous mitochondria along with good supply of capillaries. This makes them the most fatigue resistant mammalian skeletal muscle fibre type. In addition they have a unique myosin isoform profile.

2. **Orbital multiply innervated fibre (OMIF):** They are multiply innervated and have less mitochondria (oxidative capability). The central part appears to be similar to fast-twitch type of skeletal muscles, while the proximal and distal parts show characteristics of slowly contracting fibres. They represent the rest 20% of orbital muscle fibres.

3. **Global red singly innervated fibre (GRSIF):** They constitute one third of the global fibres. They are similar to the orbital singly innervated fibres in mitochondrial content, making them more fatigue resistant, but differ in the myosin isoform. Functionally they are fast-twitch and highly fatigue resistant.

4. **Global intermediate singly innervated fibre (GISIF):** These constitute about one fourth of global fibres. They are fast twitch fibres with intermediate level of fatigue resistance, as evident from their numerous mitochondria which are distributed in clusters *and* myofibillar size and sarcoplasmic reticulum which is intermediate between the other types.

5. **Global white single innervated fibre (GWSIF):** They constitute another one third of the global layer. They have few small mitochondria. They are fast twitch with low fatigue resistance and so used sporadically.

6. **Global multiply innervated fibre (GMIF):** This constitutes the remainder 10% of global layer. They have multiple grape **(en grappe)** like nerve endings distributed along the length. They have few small mitochondria arranged singly, with slow-twitch myosin profile. They show a slow graduated nonpropagated response following an activation by neural or pharmacological stimulation.

Thus a variegated assortment of different muscle types is available to subserve the diverse functions they are called upon to play.

The older classification of extraocular muscles of **Fibrillenstruktur** (fine fast twitch fibres) and **Felderstruktur** (thicker slow sustained fibres with multiple innervation) was too simplistic for the eye muscles. It now appears that all fibre types participate in all activities though to a different extent, based on the amount of work and are recruited in a sequential order.

Table 3.1: Functional properties of extraocular muscle fibre types						
Functional	Orbital			Global		
Property	1	2	3	4	5	6
	OSIF	OMIF	GRSIF	GISIF	GWSIF	GMIF
Percentage	80%	20%	33%	25%	32%	10%
Contraction mode	twitch	mixed	twitch	twitch	twitch	sustained
Speed	fast	slow	fast	fast	fast	slow
Fatigue resistance	high	variable	high	interminable	Low	high
Recruitment order	1st	3rd	2nd	5th	6th	4th

(Adapted from: *Porter JD, Baker R'S, Ragusa RJ, Bruckner JK Extraocular muscles: basic and clinical aspects of structure and function. Surv. Ophthalmol. 1995, 39, 451–84.*)

It may be noted that the fine structure of **levator palpebrae** differs, lacking the orbital, global differentiation and also lack the multiply innervated fibres. The levator subserves to maintain eyelid position and terminates blinks. It has a true slow twitch fibre not seen in other extraocular muscles plus the three singly innervated fibre types of global layer.

EMBRYOLOGICAL DEVELOPMENT

All the extraocular muscles develop from **three** distinct masses of **primordial cranial mesoderm**. The three masses correspond to the rhombomeres and the **three cranial nerves** innervate them accordingly. The **premandibular condensation** gives rise to the eye muscles innervated by the oculomotor nerve (superior, medial and inferior recti and inferior oblique). The lateral rectus and superior oblique each arises from its own adjacent tissue mass in the **maxillomandibular mesoderm**. These anlage lie as bilateral masses close to the stalk at **6 weeks gestation** (13.5 mm stage).

The four recti differentiate at 20 mm stage **(7 weeks)** and the levator palpebrae superioris differentiates from the superior rectus from its medial part at **8 weeks**. Later it grows laterally on a higher plane than the superior rectus at **3 months**.

The extraocular muscles develop in at least **two waves of myogenesis** forming primary and secondary generation fibres. The global multiply innervated fibres are phylogenetically 'old' and form first while the orbital layers mature last.

The critical development occurs at 6–8 weeks (may be up to 12 weeks). The close proximity of the anlagens may facilitate development of anomalous innervation of eye muscles. Duane's retraction syndrome is an example where the congenital absence of the abducens nerve, causes the abnormal innervation of the lateral rectus by the oculomotor nerve.

Even after birth, **postnatal maturation** continues and definitive muscle characteristics are established. This period roughly corresponds with the period of visual maturation. Eye muscle characteristics are therefore liable to be abnormally developed or may have developmental delays. The immaturity of the muscle fibres is also responsible for the effect of botulinum toxin used in early infancy, becoming more longer lasting than in adults, because of permanent changes in muscle characteristics.

Extraocular Muscle Pulleys

The EOM pulleys are sleeves of collagen, elastin and smooth muscle that encircle an EOM and are also attached to the orbital wall and adjacent connective tissues. The muscle along with its sheath passes through these pulleys. They are located near the equator of the globe they seem to deflect the anterior part of the muscle in gazes other than the primary gaze and act as the functional origin. In abnormal situations the pulleys may be heterotropic and may cause ocular motility problems (Joseph L Demer and Joel Miller, 1995).

ACCOMMODATION AND CONVERGENCE

The two eyes coordinate between themselves, when looking at a near object. The near vision complex comprises of:

i. **Accommodation:** Contraction of ciliary muscle

ii. **Convergence:** Contraction of both medial recti

iii. **Miosis:** Constriction of sphincter pupillae.

As would be desired, the accommodation and convergence are linked for viewing near objects. This implies a more or less fixed relationship between accommodation and convergence and is called Accommodative Convergence and Accommodation (AC/A) ratio. That is for any given change in dioptric power of accommodation, there is a fixed accommodative convergence. An object at 1 metre distance requires 1 Dioptre accommodation (of each eye) as also a convergence of 1 metre angle between the two visual axes. In degrees, it is 1° 50' min (roughly 2°) and in terms of prism dioptre it is about 6.5 p.d. for an interpupillary distance, (IPD of 65 mm). Actually the convergence in degrees and p.d. will depend upon the I.P.D., which determines the vergence required between the two eyes at 1 metre distance,

Metre Angle

The vergence of the two eyes for an object at 1 metre distance is 1 metre angle. The angle formed between the visual axes of one eye and the median line is the **Nagel's metre angle**, or **small metre angle (ma)**. Generally we talk in terms of vergence between the two visual axes, this is referred as **large Metre angle** (Ma) (Fig. 3.3). This would imply a convergence of 6.5 pd (for 65 mm IPD) at 1 metre distance.

The amplitude of accommodation can be measured by the **near point ruler** a ruler with a card on which a line is drawn. The nearest point before the line appears blurred is noted. If it is 8 cm, the **near point of accommodation** (NPA) is $100/8 = 12.5$ Dioptres. For 10 cm, NPA would be 10.D.

The normal amplitude of accommodation at any age can be empirically deduced from this formula of fours:

$$A = 4 \times 4 - \frac{\text{Age (in years)}}{4}$$

Also remember that any time one third reserve should be available for comfort.

Similarly the near point of convergence can be measured by seeing the nearest point before the line becomes double. If this is 8 cm the near point of convergence is $= 100/8 = 12.5$ Ma. If one knows the IPD, the exact convergence can be estimated in degrees or prism dioptres. For a 65 mm IPD, it would be 19.5 pd. for an object at 33 cm and 78 pd. for one at 8 cm (Fig. 3.4).

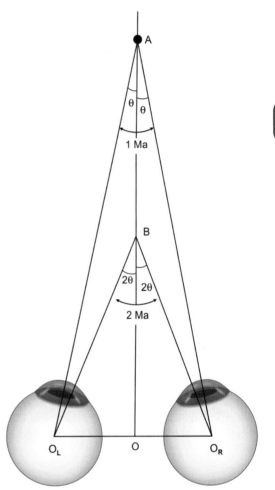

Fig. 3.3: Convergence in metre angles. O_L, O_R are the centres of 'rotation of left and right eyes. Point A is 1 metre away and point B ½ metre away convergence at A (1 m) = θ = 1 ma (small metre angle of Nagel) for each eye (angle between visual axis and median line). Convergence between the two eyes (between the two visual axis is 1 Ma (large metre angle). The latter is used commonly. For ½ m distance, point B the convergence is 2 Ma. Distance O_L-O_R is approximately equal to the interpupillary distance.

Types of Convergence

Convergence can be of involuntary or voluntary type. Involuntary or reflex convergence can be of four types:

i. **Tonic convergence:** A resting tone which is always present in the waking stage and

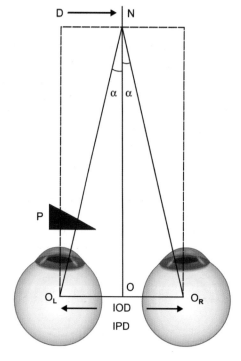

Fig. 3.4: Convergence in prism dioptres. If eyes move to N (1 metre away) from distance D (infinity) the convergence DN will be ½ IOD/IPD as a linear deviation. The angular deviation (α) would be ½ IPD (in cm) prism dioptres. (1 prism dioptre = 1 cm linear deviation at 1 metre distance).

also during various stages of sleep. Only during deep anesthesia or death does the tonic convergence subside. A relaxation of tonic convergence under general anesthesia causes the relative divergence of eyes. The tonic convergence varies in different individuals and at various ages. It is more strong in early childhood and has been supposed to be responsible for sensory esotropia in post-infancy childhood.

ii. **Proximal convergence:** A reflex increase in the tone of medial rectus due to the psychological feeling of the target, being near causes the proximal convergence. This is responsible for the synoptophore convergence being more in spite of the targets being optically placed at distance.

iii. **Fusional convergence:** This is the active effort to align the two eyes so that fixation can be maintained in spite of a tendency of exodeviation. This requires the retinal images to fall on the temporal hemiretina (bitemporal disparity). The fusional convergence converts an exotropia into an exophoria. It is also called positive convergence, as against the fusional divergence which is called negative convergence.

iv. **Accommodative convergence:** This is the additional tone the medial rectus receives as it changes the focus of the eyes from a distant to a near object. This is linked to the accommodation and is a part of the near vision complex, along with the pupillary constriction.

Accommodation–Convergence Relationship

The relationship of the accommodation and convergence are linked and supposed to be stable, unchangeable for an individual. This is defined as **AC/A ratio,** which is the convergence amplitude for a unit accommodation. However, changes can be brought about in one relative to the other and is called **relative convergence** or **relative accommodation.** The orthoptic treatment in accommodative esotropia is based on the relative dissociation of these two functions.

Stimulus and Response AC/A Ratio

Mostly in clinical studies, the change in the convergence is related to the change in the stimulus (change of lenses or change in the fixation distance). This has been called the **stimulus AC/A ratio.** In research settings the response of the eye in the change of the refractive status, to a change stimulus can also be studied. If that is taken into account for unit accommodational change a **response AC/A** can be evaluated. The latter is about 8% more than the stimulus AC/A ratio. Clinically however the stimulus AC/A ratio is more practical to determine, though efforts must be taken to ensure sufficient time has been given for a response change to occur for a given stimulus.

The Changes in the AC/A Ratio

Agents like miotics, convex glasses, prisms, or surgery artificially change the AC/A ratio. Strictly speaking the intrinsic AC/A ratio is not changed, the change is due to a change in the required accommodative effort or the manifestation of convergence.

For example: In accommodative esotropia, a child with uncorrected + 4D hyperopia, with normal AC/A ratio of 5:1 would have accommodative esotropia of 20 pd base out for distance and 35 pd base out for a near target at 33 cm (+3D accommodative effort). If he is given his proper distance correction he would have no deviation for distance, but still have the physiological 15 pd esodeviation for near. If he had a high AC/A ratio of 8:1 he would have had distance esodeviation of 32 pd base out and 56 pd base out for near. Giving him his proper correction would correct his esodeviation for distance but still leave 24 pd base out for near, more than the required physiological convergence. If he be given bifocals with additional near add, this excess near esodeviation can also be corrected.

In case miotics were used, the miotics by acting on ciliary muscle will cause facilitation of accommodation. This means less accommodational effort will be required, reducing the manifestation of the esodeviation. Thus glasses and miotics work to reduce the accommodative effort and thus 'artificially' reduce the AC/A ratio. Base out prisms or recession of medial recti act on the effector organ (the medial recti), masking the effect of convergence in response to the accommodation, the effort remaining the same, will not relieve the asthenopia, though giving a cosmetic correction of deviation.

Estimation of AC/A Ratio

The AC/A ratio can be measured by measuring the change in convergence for a change in accommodation which can be done by

a. Changing the distance of fixation, from 6 m to 33 cm **(Heterophoria method)**.
b. Changing the spherical lenses to increase' or decrease the accommodational effort, while the fixation distance is kept constant **(Gradient method)**.
   The gradient method may be done with prisms or on the synoptophore.
c. In addition a **Graphic method** can be used whereby a plot is made for the convergence against the different spherical glasses.
d. Another method used in experimental setting is the **Fixation disparity method**.

Heterophoria Method

- The interpupillary distance is measured in cm (IPD).
- The patient is made to wear his required refractive correction.
- The deviation is measured by PBCT as the patient fixates at 6 m distance (supposedly infinity) and then again as he fixates at 33 cm distance to a target that controls his accommodation (supposedly a + 3 D accommodational effort)

$$\text{Then, } \frac{AC}{A} \text{ IPD} + \frac{N-D}{3}$$

where IPD is in cm, N is the near deviation and D the distance deviation in prism dioptres, the esodeviations have a plus sign and exodeviations have a negative sign.

3 D is the normal accommodational effort for a 33 cm target and 0 being the accommodation for distance.

The AC/A ratio is expressed as a ratio 5:1 or 6:1 or actual units as prism dioptres per dioptre of accommodation.

Gradient Method

This is done at a fixed distance whether for distance at 6 m with concave lenses (to stimulate accommodation) or at 33 cm with convex lenses (to relax accommodation).

The IPD is not important as the vergence is measured at the same fixation distance.

i. For 6 m with concave lenses

- The subject is made to wear his proper correction and the deviation is measured with PBCT for distance (= D)
- The deviation is again measured after giving him—3D concave lenses and asked to fix on an accommodative target (6/9 size) (= N).

ii. For 33 cm with convex lenses

- The subject with his proper correction is asked to fix at an accommodative target at 33 cm and the deviation is measured (=N).
- The deviation is measured again with the patient fixing at the same target but through + 3.0 D (convex) lens. This should be worn for sufficient time to allow for 'fogging' (=D)

$$\text{Then,} \quad \frac{AC}{A} = \frac{N-D}{3}$$

(The sign of esodeviation is plus and for exodeviation it is minus)

Note: If other than –3D lens is used the denominator is changed by that.

Graphic Method

This is a more elaborate method which can be done with prisms or on the synoptophore. The cooperation and time required make it unsuitable for children.

The measurement of deviations are made sequentially with addition of concave lenses starting from –1.0D increasing to –4.0D. with 0.5D steps. The convergence is plotted against the accommodative effort (spherical lens power). The graph gives the AC/A ratio. (Convergence corresponding to 1.0 D accommodation).

Fixation Disparity Method

This is based on the principle that the amount of fixation disparity is altered when the positive or negative convergence is induced

by base-out or base-in prisms and again when fixation disparity is altered for the accommodative stimulus changed by concave or convex lenses. The two sets of readings are compared to give the AC/A ratio.

The subject views two centrally placed lines: the upper line, which can be moved by one eye and the lower line, which is fixed by the other eye. The subject adjusts the upper line until it is seen directly above the lower line. The amount of adjustment gives the fixation disparity. Such measurements are made for change with prisms and then with spherical glasses. The AC/A ratio is derived by finding the convergence and accommodation corresponding to the same fixation distance. This is a time consuming method, requiring special apparatus and a laboratory setting not applicable for clinical purposes.

Uses of AC/A Ratio

The AC/A ratio is useful to study in cases of

i. Accommodative esotropia to understand the different types and manage them differently

ii. Exodeviations with simulated divergence excess exotropia, to be differentiated from true divergence excess exotropia.

Types of Eye Movements

The eyes express themselves in different ways. The different types of eye movements are (Table 3.2):

1. **Saccadic** or fast eye movements (refixation and corrective movements).

2. **Pursuit** or follow or tracking movements (following a target moving regular speed).

3. **Vergence** eye movements (convergence and Divergence eye movements).

4. **Vestibular** and **tonic neck reflexive** eye movements.

5. **Optokinetic** eye movements

6. **Position maintenance system (fixation)**

Table 3.2: Types of eye movements

Parameter	Saccades	Pursuit	Vergence	Reflex (vestibular TNR)
1. Controlling pathway	Contralateral cortex or I/L PPRF	I/L parieto occipital cortex and I/LPPRF	Temporo parietal cortex/pretectal midbrain	Contralateral vestibular N and I/L PPRF
2. Function	Quick placement of object on fovea	Maintain moving object on fovea	Maintain alignment of both visual axes	Adjust eye position to head and neck position
3. Stimulus	Object of interest on peripheral retina	Moving object on fovea	Binasal/bitemporal disparity	Stimulation of semicircular canals otoliths, or neck receptors
4. Latency	200 m Sec	125 m sec	160 m sec	10 m sec
5. Velocity	300–700/sec	30–60/sec	20/sec	300/sec
6. Feedback	Sampled with suppression during saccade	Continuous	Continuous	Continuous

They are aimed to:

i. Direct the fovea on the object of interest

   a. Refixation on a new object (saccade)

   b. Following a regularly moving target (pursuit)

ii. Maintain the fovea on the object of interest (fixation).

iii. Maintain the proper alignment of eyes with respect to each other (vergence).

iv. Maintain the alignment with respect to head position or neck position (reflex eye movements).

The pathways for different eye movements are different as also, their characteristics (Fig. 3.5). A study of different eye movements

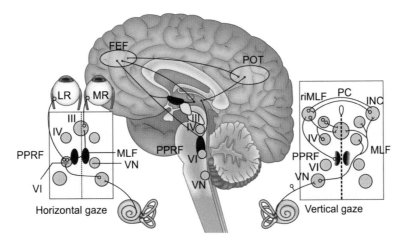

Fig. 3.5: A schematic diagram of the neural pathway of horizontal gaze and Vertical gaze. FEF = Frontal eye field; POT = parieto-occipital temporal area; PPRF = Para-median pontine reticular formation; MLF = medial longitudinal fasciculus; ri MLF = rostral interstitial nucleus of MLF; PC = posterior commissure; INC = interstitial nu. of Cajal; SC= superior colliculus; VN = vestibular nu.

(Adapted from: *Miller N.ed Walsh and Hoyt's Clinical Neuro-ophthalmology, 4th ed Baltimore Williams & Wilkins, 1983*)

can help the examiner to detect neurological lesions.

RELEVANT NEUROANATOMY

The details of neuroanatomy of the various eye movements, and of the various nuclei of the cranial nerves dealing with the eyes is beyond the scope of a book on strabismus. A brief outline is however provided and details may be obtained from any book on neuro-ophthalmology.

Salient Features

a. *Supranuclear Pathway*

1. The cortical control of voluntary saccades is contralateral frontomotor cortex. In the event of injury of one, however, the ipsilateral cortex can take over the function after some time.

2. The pursuit eye movements are controlled by then ipsilateral parieto-occipital cortex.

3. The vergence eye movements by the **temporoparietal cortex**.

4. The common pathway for most horizontal eye movements lies through the para-median **pontine reticular formation (PPRF)**. Which receives connections from frontal, parieto-occipital cortex and vestibular nuclei.

5. The **mesencephalic reticular formation (MRF)** executes the commands for the vertical eye movements. Bilateral cortical commands are required for vertical movements at the higher level. It is not exactly clear which is the vertical gaze centre.

   The **rostral interstitial nucleus of median longitudinal fasciculus and posterior commissure** are supposed to be subserving this function. A monocular elevator paresis (double elevator palsy) has raised the possibility of separate monocular vertical gaze centres.

6. The reflex eye movements, mediated through the **vestibular nucleus** communicate

through the PPRF or MRF for the requisite horizontal or vertical eye movements.

7. The convergence centre is supposedly the **central nucleus of Perlia** and not clearly seen in all humans or primates. The divergence centre is still more illusory. However, the presence of convergence in the absence of adduction on a version in cases of inter nuclear ophthalmoplegia, does indicate two separate pathways.

b. *Nuclear and Infranuclear Pathways*

The nuclear and infranuclear pathways are more clearly defined. The oculomotor nucleus consists of subnuclei for each muscle supplied by it as two lateral masses, with all extra ocular muscles receiving ipsilateral inner-vation except superior rectus (which receives contralateral innervation). Levator on both sides is supplied by a single central nucleus (therefore ptosis whenever due to a nuclear lesion is always bilateral). The Edinger Westphal's accessory nuclei supply the parasympathetic innervation to the sphincter pupillae and accommodational tone to the ciliary body the latter by the anterior masses. The parasympathetic involvement is always bilateral if due to nuclear damage or it does not present. Thus a unilateral ptosis or anisocoria excludes a nuclear oculomotor nerve palsy. The nucleus of the trochlear or IVth cranial nerve lies at the level of inferior colliculus in the midbrain. This is caudal to the oculomotor nucleus. **The trochlear nerve supplies the superior oblique contralaterally after the crossing of the nerve dorsal to the midbrain** (All the other nerves are ventro-lateral. **The long course of the nerve and the dorsal decussation makes it vulnerable in head injuries, which may be bilateral though asymmetric, causing the lesser involvement to be missed**.

The **abducens nucleus** lies close to the paramedian pontine reticular formation, near the midline in the floor of fourth ventricle. The abducens nerve fibres loop around the nucleus of facial (VII) nerve and leave the pons in the groove between the pons and medulla.

The abducens nucleus is supposed to have:

i. Motor neurons which supply the ipsilateral lateral rectus muscle and

ii. Internuclear neurons which communicate to the medial rectus subnucleus of the contralateral oculomotor nerve.

iii. This communication is the **medial longitudinal fasciculus**. Involvement of these fibres in demyelinating diseases like multiple sclerosis or ischemic infarcts cause **internuclear ophthalmoplegia** (ipsilateral adduction deficiency with contralateral abduction nystagmus with usually preserved convergence).

Suggested Reading

1. Porter JD, Baker RS, Ragusa RJ, Brueckner JK. Extraocular muscles basic and clinical aspects J structure and function. Surv. Ophthalmol. 39.451–484. 1995.
2. Dodge R. Five types of eye movements in the horizontal meridian of the field of regard. Am. J. Physiol 8. 307. 1903.
3. Newman NM. Neuro-Ophthalmology. A practical text. Appleton and Lange. Norwalk, Connecticut! 1992.
4. Miller N. ed. Walsh and Hoyt's Clinical Neuro-ophthalmology 4th Ed. Baltimore. Williams & Wilkinsj 1983. 2.
5. Warwick B. Representation of the extra-ocular muscles in the oculomotor nuclei of the monkey. Jl Comp. Neurol. 1953. 98, 449–504.
6. Jampolsky A: Ocular divergence mechanisms. Trans. Am Ophthalmol Soc. 68. 730. 1970.

The Physiology of Binocular Vision, Amblyopia and Anomalous Retinal Correspondence

Binocular vision is the nature's gift to man that has established his supremacy in the animal kingdom. Even a cursory look will show that the predator birds or animals like eagle, owl, lion or cat have the two eyes **frontally placed**. Compared to this their prey like sparrow, deer, cattle or lower animals have their eyes **laterally placed** (Fig. 4.1). The eyes on their sides offer an advantage of a larger panoramic field but it lacks in depth appreciation. This may suit the lower animals to guard them-selves from their hunters. But the frontally placed eyes offer a piercing precision of depth to pounce upon the prey. Man and to some extent the other apes have a still better

binocular vision. This in addition to their ability to stand erect with head that can turn around gives them the strategic advantage to be on top of the animal hierarchy (Fig 4.2). Let us understand the aspects of this so-impor-tant binocular vision. Because the binocular vision, which is an **asset** with normal alignment of the two eyes, becomes a **liability** when the alignment is lost.

Sensory Aspects

Objects in space are localized by us in two ways: one is relative to one another and is called **relative localization** and the other is in relation to ourselves and is called

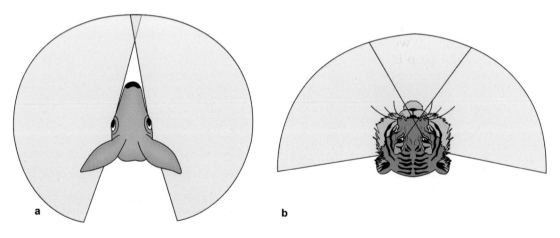

a   b

Fig. 4.1: (a) Field of vision in birds and animals which are preyed or hunted is large (panoramic) on both sides with a small binocular field, if any (b) Field of vision in birds and animals which hunt have good binocular fields with stereopsis for precision of depth.

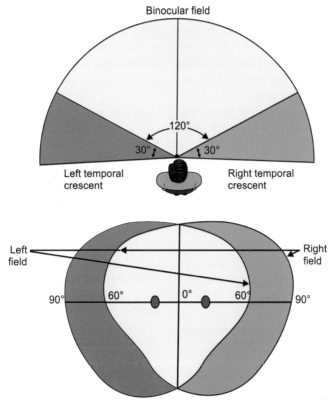

Fig. 4.2: Diagram showing binocular fields of vision. The central 120° are seen binocularly having stereopsis. At each end are 30° monocular temporal crescent. The blind spots of each eye are normally not seen as they fall in binocular area (other eye sees).

egocentric localization. Egocentric localization is being used when we say: the table is in front of me or the lamp is on my right side and so on, this is in reference to our "self". Similarly each eye has a **straight ahead localization** centred at the fovea. All the other areas of retina have localization value relative to the fovea and can change, but the foveal localization is the guide and determinant (Fig. 4.3). This straight ahead localization from fovea is the **primary visual direction**. But each eye being separated horizontally by the interpupillary distance would have its own primary visual direction. So for the sake of unification a **common visual direction** is computed from these two visual directions, which is centred at the imaginary **cyclopean eye**. The importance of this knowledge is: **any**

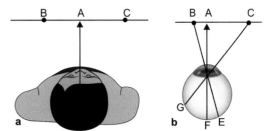

Fig. 4.3: Spatial localization. (a) Localization in space is egocentric (in relation to self) straight ahead, A or to the right of A, C, or left of A, B, (b) Eye localization is in relation to fovea for each eye in a similar manner.

object imaged on the two primary visual directions are perceived as superimposed and as if in the same line though in reality they are separated in space (this is the basis of the haploscope).

All the other retinal points in the two eyes, which have a localization relative to its own fovea, will also have to relate to the overlapping points of the other eye (because of the overlapping fields of the two eyes). These are called the **corresponding points**, because they correspond or transmit information to and fro, between the two eyes (Fig. 4.4). Each such point will correspond with only its own corresponding point. All the other points are called **disparate points** with its reference. The applied aspect is that: **the images on corresponding points are perceived as binocularly single, and an object imaged on the disparate points is perceived as binocularly double.**

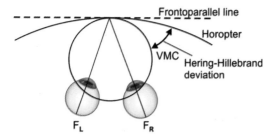

Fig. 4.4: Horopters: Geometrical, Theoretic or Vieth-Muller circle and the Empirical horopter. The deviation of the practically charted empirical horopter from the theoretic horopter is Hering-Hillebrand deviation. The Frontoparallel line is shown for reference.

If all the corresponding points are projected in space at any particular distance they form the **horopter**. It is actually a plane and is like a flattened dome. **A theoretical or geometric horopter** is geometrically constructed by drawing a circle which passes through the corresponding points of the two eyes, this is referred as the **Vieth-Muller circle.** But in actual practice it is not circular or spherical but some what flattened. This difference between the geometric and the actual horopter is called the **Hering-Hillebrand deviation**. The actual horopter can be charted by using longitudinal bars positioned such that they appear equidistant, and because this resembles the longitudes of the globe, it has

also been referred as the **longitudinal horopter**. One should remember that the horopter is with reference to our point of fixation and varies with it. And all the points on the horopter at that distance appear as equidistant.

Having the two eyes frontally placed and thus having overlapping fields, nature solved the problem of confusion of perception between the two eyes by having a system of binocular perception. The interesting part is that very small areas around the corresponding (though in reality disparate) can be binocularly fused to see singly. These are called **Panum's area of binocular fusion** (Figs 4.5 and 4.6).

But though the fusion occurs, a perceptual effort has been made. This effort is computed by the cortex to give us the **appreciation of depth**. The two eyes separated by the IPD, view the same object (that is three-dimensional and has depth of space) slightly differently. The two images lying within the Panum's area are fused and the effort recreates the depth in our perception. **Thus the Panum's area is the physiological basis for our depth perception.**

Stereopsis or the binocular faculty of depth perception is the crowning glory of our binocular vision. Though we do have monocular cues for depth perception, they are

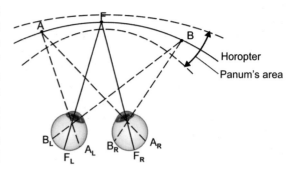

Fig. 4.5: Horopter and Panum's area F_R- F_L, A_R A_L, B_R, B_L are corresponding points. They are seen binocularly single in the same subjective frontoparallel plane as equidistant as foveal points within Panum's area are, single but create depth perception.

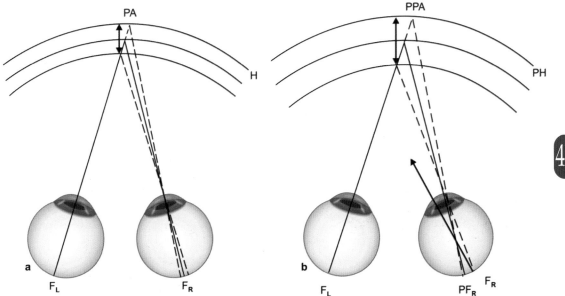

Fig. 4.6: Relationship of horopter (H) Panum's area (PA) in normal retinal correspondence (a) and anomalous retinal correspondence (b) F_L F_R are fovea of left and right eye PF_R is the pseudofovea. PH and PPA are pseudohoropter and pseudo Panum's area.

not always dependable, as they are based on certain learned experiences. They also do not operate in free space, as can be demonstrated by the **two-pencil test:** Cover one of your eyes and ask your friend to hold a pencil horizontally. Now try to align the tip of a pencil in your hand with that in your friend's hand. Observe how difficult this simple task becomes. Now try doing the same with both eyes open. Binocular vision makes it so simple! Doing the same experiment with two pencils in your own two hands is a test of proprioception and not of stereopsis. Also the tips of the pencils should not be visible end-on, aiming that is a plain monocular task.

The **monocular cues** (Fig. 4.7) that give a three-dimensional effect to a two-dimensional painting are:
- Change in apparent size
- Overlap and interpositioning
- Shadows and highlights
- Geometric perspective
- Aerial perspective
- Motion parallax
- Looming
- Relative velocity flow.

Binocular Vision and Squint

When the two eyes are in alignment, the binocular vision is an *asset* as seen above. But when squint occurs the same mechanism becomes a *liability*. It is like the husband and wife team with a common viewpoint (common visual direction) working in harmony. Then they can also fuse small differences in viewpoints **(Panum's area of fusion)** to have a more comprehensive outlook (stereopsis). But when there is a mere lack of common understanding, the two viewpoints can lead to quarrels and misunderstanding, making the life miserable. Then the marriage (binocular vision) becomes a liability rather than an asset.

When squint occurs the two fovea's view two different objects, and send two different images to a single cortical perceptual area. This leads to confusion (*more than one option*

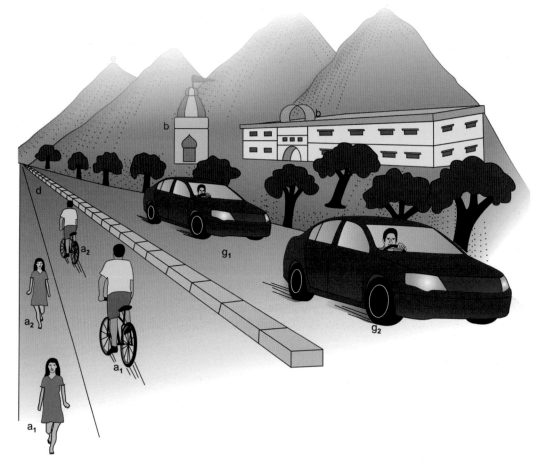

Fig. 4.7: Monocular cues used in two dimensional drawings to impart a sense of depth: (a) change in apparent size (a_1, a_2), (b) overlap and interpositioning, (c) shadows and highlights, (d) geometric perspective, (e) aerial perspective, (f) motion parallax, (g) looming (g_1, g_2).

causes confusion). However, the cortex immediately settles for one image with its inherent strong **cortical or retinal rivalry**. Therefore, confusion is never complained of.

When squint occurs an object in space is perceived by the fovea of one eye and some other extra foveal point of the other eye, which has a different projection or localization value in space. Thus an object would be localized twice in space causing **diplopia**. In diplopia, an object that has one physical location has two physiological localisations. And what we perceive is not what is located in space but what is localized physiologically. So due to squint we would see double, that becomes single on closing one eye. This is therefore binocular diplopia as against monocular diplopia which persists on covering the other eye. **Monocular diplopia** could be due to marked astigmatism or artifacts in the media or some neurological aberration.

Thus the two bugbears of squint are **confusion** (two different objects perceived by the two foveas) and **diplopia** (one, object perceived double by the two eyes).

Adaptations to Squint

While confusion is immediately controlled by strong foveal rivalry, some adaptations are required to tackle diplopia. The adaptations can be **motor** or **sensory**.

Motor Adaptations

The motor adaptations are:
- Fusion
- Head posture
- Blind spot mechanism.

Fusion

Fusion is the ability of the two eyes to check a tendency for squint. And as long as the fusion is strong a squint remains latent (heterophoria) and does not become manifest (heterotropia). The fusion requires binocular input and covering one eye breaks fusion. Fusional convergence is stronger than fusional divergence, so that a divergent tendency (exophoria) is better controlled. This fusional effort, if taxed more than its tolerance gives rise to **asthenopia**.

Head Posture

To tackle a manifest squint which has variable deviation in different gazes **(incomitance)**, **head posture** comes handy. It is that position or posture of head, by assuming which the eyes are in a position of no deviation, or such a small deviation that can be fused. Head posture has three components:
- **Chin** elevation or depression
- **Face turn** to right or left side
- **Head tilt** to right or left shoulder

Rarely when the deviation does not permit fusion a head permit may be assumed so as to increase the deviation such that the other image of the far retinal periphery, being weak can be ignored or suppressed.

Blind Spot Mechanism

In esotropias of 15° (25–30 prism-dioptres), the other image falls on the blind spot of the other eye and so does not cause diplopia. This is the blind spot mechanism described by Swan. In incomitant squint a primary or secondary deviation is chosen by fixing with either of the two eyes to take advantage of this mechanism, (Fig. 4.8).

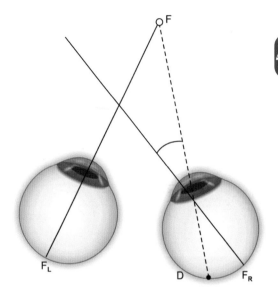

Fig. 4.8: **Blind spot mechanism.** Diplopia point falls on the blind spot of an esodeviation of about 15° (23–30 pd).

Sensory Adaptations

In young childhood during the plasticity of neurophysiological development certain changes in the sensory mechanism are possible to tackle the problems of squint (Fig. 4.9). We noted that confusion is tackled by the foveal rivalry which is actually a suppression of the image of the other fovea. In addition to tackling diplopia the extrafoveal image in the squinting eye is also suppressed. This occurs readily if the visual potential of this extrafoveal point is poor, that is when the angle of squint is large. **Suppression** is a cortical mechanism of ignoring the image of one eye from cognisance. It is more than the **visual ignorance**, which we can learn to do at any age by active denial of perception (example: learning to view through a monocular

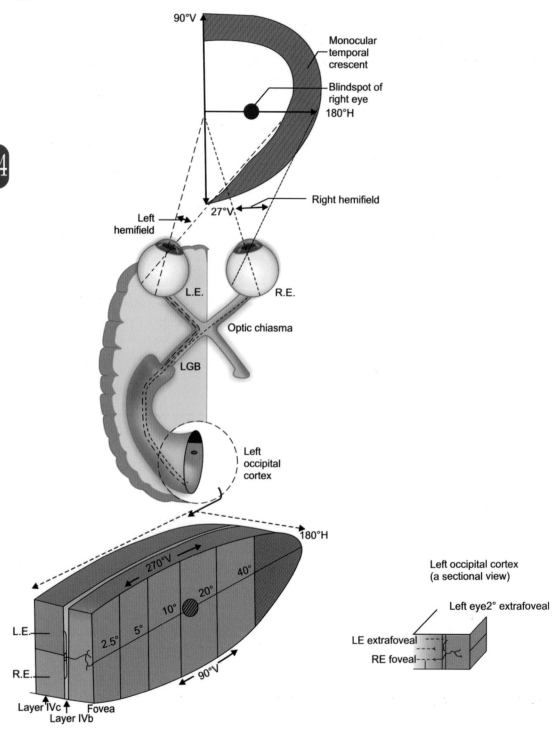

Fig. 4.9a: Normal binocular connections of right hemifield.

Fig. 4.9b: Abnormal binocular correspondence in microstrabismus.

microscope without closing the other eye). **Suppression requires** for its development: a large **angle deviation, that is constant and occurs in early childhood** (Fig. 4.10).

Suppression can be **facultative** or **obligatory**. Facultative suppression is only under binocular conditions offering the advantage but with no persisting "hang-over" under monocular conditions. Thus the visual acuity is not reduced under monocular conditions and there are no uniocular scotomas in the visual fields. Obligatory suppression is the effect which carries on even under monocular conditions resulting in diminution of visual acuity. **Amblyopia is the fallout of this obligatory suppression.**

Anomalous Retinal Correspondence

We noted that suppression is easy if the visual potential of the extrafoveal area is poor but what if it is fairly good? This happens if the angle of squint is small and the extra foveal point is close to the fovea. Just like a weak opponent can be easily ignored, but a strong opponent has to be reconciled with. Another mechanism would be required in such cases. **Anomalous retinal correspondence (ARC)** is the establishment of a new working relationship between the fovea of one eye and the extra foveal point of the squinting eye. **It is the attempt to regain the binocular advantage, although anomalous (because it is foveo-extrafoveal and not foveo-foveal).** In ARC under binocular conditions the fovea and the extra foveal point share the common subjective visual direction. But when the normal eye is closed, the extra foveal point loses any advantage over the fovea of that eye, which retains its primary visual direction or straight ahead gaze. Thus under monocular conditions the central fixation is retained by the fovea, which shows up as a manifest tropia when a cover test is conducted (Fig. 4.11).

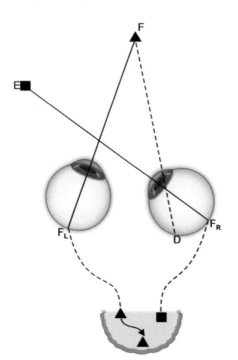

Fig. 4.10: Right foveal suppression in right esotropia at the cortical level.

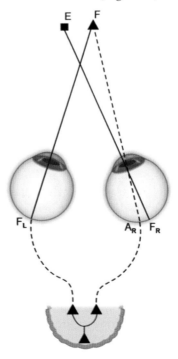

Fig. 4.11: Anomalous retinal correspondence in right esotropia between F_L and A_R.

This results in the eyes seeing binocularly single in spite of a manifest squint (Figs 4.9a and 4.11). It may also be understood that the **subjective angle would be zero**, though the objective angle would be equal to the angle of squint. Such a situation is called **harmonious ARC**. Harmonious ARC is in a way a **subjective readjustment of the zero-error**. This can occur only in a small angle squint, with constant deviation and in young childhood. A condition called **unharmonious ARC**, referred in the older textbooks may be only an artifact of the more dissociating testing conditions. A more physiological test like Bagolini's striated glasses will reveal a harmonious ARC, while more dissociating tests like synoptophore or red-green glasses show an unharmonious ARC. In unharmonious ARC the angle of deviation has not been fully accounted for in the subjective or sensory adjustment.

However, a situation may result when the fovea of the other eye loses its property of primary visual direction or straight ahead gaze, which is usurped by the extrafoveal point. This point then becomes the point of **eccentric fixation**.

AMBLYOPIA

Clinical Features, Pathophysiology and Management

Amblyopia is a condition with unilateral or bilateral decrease of visual functions, caused by form vision deprivation and/or abnormal binocular interaction, that cannot be explained by a disorder of ocular media or visual pathways itself. In appropriate cases it is reversible by therapeutic measures.

It is a condition caused by abnormal visual experience during early childhood - the critical period of visual development. Over the years a lot of work, experimental as well as clinical has been done in the study of central visual pathways, which has removed some cobwebs but the suspense still remains.

Prevalence: The prevalence of amblyopia in general population can be estimated to be 2–2.5% from the various surveys conducted in selected populations. In pre-school and school children it has been reported to be 1.3 to 3.5%, in recruited soldiers it is 1–4% and in ophthalmic patients it is 4–5%.

Classification of Amblyopia

1. Strabismic amblyopia
2. Anisometropic amblyopia (unilateral or asymmetric)
   a. Anisohyperopic
   b. Anisomyopic
3. Form Vision Deprivation amblyopia (unilateral or bilateral)
   a. Stimulus deprivation amblyopia or asymmetric amblyopia ex anopsia) due to ptosis (covering pupil), media opacities (cornea, lens or vitreous), unilateral occlusion or penalisation,
   b. **(Ametropic amblyopia)** An uncorrected bilateral high refractive error
      i. Hyperopia
      ii. Myopia
      iii. Astigmatism (meridional amblyopia)
4. **Nystagmus related amblyopia**
5. **Organic amblyopia**
   a. Sub-clinical macular damage
   b. Malorientation of cones
   c. Cone deficiency syndrome

Clinical Features

Amblyopia is a disorder of visual perception, only one of which is the visual acuity on the standard vision charts (Snellen acuity). But there are other visual functions too that are affected.

The **amblyopia syndrome** shows the following abnormalities:
1. Decreased visual acuity (e.g. Snellen's)
2. Decreased grating acuity (e.g. Teller's)
3. Decreased Vernier acuity
4. Decreased or lost stereo-acuity
5. Decreased contrast sensitivity
6. Decreased brightness perception

7. Abnormal contour interaction
8. Increased perception and reaction times
9. Naso-temporal asymmetries in resolution of vertical gratings
10. Motility defects in pursuit, saccades and fixation.

While the hallmark of amblyopia is decreased visual acuity, it is important to understand that **recognition acuity** (Snellen's or similar charts) is or more affected than either **resolution acuity** (Teller's, VER, etc.) or **detection acuity** (Catford drum or Bailey-Hall cereal test). Secondly the anisometropic and strabismic amblyopes behave differently. The Snellen letter or recognition acuity is affected more in strabismic or mixed (strabismic + anisometropic) amblyopes compared to anisometropic amblyopes. Both Snellen's acuity and grating acuity are affected equally in anisometropic amblyopes, whereas in strabismic amblyopes the grating acuity is affected to half the extent of Snellen's acuity. Thus strabismic amblyopia is underestimated on grating tests.

For **diagnosis of amblyopia** any diminution of vision: Difference between two eyes in case of both eyes being affected, difference from the age-related norm is taken to indicate amblyopia. Clinically a **two-line on Snellen's chart** (one octave difference) is considered significant.

The visual apparatus is capable of making much finer spatial discriminations than resolving capability of the retina may suggest (by Snellen's or grating acuity), this is termed the **hyperacuity**. Two common types hyperacuity are **Vernier acuity** and **Stereo acuity**. Vernier acuity includes a variety of tasks that involve sensing the direction or spatial offset of a line or a point to a reference. Vernier acuity can have an accuracy of 3–6 seconds of arc or better. This processing is technically of "sub-pixel" resolutions and is done at higher cortical areas. These are not easily influenced by retinal image motion or optical blur, implying there less likelihood of deterioration

by uncorrected refractive errors or light media opacities. The latter aspect has been utilised in predicting visual potential in the presence of cataract.

Another well recognized feature of strabismic amblyopic vision is that it is not degraded by **neutral density filters**, it may even show some improvement. However, in anisometropic amblyopes, an equal deterioration was seen in amblyopic and normal eyes. Other organic retinal pathologies causing diminution of vision are susceptible to deterioration by neutral density filters. This test can thus distinguish functional amblyopia from these conditions.

Abnormal contour interaction is seen in the form of degradation of visual acuity for objects placed in a row or line (linear acuity), compared to the acuity of the same object viewed separately (single letter acuity). This phenomenon has been described as the **crowding phenomenon.** Crowding phenomenon is present to some extent even in normal subjects (critical area of separation=1.9 to 3.8 min. of arc). In amblyopes it is even more pronounced, similar to the critical area of separation of peripheral retina of normal subjects, (=8.4 to 23.3 min. of arc). The crowding phenomenon has also been attributed to the poor visual acuity that is there in amblyopes. But its importance in prognosticating progress in amblyopia therapy should be remembered. The **single letter acuity** improves more rapidly during the course of treatment. Finally both the **single letter** and **line acuity** should approach each other, if it is not so there is always a risk of recurrence of amblyopia. For children untestable with line charts single **letter optotypes with "surrounds"** can be used to cause contour interaction.

In the normal charting of Snellen vision, high contrast (80%) letters are used, but in amblyopia **abnormal contrast functions** have been recorded both in strabismic and anisometropic amblyopes, particularly at high spatial frequencies. Thus, though at low spatial frequencies the contrast sensitivity is the same as normal, at high spatial frequencies the contrast sensitivity in amblyopes is deteriorated, more so with severe amblyopia. This is due to a neural loss of foveal function and not due to optical factors, or unsteady fixation movements or eccentric fixation. Contrast sensitivity has been observed to differ in strabismic and anisometropic amblyopes. It became normal in strabismic amblyopes when the luminance levels were reduced, while the deficit persisted in anisometropic amblyopes.

Other **psychophysical functions** are also affected. While primarily it is the form vision which is affected in amblyopia, **brightness perception** is also affected. Dark adaptation curves are essentially normal and even if there is an effect on the **light sense** there is clearly a dissociation between the effect on the light sense and the acuity. While recovery time after a glare stimulus to fovea is normal, the **perception time** and reaction time is 6 times longer. The **critical flicker fusion frequency** (rate at which a flicker just disappears) is generally normal compared to maculopathies. Pupils are generally normal and briskly reacting though **afferent pupillary defect and raised edge light pupil cycle time** has been reported by some workers. It may be generalised that:

1. **In amblyopia the visual perception in fovea simulates that of the peripheral retina.**
2. **The amblyopic visual system contains abnormally large receptive fields.**
3. **Functionally the amblyopic eye is at its best in mesopic and scotopic conditions and at its worst in photopic conditions.**

Binocular Development and Amblyopia

Though practical difficulties have limited the data pertaining to the visual development in humans, elegant and methodical experiments conducted by investigators on kitten and baby monkeys have revealed a lot. The periods mentioned in human is by extrapolation from experimental work.

Intrauterine Development

In the human retina most of the ganglion cells are generated between the eighth and fifteenth week of gestation, when the ganglion cell population reaches a plateau of 2.2 to 2.5 million. This is maintained till the thirtieth week, when it starts to fall drastically due to rapid cell death for about 6–8 weeks. Thereafter this process continues at a rapid rate through birth for the first few months of infancy. The ganglion cells at the final count are about 1 million. The loss of more than a million cells and their axons serve to fine tune the topography and specificity of the retinogeniculate projection by elimination of inappropriate connections. The geniculate body in humans is generated between gestational 8–11 weeks and by 10th week the first retinal ganglion cells start invading the LGB. The geniculate laminae emerge between 22 and 25 weeks. From an initial intermingling of inputs from each eye, the segregation of afferents occurs by pruning.

The striate cortex cells appear at the age of 10–25 weeks of human fetus. The geniculate afferents begin to innervate the striate cortex by 26th week. This has been demonstrated by injection of anatomic tracers. Initially geniculate afferents representing each eye overlap extensively in layer 4c. The segregation of inputs into **ocular dominance columns** occurs during the last few weeks of pregnancy and is almost complete by 4–6 weeks of birth. Until shortly before birth there is a sort of loose wiring, which is extensive and expansive, providing enough of material for fine tuning, which occurs by a method of making new usable synapses and breaking old unused synapses, **synaptogenesis**.

In the retina two streams of ganglion cells: **alpha (a) cells and beta (b) cells,** are present. The A cells communicate via the magnocellular layer of the LGB (large cell layers: 1

Table 4.1: Parallel visual pathways

Retinal Ganglion cell	LGB Lamina	V_1	V_2	Cortex Other
Alpha	Magno-cellular	4B	Thick stripes	V_3 MT, motion
Beta	Parvo-cellular	4A interblob	Inter-stripes	V_4, static stereopsis
Beta	Parvo-cellular	4A blob	Thin stripes	V_4, colour

Note: V_1 - Striate cortex primary visual area (A-17) V_2-V_3 V_4 are in Area 18, 19 and more anterior temporoparietal cortex.

and 2) to the cells of 4-alpha of visual cortex, area 17. The B cells of retina communicate via the **parvocellular layer** of the LGB (small cell layers: 3–6) to 4-c-beta cells of the visual cortex, area 17 (Tables 4.1 and 4.2).

The modular organization of columns in the cortex is tuned to a variety of stimulus specifics such as orientation, binocular disparity, motion perception, colour perception, etc. Each has very discrete inputs and outputs (Fig. 4.12).

The basic applied aspect of all this development process is that the visual development is occurring by changes in the connections over a period of 0-5 years or more up to 9 years, during which it is plastic until it reaches visual maturity. Later, all these inter connections are difficult to be changed. The two pathomechanisms for different types of amblyopia are (i) **form vision deprivation** and (ii) **abnormal binocular interaction** (Fig. 4.13).

The Role of Visual Stimulus

Visual experience has a significant role to play in the aforementioned synaptogenesis. In monkeys born by Cesarean section with closed eyes, precisely oriented simple and complex cells similar to the adult animal are seen, even with the orderly sequence of ocular dominance and orientation columns. These are maintained in utero by spontaneous action

Table 4.2: Comparison of visual processing systems

	Magnocellular	Parvocellular
I. Perception	Thick stripes • Motion • Flicker • Transient luminance	a. Interblob-interstripe • High spatial frequency acuity • Some colour b. Blob thin stripe • Colour • Low spatial frequency acuity
II. Stereopsis	• 40"–80" • Local • Non cyclopean • Coarse • Motion	a. Interblob-interstripe • 6"–1000" • Global • Cyclopean • Fine • Static b. Blob-thin stripes • Depth tilt
III. Ocular motor	• Pursuit • Vergence initiation	• Vergence maintenance

Ref. (1) Tyler CW Sensory processing of binocular disparity in Schor CM, Ciuffreda KJ eds Vergence Eye Movements Basic and Applied Aspects. Boston, Butterworth, 1983.
(2) Tyler CW A stereoscopic view of visual processing streams. Vision Res. 30. 1877–1990.

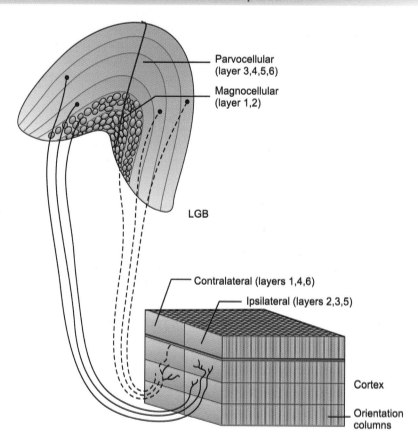

Fig. 4.12: Organization of visual cortex and lateral geniculate body LGB. The relationship of ipsilateral and contralateral fibres which compete in layer IVc of cortex (after Hubel and Wiesel, 1965).

potentials discharged by mammalian retinal ganglion cells. Abolition of these action potentials by tetrodotoxin, prevents the normal prenatal segregation of retinogeniculate axons into appropriate laminae of the LGB. The same is observed after intraocular administration of tetrodotoxin. If a new born monkey is reared in dark or with both eyes sutured, cells in striate cortex develop bizarre receptive field properties, losing sharp orientation tuning and normal binocular responses. After a prolonged period of deprivation, if the monkey is reintroduced to normal visual environment (lids reopened), the animal is profoundly blind with minimal potential for recovery. These observation stress the role of visual stimulus for normal binocular development, and are corroborated by good visual recovery only if early surgery and rehabilitation is done for bilateral or unilateral cararacts.

The Role of Monocular Deprivation

The experiments of Hubel and Wiesel have established the role of cortical competition in binocular visual development. To start with at birth all cortical cells have potential connections with both eyes. If both eyes are functioning equally, the cortical cells driven by each eye are equal. About 10% cells are driven by right eye alone and a similar number by the left eye, the rest 80% cells are driven binocularly (the central 20% of these equally by both eyes and the rest have a

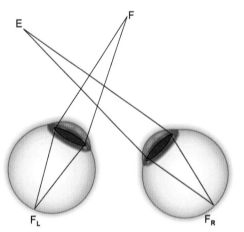

Strabismic amblyopia. Right fovea suppressed in right esotropia (abnormal binocular interaction)

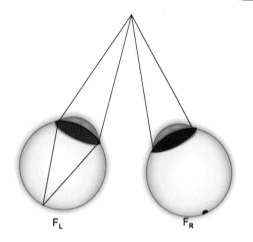

Stimulus deprivation amblyopia. Right fovea suppressed due to cataract right eye (form vision deprivation) plus abnormal interaction

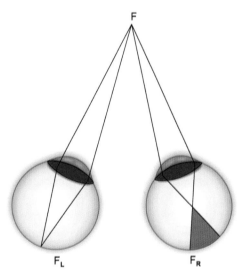

Anisometropic amblyopia. Right fovea suppressed due to uncorrected refractive error in right eye (form vision deprivation + abnormal interaction

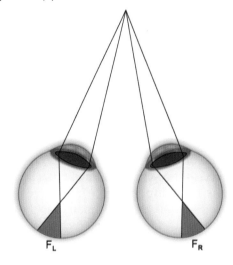

Ametropia amblyopia. Both fovea suppressed due to bilateal uncorrected refractive error (form vision deprivation)

Fig. 4.13: Pathomechanism in different types of amblyopia (after von Noorden, 1974).

predominance of one eye or the other) If by any chance one of the eyes is not functioning properly, the cortical cells of one eye are stolen or usurped by the other. This process of competition is entirely reversible in the initial period of plasticity, (Fig. 4.14). Monocular deprivation produces a radical alteration in the ocular dominance columns in the striate cortex in favour of the normal eye. It is believed that the two eyes compete for synaptic contacts in **layer 4-c of visual cortex**. Monocular eyelid closure imposes a severe handicap in this contest. As a consequence the deprived eye loses many of the connections

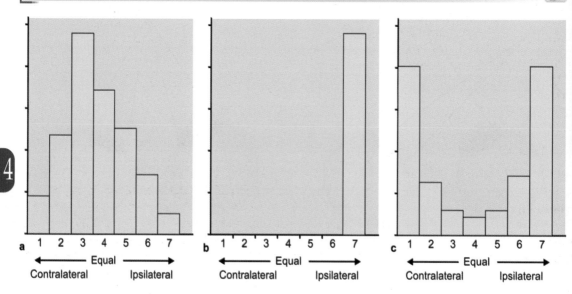

Fig. 4.14: Responses of cortical cells to stimulation by ipsilateral or contralateral eye. (a) Normal groups of cells numbered 1–7 with extremes being stimulated by contralateral or ipsilateral eye only. Group 4 stimulated equally by both sides. In normals equal dominance of two sides seen with 80% cells binocularly driven, (b) In unilateral squint with amblyopia, predominant stimulation seen by normal eye, (c) In alternating squint with no amblyopia both ends have monocular dominance with few binocularly driven cells. (Made from data from: Hubel & Wiesel and Von Noorden).

already formed at birth. The ocular dominance columns of the deprived eye shrink and those of the favored eye swell. A similar change is observed in the laminae of the LGB, although there is no competition at this level. The deprived of LGB cells are smaller as they are required to sustain a lesser arbor of axons in layer 4-c of cortex.

Important Conclusions

Some important conclusions from these studies are:

1. The loss of binocularly innervated striate neurons is not specific for amblyopia, it occurs after any brief disruption of binocular input early in life. This has been correlated with stereopsis.

2. The decrease of cells responding to the stimulation of the amblyopic eye is highly specific for amblyopia, regardless of the etiology and correlates quantitatively with the decrease of visual acuity.

3. Even one week of disruption is sufficient to cause amblyopia in the sensitive period. Occlusion amblyopia develops rapidly in children upto 4 years, but can occur later also.

4. Recovery of the neurons connected with amblyopic eye does occur on treatment, but impairment of binocular cells appears to be permanent, at least in monkeys, after disruption of binocular vision early in life. Infantile esotropia of early onset does not allow good stereopsis.

5. In anisometropic and visual deprivation amblyopia both monocularly and binocularly innervated portions shrink, but in strabismic amblyopia only the binocularly innervated part shrinks, in the LGB. In the cortex the same is observed for visual deprivation amblyopia but need to be confirmed for strabismic and anisometropic amblyopia.

6. Nerve growth factor (neurotrophin) seems to prevent shrinkage in LGB in rats in

strabismic and visual deprivation amblyopia, yet to be confirmed in primates.

The applied aspect in clinical practice is: the same process occurs during occlusion therapy. In the initial period of therapy the vision improves in the amblyopic eye by the "take over" of the selected cells of the other eye and is reflected in the drop in visual acuity of the normal eye. However, gradually the earlier "unselected" cells are recruited for the amblyopic eye. Thus all the gain of the amblyopic eye is not due to a loss of the good eye. But a loss is possible if the normal eye is not given a chance intermittently, a breather. Then it results in occlusion amblyopia, which is a type of visual deprivation amblyopia and has grave prognosis.

The Critical Period

The critical period corresponds to the time phase when the wiring is still malleable. It should be clear that when amblyopia is likely to be corrected, occlusion amblyopia is also possible. For good effect this period is 6–8 years in humans. It has been observed to differ for different types of amblyopia. For visual deprivation amblyopia the upper limit is 6 years, and for anisometropic amblyopia it is 8 years. The latter cases do respond even in the teenage, whereas the strabismic amblyopes do not respond after 12 years. It depends on the presentation vision and the motivation and compliance of the subject to do the occlusion, which is more and more difficult as age advances but not impossible.

ANOMALOUS RETINAL CORRESPONDENCE

Anomalous retinal correspondence (ARC) is a binocular functional adaptation to strabismus at the cortical level. The fovea of the fixing eye develops a correspondence (binocular relationship) with an extrafoveal point of the other eye. Thus the two eyes become functionally linked binocularly albeit in an anomalous (abnormal) connection. The

shift from the fovea to the extrafoveal point of the other eye is the angle of anomaly. The latter may be considered as a zero-error correction at the perceptual level in order to restore binocularity in spite of a manifest strabismus.

At the **cortical level there is a change in the synaptic connections from the foveo-foveal to the foveo-extrafoveal**. This automatically implies that the extra-foveal point should not be anatomically far-off, this puts a limit on the possibility of the connections (clinically it is for up to 8 pd (4°) Esotropia). The extrafoveal point should have good visual potential in order to have an association with the fovea of the fixing eye.

To give an analogy: The squint may be equated to a quarrel or misunderstanding between two friends, if one of the two is weak or of less importance (=poor vision), he can be easily ignored (=suppressed), but if he be of equal importance or influence (=good vision), a reconciliation is attempted. The reconciliation (=ARC) will never be as good as a normal friendship (=normal bifoveal correspondence).

Requirements for ARC

ARC is possible in the following situation:
- Early onset squints (good neural plasticity is required for new synaptic connections),
- Constant angle of deviation (constancy of stimuli required for the new connections).
- Small esodeviations mostly, but rarely small angle constant exodeviations also develop (exodeviations are generally intermittent if variable due to good fusional convergence).

On the contrary variable angle deviation, or intermittent deviations or late onset squint do not develop ARC.

Diagnosis of ARC

The basic requirement in diagnosis of ARC is to **assess the angle of deviation by the subjective and the objective methods**. ARC present when the subjective and objective deviations differ. If there is normal retinal correspondence (NRC) the objective and subjective angles are the same. If the subjective angle is zero (no subjective squint) in the presence of objective angle showing a squint, it is **harmonious ARC**. If the subjective angle is not zero but is still less than the objective angle of deviation, it is unharmonious ARC. If subjective angle is SA, objective angle is OA and angle of anomaly is AA, then:

In HARC: OA-SA =AA, SA=0, $\therefore$ OA=AA

In UHARC: OA-SA=AA, OA is more than SA

In NRC: OA = SA $\therefore$ AA = 0.

The **objective angle** of deviation can be measured by Prism Bar Cover Test (PBCT) or by cover-uncover test on the synoptophore, with the alternate on-off method.

The **subjective angle** of deviation can be measured by various methods depending on the method used for dissociation. In order of most dissociating to the least dissociating they are as follows:

1. After-image test
2. Synoptophore
3. Worth four dot test (red-green dissociation)
4. Maddox rod or red filter test
5. Polaroid dissociation
6. Phase difference haploscope
7. Bagolini's striated glasses

It should be understood that the abnormal coordination could be "fragile" which may breakdown in case of more dissociating tests. And it has been observed that there may be **two levels of correspondence**. One working at a finer level (more physiological and real situations, seen by less dissociating tests) and other at a coarser level (manifesting with the more dissociating tests). This can result in different responses with different tests. A finer test like Bagolini's test would give more often a harmonious ARC whereas a more dissociating test like synoptophore or after-image test would give an unharmonious

ARC or a suppression response of the deviating eye.

Bagolini's Striated Glasses

The squint is measured first by cover test using PBCT, (=objective angle—OA.). Next with the squint manifested, the patient looks through the Bagolini's striated glasses. If he sees a cross response (seen by a person with normal retinal correspondence with no squint), in the presence of a manifested squint, it implies a HARC. In the presence of squint with NRC he sees two oblique lines crossing asymmetrically to form a V or A instead of the normal X response. In the presence of suppression he sees only one line, the other line of the other eye suppressed is not seen. In case of a central (macular) scotoma the eye with the scotoma sees a line with a break in the centre.

If the patient does not see a cross (X), the prisms are added to get an X response, the prism power required is the subjective angle of deviation (=SA).

For example, if the deviation is 25 pd base-out (BO), (OA = 25 pd), and with the Bagolini's glasses it neutralizes with 15 pd BO (SA = 15 pd). It is an unharmonious ARC with the angle of anomaly being 10 pd. If it was HARC the neutralization would have been with zero prisms, and in case of NRC it would have required 25 pd.

Worth's Four Dot Test

In this test also the objective angle is measured by PBCT, but the subjective angle is measured with the patient wearing red-green glasses. The prisms are added till the patient sees the normal (no squint) response, that is the four dots in a normal rhombic pattern.

Synoptophore

The objective angle is measured by the patient alternately fixing till there is no movement of eyes on alternate on-off. The subjective angle is measured by the patient aligning the two images by his perception of simultaneous perception slides.

After Image Test

This also tests the subjective angle. Each eye is monocularly flashed with a self-flash to create a horizontal after image in right eye and vertical after-image in left eye. Each after image is centred at the fovea (even in cases of ARC, due to central fixation). A case of paralytic squint with esodeviation or exodeviation also sees a **symmetric cross**. But a case of anomalous retinal correspondence sees an **asymmetric cross**. The displacement between the centres of the two after images is proportional to the **angle of anomaly** (tan q = displacement/distance of testing). The angle of anomaly can thus be calculated.

Suggested Reading

1. Tychsen L. Binocular Vision/In Hart WM. ed. Adler's Physiology of the Eye: Clinical Applications. 9th Ed. St. Louis, Mo. CV Mosby. 1992 pp 773–853
2. Bagolini. BI Sensorial anomalies in strabismus (suppression, anomalous correspondence, amblyopia) Doc Ophthalmol. 41:1, 1976.
3. Bagolini B. II Sensorio-motorial anomalies in strabismus (anomalous movements). Doc. 41: 23. 1976.
4. Campos. EG. Amblyopia Surv. Ophthalmol. 40: 23–39. 1995.
5. Demer JL, Noorden GK von, Volkow ND, Gould KL. Imaging of cerebral blood metabolism in amblyopia by positron emission tomography. Am. J Ophthalmol 105.
6. Hubel DH and Wiesel TN. Receptive fields of cells in striate cortex of very young inexi kittens J. Neurophysiol, 154. 572, 1960.
7. Hubel DH, Wiesel TN and Le Vay S. Plasticity of ocular dominance columns in monkey cortex. Philos. Trans. R. Soc. London (Biol.) 278. 377, 1977.
8. Noorden GK. von. Mechanisms of amblyopia. Doc. Ophthalmol. 34. 93. 1977.
9. Noorden GK von. Amblyopia: A multidisciplinary approach (Proctor Lecture) Invest. Ophth Vis. Sci. 26. 1704, 1985.
10. Noorden GK. von. A reassessment of infantile esotropia (XLIV Jackson Memorial Lecture) Ophthalmol. 105, 1, 1988.
11. Demer JL, Noorden GK von, Volkow ND and Gould KL Brain activity in amblyopi Orthopt. J. 41. 56, 1991.
12. Crawford MLJ, Smith EL Ill, Harwerth RS and Noorden GK von, stereoblind monkey few binocular neurons Invest. Ophthalmol. Vis. Sci. 25. 779, 1984.
13. Fells P. Richardson Cross Lecture 1989. Amblyopia an historical perspective. Eye. 4:775.
14. Flynn JT. Amblyopia revisited. (17th Annual Costenbader Lecture) J. Pediatr. Ophthalmol. Strab 28. 183, 1991.

4

5

The Preliminary Examination and Assessment of Visual Acuity

HISTORY

The history given by the patient, his parents, or other peers is more important than the examination by the clinician. A well controlled deviation, without symptoms may be of no consequence whereas a small deviation that is symptomatic may require treatment. It is not the deviation per se but the discrepancy between the deviation and the motor amplitudes of fusion, that is of clinical importance. In recording the history it should be noted, that it is not just a verbatim patient's "story" but it is a clinician's record of "history". The clinician is like an historian, who should put the right questions and correctly interpret the patient's story to make it a history.

Presenting Complaints

First of all, the presenting complaints (Table 5.1) must be recorded in the patient's words. They may be **asthenopia or eye-strain**, associated with redness, heaviness, dryness and soreness of eyes, pain in and around the eyes or localized occipital and frontal headache. It should be enquired if these are on near work or on gazing at moving objects at a distance, as on seeing movies or at near, as working at the computer terminals. Asthenopia may be **uniocular** or **binocular**. Uniocular asthenopia is due to an uncorrected refractive error, including astigmatism or accommodative problems. **Extraocular muscle**

Table 5.1: Common presenting complaints

1. Eye strain
2. Associated redness, heaviness dryness, soreness
3. Pain in and around eyes
4. Headache*: occipital/frontal
5. Diplopia (binocular)
6. Deviation of eyes
7. Past pointing
8. Vertigo
9. Head posture

*All of these aggravation near work

weakness causes binocular asthenopia. It is relieved by occluding one eye. Patients with a neurotic disposition may have exaggerated symptomatology, even gastric symptoms and nervous exhaustion. Generalised weakness due to debilitating diseases may cause difficulty in maintaining fusion.

Cases with recent onset squint may present with **diplopia, past-pointing, vertigo** and **rarely prostration**. Diplopia may not be complained of in case of adoption of head posture or when sensory adaptations have occurred in the form of suppression-amblyopia or anomalous retinal correspondence. At times it may be just a cosmetic problem: a deviation or abnormality of eyes. Then it is of importance to know: who first noticed it and when? A cosmetic defect observed by the clinician but which does not bother the patient or his parents, should not be given undue significance. On the contrary a cosmetic defect perceived by the patient, or his parents though not observed by the clinician should be noted and checked on a repeat examination. About some cosmetic defects the patient may just require to be reassured.

The **age of onset** and the **duration of squint** have a tremendous bearing on the prognosis for attainment and maintenance of binocular vision. An early onset, long duration, constant angle squint has a poor prognosis. It is pertinent to ask about the precipitating event: injury, illness, shock or intimidation. A patching of an eye for a lid or anterior segment problem that breaks fusion can also precipitate a squint. In case it dates since birth, **antenatal factors like:** drugs taken or illness during pregnancy, and **perinatal factors like:** type and the length or any peculiarities of the labour, the birth weight, and the term duration should be enquired.

Regarding the **deviation** it should be noted whether it is **intermittent or constant, unilateral** (left or right) or **alternating**. An intermittent deviation, even of a longer duration, has a better prognosis, as at some time binocular stimulation was available. A constant deviation indicates poorer vision for the deviating eye, and a poorer prognosis for binocularity. A deviation may have been variable, and if it is so, note whether it is due to fatigue or near work (fusional or accommodative weakness). At times the deviation may be periodic or cyclic recurring at regular intervals. A history of head posture or a more specific history of no deviation with head posture, confirmable by old photographs, may indicate good binocular potential in spite of a congenital squint.

The **history of treatment** should be taken in detail and interpreted. A history of prescriptions of **glasses** should trigger queries: regularity of use, power of glasses being used, whether refracted under **proper cycloplegia for his age**? Also note if any **prisms** were prescribed at any time? Any history of undergoing **convergence exercises**? Any history of use of **occlusion**: its type, duration, compliance and at what age? Any history of surgery? If yes, one or both eyes? Which muscles, how much and what surgery? Such questions should be asked and if possible corroborated with accompanying papers.

REFRACTION

Whether or not a proper a visual assessment is possible in a young child, a proper cycloplegic refraction is indispensible. It is a serious blunder to operate a case without assessment of ocular deviation with his proper glasses, irrespective of a convergent or divergent squint. **All cases of squint under 6 years of age should be refracted under atropine cycloplegia, and preferably also all cases with eso deviation under 12 years of age.** Atropine sulphate 1% ointment should be applied in **rice-grain size**, three times a day, for three days, prior to the day of refraction. Instillation of atropine drops should be avoided for the risk of systemic absorption via nasal mucosa. Allergy to atropine is rarer than feared and is usually a toxicity due to an overdose by an over-enthusiastic parent, not properly guided by the clinician. However, mild rise of body temperature or skin rash may be forewarned to the parent.

During refraction if necessary, **sedation** by phenergan syrup (one tea-spoon) or chloral hydrate (50–100 mg/kg of a 500 mg/10 ml solution) may be used. Rarely a general anesthesia may be required, but mostly withholding feeds until refraction time should suffice. In small children uncooperative for post cycloplegic testing, the prescription should be done under the effect of cycloplegia itself, on the basis of retinoscopy. This is better accepted by hyperopic children. The effect of wearing of glasses cannot be assessed immediately and may take weeks for the accommodative mechanism to relax. Therefore a **proper time should be allowed** for the prescribed glasses before any deviations are measured.

Refractions in children are notorious to change from time to time. Majority of neonates are hyperopic at birth, which increases till about 7 years, when it starts decreasing till teenage, The trend is of **emmetropization** though all cases may not become emmetropic. Refractions are therefore required from time to time. It may be desirable every 6 months in first two years and then annually till about 6–7 years or whenever necessitated, as determined by the change in vision or other symptoms due to poor vision.

EXAMINATION OF ANTERIOR AND POSTERIOR SEGMENT

The examination of associated **lid problems**, **ptosis** or **media opacities** in the anterior segment is of direct importance. The examination of **pupillary reflexes** may reveal the underlying **optic nerve** or **retinal pathologies** which may be responsible for poor vision. Similarly an organic pathology in the fundus seen by the ophthalmoscope may avoid an occlusion which would be of no use. A good, sharp foveal reflex is therefore a good prognostic sign to be noted prior to occlusion. A note should also be made of the **site** and **type of fixation**, whether it is **steady** or **unsteady** and whether it is **foveal** (within 2°), **parafoveal** (2°–5°), **paramacular** (5°–10°), **paracecal** or **peripheral** (or **temporal**). A **steady central foveal fixation is a good prognostic sign** (Fig. 5.1). An unsteady but central foveal fixation indicates a possibility of good vision with conventional occlusion. But a steady peripheral or paramacular or paracecal fixation generally indicates a poor prognosis. Eccentric fixation is generally unilateral, with the other eye showing central fixation. But sometimes one may encounter

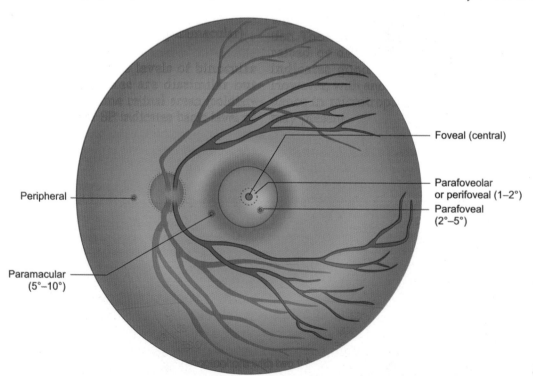

Fig. 5.1: Eccentric fixation. Some people also use a term "paracecal" for fixation close to blind spot, and 'Temporal' for exodeviations (beyond paramacular).

bilateral eccentric fixation. This is usually vertical, i.e. the fixating points are above or below the fovea in both the eyes. It indicates a macular pathology, which may be being missed clinically. Electrophysiological tests: ERG and EOG, done in such cases confirm and prognosticate such cases.

The examination of the fundus has assumed more importance, recently, in light of objectively observing **torsion of the eyes**, (Fig. 5.2). In normal individuals a horizontal line drawn through the fovea cuts the disc midway between the centre of the disc and the lower pole. (That's why the blind spot is 3/4 below the horizontal line in the visual fields). In significant **intorsion (incycloduction)**, the horizontal line cuts the disc in its upper half or is above its superior pole. In significant

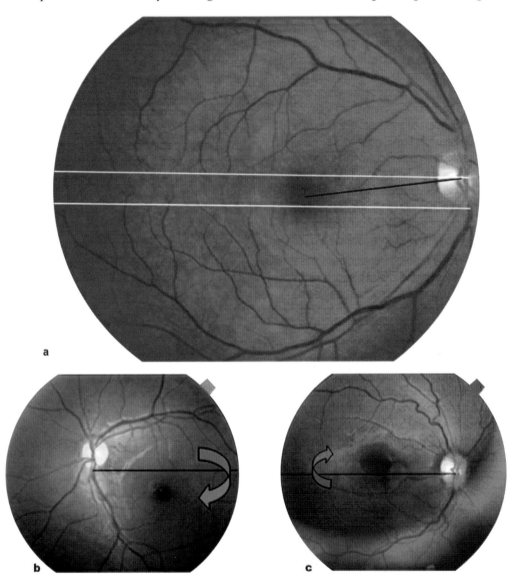

Fig. 5.2: Torsional assessment on fundus: (a) normal, (b) extorsion and (c) intorsion.

extorsion (excycloduction), the horizontal line passes below the inferior pole of the disc. This can be photographed or confirmed by charting central visual fields, with head held vertically straight.

VISUAL ACUITY ASSESSMENT

The basic function of the eyes is to see and the assessment of visual acuity deals with estimating the maximum ability to see. In adults the test is simple and standardized by using the Snellen's Charts at 6 metre distance (Fig. 5.3a). For academic and research purposes, these charts have been modified and the **log MAR** charts are used where each subsequent line differs by 0.1 log unit in the minimum angle of resolution (MAR) required for that line. They have equal number of letter in each line and are used at a distance of 4 metres as per the recommendation of National Academy of Science – National Research Council (NAS–NRC - 1980) of the Unites States (Fig. 5.3b).

The Organic Basis of Visual Acuity

The organic basis of visual acuity, or the finest optotype discrimination possible, depends[1] on

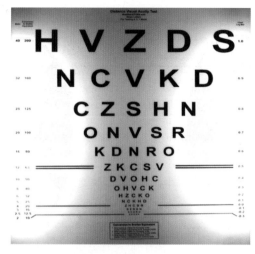

Fig. 5.3b: Log MAR vision chart showing 5 letters in each row, each row differs, with half octave difference.

the separation between the foveal cones and the size of foveal cones. **Two points can be discriminated as long as they stimulate two separate cones.** The width of foveal cones is 2.5 microns (μ). In terms of angular separation this distance is 30 seconds or half minute and thus allows a maximal visual acuity of 6/3 or 20/10 or 2.0 (in decimal notation). However, the **standard norm fixed is 6/6**, which is equivalent to an angular distance of **one minute at the fovea** (Fig. 5.4a). The 6/6 letter on any chart subtends an angle of 5 minutes at 6 metres distance and the critical separation between two parts of a letter like the gap of C

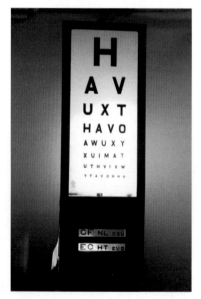

Fig. 5.3a: Snellen's vision chart.

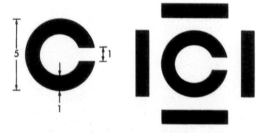

Fig. 5.4a: A Snellen's optotype subtends an angle of 5 minutes while each determinant part of the optotype subtends an angle of 1 min. of arc at the requisite distance for each optotype. Right hand side shows the optotype with surrounds for crowding effect.

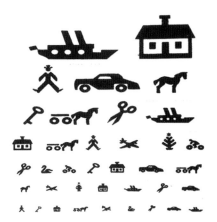

Fig. 5.4b: Allen picture optotypes.

or E is 1 minute at 6 metres. The same is true for a 6/60 letter at 60 metres distance. Picture optotypes shown in Fig. 5.4b.

Types of Visual Acuity

Visual acuity in a broad sense has been described to be of three types:

1. **Minimum visible** (which is actually a function of brightness and is about 1 second of arc).
2. **Minimum separable** (which is a hyperacuity, a function of higher cortical centres and is about 16–20 sec of arc more than the maximum potential of foveal cones therefore called hyperacuity. Vernier acuity and Stereoacuity are two examples).
3. **Minimum resolvable** and **minimum recognisable** (which is what is understood by visual acuity and is limited by the foveal configuration). The finest acuity can be of 30 sec of arc.

Tests for Visual Acuity

The tests for visual acuity can be grouped into three types:

1. **Detection acuity tests:** They assess the ability to detect the smallest stimulus, (without recognising correctly) e.g.
   i. Catford drum
   ii. STYCAR graded ball's test
   iii. Schwarting's metronome
   iv. Boeck candy beads
   v. Dot visual acuity
2. **Recognition acuity tests:** They assess the ability to recognise the stimulus or distinguish it from other competing stimuli.
   a. **Direction identification tests**
      i. Sjögren's hand test
      ii. Landolt's C
      iii. Snellen's E
      iv. Arrows.
   b. **Letter identification tests**
      i. Snellen's charts
      ii. Sheridan's letter test (STYCAR)
      iii. Lippman's HOTV test
      iv. Ffook's symbol test
   c. **Picture identification charts**/miniature toys
      i. Beale Collin's picture charts
      ii. Light house test
      iii. Allen's picture cards
      iv. Domino cards test
      v. Miniature toy test of Sheridan
   d. **Picture identification on behavioural pattern**
      i. Bailey-Hall cereal test
      ii. Cardiff acuity cards
      iii. OKNOVIS: Based on arrestovisography
3. **Resolution Acuity Tests**
   i. Optokinetic drum
   ii. Preferential looking tests
      • Forced choice or operant type
      • Teller Acuity cards,
   iii. Visually evoked responses.

A SIMPLE FORMULA FOR ESTIMATING VISION

One can estimate the visual acuity of a child, if one knows the size of the smallest object that is recognised by a child, at a particular distance by this formula, VA in decimal units (6/6 = 1.0)

5

$$VA = \frac{0.3 \times \text{Object distance in meters}}{\text{Object size in mm}}$$

a. Vision Tests in Different Ages

The commonly available tests have been grouped as used in different age groups:

Vision Tests in Infancy

1. Catford Drum Test

This is a detection acuity test devised by Catford and Oliver useful in infants and preschool children. It is based on the observation of an pendular eye movement (oscillatory eye movement not an optokinetic nystagmus) that is elicited as the child follows an oscillating drum with dots. The displayed dots are in various size: 15 mm to 0.5 mm and the test distance is 60 cm (2 feet). The dots represent 20/600 to 20/20 vision. The smallest dot that evokes the pendular eye movement determines the visual acuity. Unfortunately it is known to overestimate vision by double or quadruple times and is unreliable for amblyopia screening (Fig. 5.5).

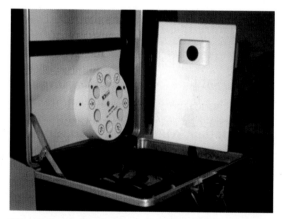

Fig. 5.5: Catford drum showing oscillating dot optotypes of different sizes, used at 50 cm distance for detection of acuity vision.

Other tests of this type are:

    i. Mc Ginnis' drum which has vertical black and white stripes,

    ii. German's canopy with striped scroll arched over infant's head,

    iii. Harcourt's OKN drum (actually tests resolution acuity by eliciting an optokinetic nystagmus).

The disadvantage of detection acuity tests or resolution acuity tests is that they do not indicate the normalcy of the parietal cortex. Also note that a moving optotype is detected better than a stationary one.

2. Preferential Looking Tests

These are based on the behavioural pattern of an infant to prefer to fixate a pattern stimulus rather than a blank, both being of the same brightness: **space average luminance**. This preference would be elicited as long as the pattern is visible or resolvable by the child. In the testing methodology it is called **Forced Choice Preferential Looking Test (FCPL)** and is usually done as two **alternative forced choice (2-AFC)**. In the operant variation (OPL), the behaviour pattern of the child is reinforced by giving him an incentive for a correct choice.

In the original system, it requires a parent in whose lap the child sits, an observer who is blind to the patterns displayed (just observes the preference), and a third person checks the correctness of the response.

Teller Acuity Cards Test (TAC)

TAC is a modification based on PLT which is designed for a simpler and rapid testing. It has seventeen 25.5 × 51 cm cards. Fifteen of these contain 12.5 × 12.5 cm patches of square-wave gratings (vertical black and white stripes) ranging in spatial frequency, from 38.0 cycles/cm to 0.32 cycles/cm. The range is in half-octave steps (Figs 5.6a to c).

It may be noted that a cycle consists of one black and one white stripe and an octave is a halving or doubling of spatial frequency (Table 5.2). **In Snellen's terms it is an halving or doubling of the denominator, e.g. 6/6,6/ 12,6/24. Half octave steps would be 6/6, 6/9, 6/12, 6/18, 6/24 and so on. There is a 'Low Vision Card' containing 25.5 cm × 23 cm**

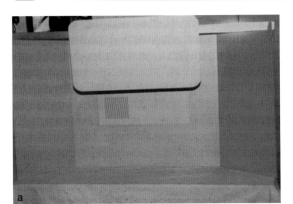

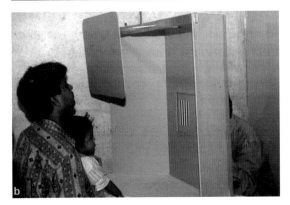

Table 5.2: Conversion of cycles/cm to Snellen's

Cycles /cm at 55 cm	Snellen's equivalents base 20 feet	base 6 metres
38.0	20/16	6/5
26.0	20/24	6/7.5
19.0	20/32	6/9
13.0	20/47	6/15
9.8	20/63	6/18
6.5	20/94	6/30
4.8	20/130	6/40
3.2	20/190	6/60
2.4	20/260	6/75
1.6	20/380	6/114
0.86	20/710	6/200
0.43	20/1400	6/420
032	20/1900	6/600

because of brightness difference. Detection of pattern alone determines the fixation preference. Proper illumination without any shadows, scratches or smudges on the screen or the charts should be ensured (10 candelas/m²).

Testing distance from patients's eyes to the cards is maintained constant as it determines the visual acuity.

- Infants up to six months of age are tested at 38 cm,
- From age seven months to three years at 55 cm and later at 84 cm.

The test is a very useful quick test for the infants and preschool especially up to 18 months after which children start having distractions. Graph shows the visual acuity by TAC.

Certain drawbacks should be kept in mind.

- It tests near acuity, not distance acuity and so can miss mild myopia (up to 3 D).
- It measures resolution acuity and not recognition acuity. Measures of resolution acuity over estimate visual acuity and can miss conditions like amblyopia.

Conversion of cycle/cm to cycles/degree for distance 20 cm or more

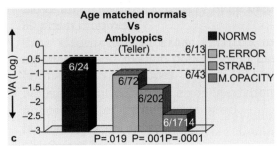

Fig. 5.6: (a and b) Show the procedure: Teller acuity cards and the screen showing grating on right side of the observing hole with blank on left side. (c) Visual acuity by Teller acuity cards in normals and amblyopics at 11 months of age.

patch of 0.23 cycle/cm (2.2 cm wide black or white stripes). The seventeenth card is a blank gray card with no grating pattern.

The gratings have 82–84% contrast and is matched to the surrounding gray card to within 1% in space average luminance. This minimises the chances of a patient fixing

$$Cycle/deg = \frac{Test\ dist. \times Cycles/cm}{55}$$

(at 55 cm dist. cycles/deg = cycles/cm)

3. OKNOVIS

This is an objective test, devised by the author with the help of Bio Medical Engineering department of IIT Delhi. It is based on the principle of arresting an elicited optokinetic nystagmus by introducing optotypes of different sizes. It is a portable hand held drum moving at 12 rpm with coloured pictures to elicit an optokinetic nystagmus. Optotypes of different sizes are then introduced to arrest the OKN. The testing distance is 60 cm. The test lacks full optotype standardization but has advantages of being a quick objective test, (Fig. 5.7). This was presented at International Congress of Ophthalmology, 1994 at Toronto, and now may be adapted in computer format.

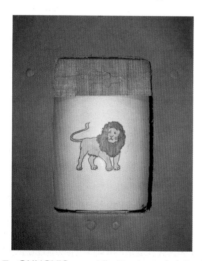

Fig. 5.7: OKNOVIS: an objective test of vision based on arrestovisography: optotype that arrests an elicited nystagmus.

4. Cardiff Acuity Cards (Fig. 5.8)

These are based on the principle of preferential fixation on cards which have a picture optotype and a blank located vertically. The picture optotypes are of the same size but have been specially drawn with two dark lines with

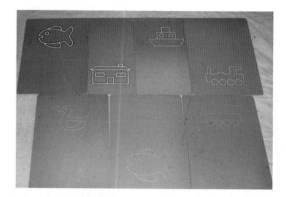

Fig. 5.8: Cardiff acuity cards based on vanishing optotype principle.

a white space (of varying width) in between, such that the picture is visible only at a particular distance or closer. These are known as **'vanishing optotypes,** as they vanish at a farther distance (Fig. 5.8).

They have been developed at Cardiff, UK. The child can identify the picture by verbalising, pointing or fixation preference. They are more likely to be in the Recognition Acuity group. The visual acuity is described in Snellen notations.

5. Visually Evoked Response (VER)

VER records the change in the cortical electrical pattern detected by surface electrodes monitoring the occipital cortex following light stimulation of the retina. The stimuli may be a pattern: checker board or stripes or an unpatterned flash. The pattern reversal type is preferred. The sizes of gratings or checks is 60, 30, 15 minutes of arc. Larger check sizes than 60 min (1°) are fallacious for visual-acuity. The P-100 amplitude and latency are noted. If the latency is not between 100 and 145 m sec it cannot be relied upon and should indicate poor vision. The VER can be recorded in two modes:

• **Transient VER**, where abrupt unique alteration of stimulus is at a relatively low rate so that each stimulus generates a separate VER output.

- **Steady state VER**, where rapid rate of stimulation causes the blending of the output into a continuous wave.

Visual acuity of 6/12–6/6 have been estimated at 6 months of age by VER. These estimates of visual acuity have not been very reliable and are higher than by other methods. They may reflect the electrophysiological changes but not truly indicate the visual characteristics which is a perceptual phenomenon. They are however useful in giving an objective record of the underlying visual pathway and do exclude organic pathology.

The Smith Kettlewell Institute, US group has described the 'Sweep-VEP' where 20 spatial frequency stimuli 0.2 cpd to 12.5 cpd are successively altered in a "Sweep" each projected for 0.5 sec, completing a test in ten seconds. The amplitude and phase measure for each spatial frequency is plotted. Acuity estimated by extrapolation of the graph of amplitude vs. check size function to zero amplitude.

6. *Indirect Assessment of*
   Visual Acuity in Infants

A knowledge of visual milestones helpful in estimating visual potential absence of any definite vision tests.

i. **Reflex responses**
The baby **blinks** at birth in response to sound, movement or touching the cornea, but not usually on the approach of an object. Menace reflex, which is a learned response, comes *by* 5 months.

The **pupil reacts** to light after 29th week of gestation. Premature babies of 26–30 gestation dislike bright light. The baby begins to turn its head to diffuse light after 32nd week of gestation.

ii. **Fixation**
The fixation reflex is a pre-requisite of normal visual development and is present at birth, even in preterm babies after 33 weeks

gestation (Tables 5.3 and 5.4). But it may not be well established, 75% of infants fixate by two weeks and 100% by **two months**. Newborns show fixation **preference** for moving stimuli, blinking lights patterned stimulus, stimuli with high contrast, stimuli with colours especially red-green or human face. Near objects are preferred, fixation may not be steady and is interrupted with refixations. The spans of fixation last seconds to minutes.

Table 5.3: Fixation and vision

Fixation pattern	Visual acuity
• Gross eccentric fixation	Less than CF 1 m
• Unsteady central fixation	Less than 6/60
• Steady central fixation but not maintained	6/60–6/30
• Central steady fixation, can maintain but prefers other eye	6/24–6/9
• Central steady fixation, free alternation or cross fixation	6/9–6/6

Table 5.4: Age of child and visual acuity

Age in months	Visual acuity
1	6/120*
2	6/60*
6	6/30*
12–18	6/48–6/12
18–24	6/24–6/7.5
24–30	6/15–6/7.5
30–36	6/12–6/6

Note: *Visual acuity assessed by OKN, PL and VER. VER has revealed 6/6–6/12 at 6 months also. There is an overlap in visual acuities indicating variation in development of different children

Other associated changes with visual attention are widening of palpebral fissure relaxation of facial features and regularity respiration with relaxation of other moltor activity.

Central steady fixation usually means good potential for vision, in newborns atleast 6/60 later this should indicate 6/9–6/6 vision.

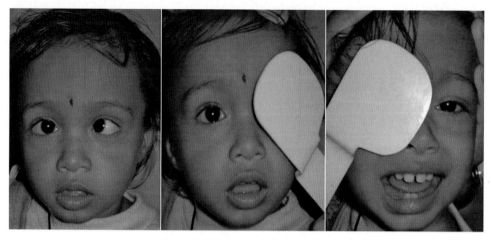

Fig. 5.9: Fixation preference test.

A preference of fixation with one eye over the other indicates poor vision in the non-preferred eye. Resentment of closure of one eye implies poor vision in the other eye (Fig. 5.9).

Induced Prism Test

Assessment of visual potential on the preference of fixation of one eye over the other is simple in the presence of a squint. In the absence of a squint a deviation can be induced by introducing a 10–15 pd prism base out, the child is forced to choose to fixate with one eye or the other.

iii. Follow-movements

Following horizontally moving targets has been seen in full term newborns and well developed by first month. Vertical tracking usually is elicited by 4–8 weeks. The movements may have jerky interruptions, and corrective movements are slow. The range of following is 45° at birth, 90° by 4 weeks and 180° by 3 months.

iv. Development of vision

The visual development occurs in two phases: rapid phase from birth to 8–9 months and a slow phase from 8–9 months to 8–9 years see graphs of Teller's Acuity Card (TAC). Visual milestones (Table 5.5).

Factors in Maturation of Vision

Several factors contribute to this development delay in maturation of vision:

i. Though rods and cones are distinguished even 15 weeks prior to birth, they do not attain adult-like dimensions until 4 months after birth.

ii. Myelination of visual pathways is completed by one month, but the amount of myelin increases in the subsequent months up to 2 years.

iii. Cortical neuronal dendritic growth and synapse formation at 25 weeks of gestational age, and is very active in the first two years.

These factors correlate with vision as well as other functions like

i. **Accommodation** which is minimal at 1 month age but well developed by 4 months age.

ii. **Fusion**, starts at 2 month age and fusional convergence developed by 6 months.

iii. **Stereopsis** is present at 1–2 months, well developed by 4 months, though adult levels may be seen at 5–7 years of age.

b. Vision Tests in 1–2 Years

Apart from the Acuity cards of Teller, Cardiff Acuity cards, some other tests become

Table 5.5: Visual milestones

Age	Visual milestones
1. 29 weeks Gestation,	Pupillary reaction to light
2. 30 weeks G to birth	Dislikes bright light (Closes lids in response)
	• Turns to subdued light
3. Birth–1 week	Fixation present
	• Follow horizontally moving targets–OKN and vestibular eye movements well developed.
	• Visual acuity on acuity cards (6/120)
4. 4 weeks–8 weeks	Fixation well developed
	• Follows vertically moving objects
	• Fusion develops
	• Watches mother's face intently for prolonged duration
	• Watches toys held in front of face
	• Doll's head eye movements present
5. 3 months	Watches movements of own hands
	• Reaches out to interesting objects
	• Prefers photographs, mirror faces to patterns.
6. 4 months	Foveal differentiation completed. Accommodation developed.
7. 5 months	Blink response to visual threat (Menace reflex)
8. 6 months	• Grasps objects and explores with fingers
	• VEP acuity adult level (6/6), Acuity cards: 6/30
	• Stereopsis on PLT well developed
	• Fusional convergence well developed
9. 9 months	Visual differentiation of objects, picks up small objects
10. 18 months	Visual acuity (Acuity cards: 6/6)
11. 3 years	Vision 6/9–6/6 on Tumbling E/HOTV (Recognition)
	• Contrast sensitivity adult level
12. 5–7 years	Stereopsis well developed (adult level)
13. 10 years	End of critical period for monocular deprivation (synapse formation completed)

(Modified from: *Greenwald MJ visual development in infancy and childhood in pediatric clinics of North America, 1983, 30 (6) 977–93*).

applicable. At the same time, as the child's attention is easily distracted after 9 months, the above tests become more difficult to perform in such older childen. The other tests are:

1. Boeck Candy Test

Small edible candies also serve as incentives are used as visual stimuli. Initially the child's hand is guided to the bead and then to his mouth. He finds it worth repeating. Each eye is alternately covered and the difference is noted.

2. Worth's Ivory Ball Test

Ivory balls 0.5" to 1.5" of diameter are rolled on the floor in front of the child. He is asked to retrieve each. Acuity is estimated on the basis of the smallest size for the test distance, (see formula on page 58).

3. Sheridan's Balls Test

These are styrofoam balls of different sizes rolled in front of the child. The quality of fixation for each size is assessed.

The same can be used as mounted balls used at 10 feet distance against a black screen fixation behaviour for each ball is observed by the examiner hidden behind the screen.

c. Vision Tests in 2–3 Years

1. **Miniature toys test:** This is a component of STYCAR test. Pairs of miniature toys are used. The child is asked to name or pick the pair from an assortment. Test distance is 10 feet.
2. **Coin test:** Coins of different sizes at different distances are shown. The child is asked to distinguish between the two faces of the coin.
3. **Dot visual acuity test:** In a darkened room the child is shown an illuminated box with printed black dots of different diameters, one at a time. Successively smaller dots are shown. The smallest dot identified correctly twice is taken as acuity threshold.

d. Vision Tests in 3–5 Years

Many vision tests using pictures, symbols, or even letters become applicable in this age group. A little training at home by the mother with the symbols to be shown is very helpful.

1. Tumbling E

This test is the preferred vision test for mass screening in preschool children. It consists of different sizes of E in one of the four positions: right, left, up, or down (Fig. 5.10) familiarising the child, he indicates in which direction the

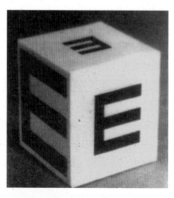

Fig. 5.10: The tumble E is an excellent vision test but tests single letter acuity.

E is oriented which he does by hand or orally. It is done at 6 metres distance and each eye is tested separately.

Single letter acuity is supposed to be better in amblyopes, in comparison to the line acuity on charts, due to crowding phenomenon. E with surrounds have been suggested to offset this disadvantage.

2. Landolt's C is used in a Similar Manner as also Sjögren's Hand and Arrows

3. Sheridan Letter Test

The Sheridan's test uses 5 letters H.O.T.V and X in the 5 letter set; A and U are added in the 7 letter set; and C & L are also added in the 9 letter set. Testing distance is 10 feet (3 metres). The child is expected to name the letters or indicate the similar letter on the card in hand.

4. Lippman's HOTV Test

This is a simpler version of the Sheridan's test using only 4 letters H,O,T,V at a test distance of 3 metres. The method is the same as above.

Other tests using pictures and symbols have been listed in the Recognition acuity in the table.

HYPERACUITY

The human eye is capable of seeing more than the ability of the retinal cones to resolve. This ability is called hyperacuity and is due to the involvement of higher cortical centres in the parietal cortex. Two examples of hyperacuity are:

1. **Vernier acuity:** This is the ability to discern the vernier separation between two lines not in perfect alignment. It is in the range of 10–20 arc seconds.
2. **Stereoacuity:** This is the ability to perceive a separation in the third dimension 3 D depth perception. It is 16 arc second.

Vernier Acuity Testing

Vernier acuity tests are of interest particularly in the screening of amblyopia as it is affected

Fig. 5.11: Figure showing gratings and Vernier gratings for Vernier acuity.

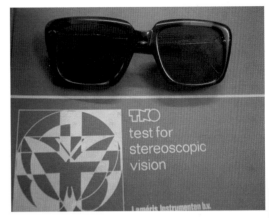

Fig. 5.12: TNO stereotest and the red and green glasses.

by amblyopia, whereas grating acuity may be fallaciously normal. It has been used in the Acuity card format for infants and small children, using the 2-AFC pattern (Fig. 5.11).

Stereoacuity

Stereoacuity has been seen to be developed and testable on the PLT by 6 months. It has been used as a screening test for binocular vision anomalies in preschool children, but with difficulty.

Stereoacuity Tests

The real-depth tests are not used as clinical tests. Most clinical tests are based on the haploscopic principle, using two two dimensional or vectographic pictures. Some elements of the two pictures have a disparity which is fused to create a 3-D image. This can be tested on:

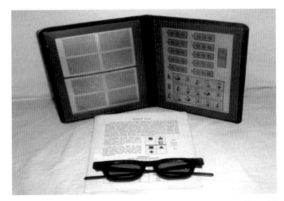

Fig. 5.13: Randot stereotest and the polaroid glasses.

i. Synoptophore: with stereopsis slides
ii. TNO test: With red-green goggles (Fig. 5.12)
iii. Randot stereotest and litmus stereotest: with polaroid spectacles (Fig. 5.13)
iv. Lang's stereotest: Using no glasses (Fig. 5.14)
v. Special 3-D pictures.

The last two are examples in which the dissociation is not achieved by glasses which may not be liked by children. The **Lang's test** is based on the principle of **"panography"**

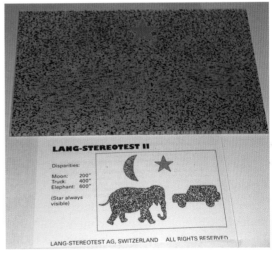

Fig. 5.14: Lang's stereotest.

where two images are printed on the same card each interrupting the other with regular linear interruptions. A prismatic film laminated over the picture ensures that one image is visible to right eye only and the other to the left eye only. The two, when fused in spite of the disparity, create a 3-D vision (Fig. 5.14).

The newer **special 3-D pictures**, much in fashion recently have two pictures specially merged in such a manner that if the two eyes are artificially diverged but controlling accommodates (as if looking for distance "through" the print), each eye sees two different images creating a 3-D image.

Randot Stereotest

This is the most popular clinical test and has replaced the earlier popular Titmus fly test. It uses Julesz' random dot background to mask monocular cues which are there with the 'animal' tests and Wirt's circle test. Geometric figures like square circle, triangle, star, etc., are also presented devoid of any monocular clues. But the latter type figures, though a better test, are usually not appreciated by small children (Fig. 5.13).

The test requires polaroid glasses to be worn by the patient. It is used at a distance of 40 cm and thus tests near binocular vision, so myopes up to 3 dioptres can be missed in a screening test. The Wirt's circles 1–10 test the stereoacuity from 400 arc sec to 20 arc seconds.

TNO Test

This test is also based on the random-dot background but uses red-green glasses for dissociation of the two images. It tests stereoacuity from 480 arc second to 15 arc seconds (Fig. 5.12).

Frisby Test

The Frisby stereotest consists of three perspex plates of differing thickness: 6 mm, 3 mm, and 1.5 mm. On one face of each plate are found squares, three of which are filled with a random pattern of blue triangles of various sizes and the fourth of which has a central, circular area that is not patterned. On the opposite side of the plate coincident with this area is a circular pattern of similar blue triangles. The plate is held in front of a white board and when viewed directly, the squares are all filled with random patterns although in one square a binocular viewer will see a circle standing up from the plate (crossed disparity) or lying below the rest of the design (uncrossed disparity) depending on which side of the plate is closest to the observer. By altering the thickness of the plate and the distance from the subject different stereoacuities can be assessed. For 30 cm viewing distance, the 6 mm, 3 mm and 1.5 mm plates represent 600, 300 and 150 arc seconds of stereoacuity, respectively. This assumes the interpupillary distance of 60 mm, but no significant change is caused by different IPD.

Distance Stereopsis Tests

Stereoacuity should be tested for distance also. A projection vectographic test or Oculus distance stereotests can be used to test stereopsis for distance. A diminished stereopsis for distance may be an early sign of decompensating exophoria. Recently Frisby Davis Disance(FD2) is used at 3,4 or 6 metres distance as a real depth test for distance stereopsis (Fig. 5.15). It has four forward or backward movable optotypes, and any one is moved keeping the rest as before and subject asked about the depth appreciation. The

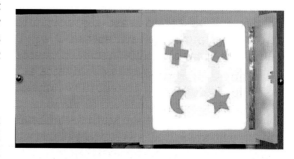

Fig. 5.15: Frisby Davis distance (FD2).

minimum difference he can appreciate is quantified. Another test is the distance Randot which is used at 3 metres distance (Fig. 5.16).

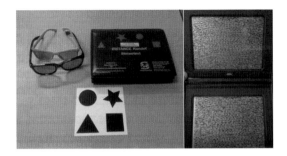

Fig. 5.16: Distance Randot test.

Normal Stereoacuity

Though adult individuals are capable of appreciating stereopsis with disparities as fine as 15–20 arc seconds. The adult-norm is 40 arc second. For children, 3–5 years old the norm is 70 arc seconds, and for 5–7 years it is 50 arc seconds. Children above 8 years have the adult norm.

Gross Stereopsis

In the absence of fine stereotests a gross estimation of stereopsis can be made by a bed side test: two pencil test of Lang and modified and popularised as horizontal pencils by the author.

A pencil is held in the examiner's hand horizontally and the child is asked to touch the tip with the tip of another pencil rapidly, coming from one side. Care should be taken to avoid giving the end on view of the pencil, as that can be accomplished even monocularly, therefore horizontal pencils are better, as they do not allow an end-on view. Always compare the binocular task with monocular task, is a gross-stereopsis test of about 400 arc disparity (Fig. 5.17).

A rough estimation of visual acuity has been made on the basis of stereoacuity.

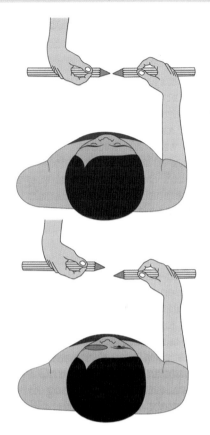

Fig. 5.17: Lang's two-pencil test to test gross-stereopsis. When tested with both eyes open (with binocularity) alignment is quick and precise. With squint or one eye closed the alignment is not easily achieved. Do not allow the patient to see the tip of examiner's pencil "end-on".

Suggested Reading

1. Bixenmann WW and Noorden GK von. Apparent foveal displacement in normal subjects and in cyclotropia. Ophthalmologica 89. 58, 1982.
2. Teller DY, McDonald M Preston, K. Sebris S.L. and Dobson V: Visual acuity in infants and children: the acuity card procedure. Dev. Med Child Neurol. 28. 779, 1986.
3. Sokol S. Visually evoked potentials: theory techniques and clinical applications. Surv. Ophthalmol 21. 18, 1976.
4. Wright KW, Kalonker F & Edelman P. 10 dioptre fixation test for amblyopia. Arch Ophthalmol 1242, 1981.
5. Fern KD and Manny RE. Visual acuity of the preschool child: a review. Am. J. Optom. Ph Optics. 63; 314-345, 1986.
6. Nongpur M and Sharma P. Horizontal Langs the pencil test. Ind J. Opthalmol.

5

Examination of a Case of Squint

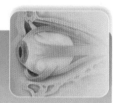

THE SQUINT EXAMINATION

Prerequisites

The examination of squint requires very few special equipment and allows for improvisation in case of absence of some others. What is indispensable is an equipped mind. Over the years the synoptophore, which for long symbolised this speciality, no more appears to be an essential outfit.

a. *Essential Equipment*

1. Prism bars: Horizontal and vertical.
2. Loose prisms set (at least 30 and 45 prism dioptre prisms).
3. Occluder.
4. Fixation targets, for distance and near to control the accommodation as desired.
5. Trial set with prisms of 1 to 8 pd. at least.
6. Bagolini's striated glasses.
7. Red and green goggles.
8. Double Maddox rod set.
9. Snellen's chart with letters and E in rows and also a single letter-E chart.
10. A protractor with a foot ruler.
11. Ophthalmoscope (direct).
12. Spielman's occluder (translucent or one-way reflecting or its equivalent).

b. *Desirable Equipment*

1. Synoptophore (basic type with antisuppression).
2. TNO or Randot stereotest for near.

3. Hess chart.
4. Perimeter (any one).
5. Camera for documentation.
6. Indirect ophthalmoscope.

c. *Additional Equipment*

1. Teller acuity cards with screen.
2. Cardiff cards and other pediatric vision cards.
3. Haidinger brushes and after images attachment for synoptophore.
4. OKN drums.
5. VER and electronystagmography system.
6. Distance Stereotests Frisby Davis Distance, Distance Randot.

THE EXAMINATION OF A CASE OF SQUINT

The examination of a case of squint will be considered in two aspects:

a. Examination of the motor status
b. Examination of the sensory status.

Examination of the Motor Status

The examination of the motor status entails looking for:

1. Head posture.
2. Ocular deviation.
3. Limitation of movements or the extent of the versions.
4. Fusional vergences.

Head Posture (Fig. 6.1)

Observation of head posture starts at the first glance of the patient, as he enters the clinic, without any instructions to him. This could be of significant importance as it reveals how much is the adaptability or handicap of the patient. A lot of information is lost after the patient becomes conscious of being examined. As noted earlier, head posture has three components:

1. **Chin** elevation or depression **(vertical)**
2. **Face turn** to right or left side **(horizontal)**
3. **Head tilt** to right or left shoulder **(torsional).**

These three components at three different joints between the head and the neck correct for the motility disturbances in the three dimensions. The patient chooses a head posture such that the ocular deviation is the least, and that can be fused. Rarely a head posture which provides for the maximal deviation is chosen so that the peripheral image can be easily suppressed or ignored. In fact if a head posture does not offer such an advantage, it may not be a clinically significant head posture, but just a habit.

Common causes of head posture should be noted.

i. **Incomitant squints** either paralytic, restrictive, or musculofascial anomalies commonly present with head posture.

ii. Apart from these concomitant squint with **A or V phenomenon** cases can also assume head posture: chin up in a V-exotropia or A-esotropia and *vice versa* in the other types.

iii. **Nystagmus** cases with a null position also have a head posture which can have any of the three or a combination thereof as the head posture.

iv. Other common causes are **refractive**, under corrected glasses in which the peripheral stronger power helps, or a wrong cylinder axis.

v. **One eyed persons** also can assume a head posture to centre their gaze to the available field.

vi. Just as the cases of **homonymous hemianopia** would also do so.

Ocular torticollis is a classic example of a head posture in cases of congenital superior oblique palsy who maintain a binocular vision in spite of the congenital defect. Such cases may present later with their head posture forcibly corrected, but old family photographs can be diagnostic and rule out a supposedly acute onset. The head posture in a case of right superior oblique (RSO) palsy will have chin depression, face turn to the left, and head tilt to the left shoulder. For comprehension it is told that: RSO being a depressor, chin depression occurs, it being an intorter, a head tilt towards the opposite shoulder occurs. And a face turn to the left brings the eyes in abduction so that the vertical movements can be executed by the vertical recti. **Head posture ensures that the eye is out of the field of action of the paralytic muscle.**

Measurement of Interpupillary Distance

The interpupillary distance (IPD) is a very important parameter that can give information about the craniofacial disorders, a true hypertelorism versus telecanthus, the vergence requirement and is helpful in proper centering of the spectacles. **Decentred lenses induce** prismatic effect and can increase or decrease an existing deviation, or induce a squint causing eye strain.

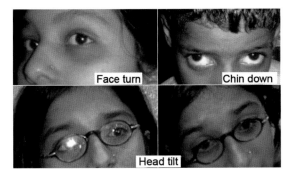

Fig. 6.1: Different head postures. Right face turn (top left); chin down (top right) and right head tilt for distance and near fixation (bottom).

a. *By an Ordinary Millimeter Scale*

A 15 mm rule, is required to measure the IPD.

The patient is seated with the examiner positioned about 33 cm in front, both in same vertical plane.

The millimeter rule is placed on the nasal bridge of the patient in the spectacle plane. The examiner closes his right eye and asks the patient to look at his left eye with his right eye (left eye may be closed). The scale reading bisecting the pupil is aligned to zero. Next the right eye of the patient is covered and patient asked to look at the examiner's right eye with his left eye. Again the scale reading bisecting the pupil of left eye of the patient is taken. The difference between the two readings gives the IPD.

It is better to note the scale reading aligned with the midline of the patient as zero reference point. This gives the pupillary distance of each eye from the midline and helps in detecting **asymmetry** of the face. An asymmetric face requires an asymmetric adjustment of the optical centres of the spectacle. The IPD should also be taken with the patient looking at the distant target (6 m) and IPD similarly measured. There may be slight (2–3 mm) addition of these near and distance measurements.

b. *Using the Pulzone-Hardy Rule*

This is a special device for measuring the pupillary distance of each eye. It has a slot for the nose and the central line is aligned with the midline of the patient. With the patient and examiner seated as in the above method, with the left eye occluded the patient fixates with his right eye at the examiner's left eye. The vertical wire is moved till it bisects the pupil. The reading is taken (half IPD). Similarly, the left half IPD is taken. Adding the two gives the interpupillary distance. Difference between the two readings indicates asymmetry.

c. *Using the Synoptophore*

The IPD can be simply determined on the synoptophore and is in fact the very first step before the synoptophore can be used for any measurement. This is done by adjusting the distance between the two eye pieces each of which can be separately adjusted and the distance between them read on a millimeter scale.

The arms of the synoptophore are kept at zero and the patient asked to look at the centre of the slide in the right picture tube with his right eye. The examiner with his right eye closed, aligns the central white line on the top of mirror unit of the tube with the reflection of the light in the centre of patient's pupil. The procedure is repeated with the left eye of the patient similarly and the IPD read from the millimeter scale. This once set is locked for the different procedures for one patient.

Ocular Deviation

The examination of ocular deviation is the most important part of our examination. First to establish the existence of a squint and next to quantify it. A squint complained of by the patient or parent may not be true, it may be an apparent squint. Looks can be deceptive! A cover test is required to establish the existence of a squint. But before we talk of cover test, let's consider apparent squint.

Pseudostrabismus

A **true squint** is a misalignment of the two visual axes, so that both do not meet at the point of regard. An **apparent squint** is just an appearance of squint in spite of the alignment of the two visual axes. Apparent squint or **pseudostrabismus** can be due to an abnormality of adnexal structures like the lids, canthi or orbits, or due to abnormal relationship between the visual axis and optical axis of the eyes.

A **telecanthus** or a broad nasal bridge covers the nasal bulbar conjunctiva and gives the appearance of a convergent squint (**pseudoesotropia**) (Fig. 6.2). This becomes

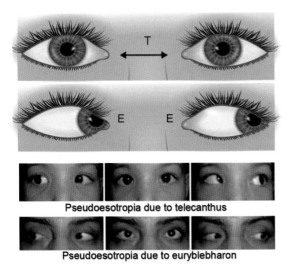

Fig. 6.2: Pseudoesotropia, marked on levoversion in right eye, due to telecanthus (T) and epicanthus (E) seen in mongoloid races and in infants.

Pseudoesotropia due to telecanthus

Pseudoesotropia due to euryblebharon

more prominent whenever a lateral gaze is attempted, the adducting eye getting covered by the telecanthal fold. Similarly, the **epicanthus** covers the nasal bulbar conjunctiva to cause a pseudoesotropia. Neonates and young infants are commonly suspected to have such a squint. A proper examination can exclude this and reassure the mothers.

A **hypertelorism** is a condition with greater interorbital separation and gives the appearance of a divergent squint (**pseudo-exotropia**) (Fig. 6.3). This appearance may well be compatible with beauty as testified by some actresses and models. Similarly, bilateral or unilateral lateral canthoplasty will give the look of a pseudoexotropia. On the other hand, **euryblepharon**, a condition with horizontally large palpebral apertures gives a look of pseudoesotropia.

Similarly, a **ptosis** or **lid retraction** can masquerade as a vertical squint. A ptosis may also mask an existing hypotropia or aggravate an hypertropia. And a telecanthus may mask an exotropia and highlight an esotropia. These appearances, therefore, assume importance even in a case of squint for surgery. The patient

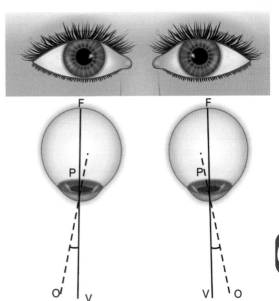

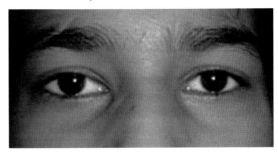

Fig. 6.3: Angle kappa. The angle formed between the visual axis VPF (joining the object of fixation and fovea) and the optical axis at the pupillary reference, OP. The angle is OPV is seen as the decentered corneal light reflex in reference to the pupil. The figure shows positive angle kappa (optical axis temporal) and gives a look of pseudoexotropia.

should be explained of the consequence of a surgery in advance to avoid any discontentment later.

Angle Kappa

The **visual axis** (the line joining the fovea and the target) is not the same as the optical or **geometric axis** (the line passing through the centre of the pupil or cornea). They differ normally by about + 5°, that is the eye would appear to be looking 5° out (exotropic) when it looks at any object. This is called as **angle** kappa (Fig. 6.3): **the angle between the visual axis and the optical axis.** This is nature's mechanism to offset some optical aberrations. But they give a look of exotropia in spite of perfect alignment but it is within our limits of acceptance. When it is more than this amount, as in hyperopes, this causes **pseudoexotropia.** On the other hand an angle kappa less than this amount or a negative angle kappa, as in some myopes, causes **pseudoesotropia.** Angle kappa can be measured on the synoptophore with a special slide.

Detection of a Squint

As we have noted that appearances can be deceptive, due to angle kappa or adnexal features, a **cover-uncover test** is required to confirm a squint. It has two components:

1. Observations to be made during covering **(cover test)**
2. Observations to be made during uncovering **(cover-uncover test)**.

Cover Test

It is important to have a proper **fixation target.** It should be a figure or letter of size 6/9 of Snellen's chart. This is to control accommodation. A fixation achieved by torch light is not desirable. The fixation distance should be 33 cm for near and 6 meters for distance. Thirdly an occluder is required and in case of children it is the hand or a thumb which can be used to avoid scaring him.

The subject is asked to fixate on the target at the requisite distance and an observation is made whether both eyes appear to fixate (no apparent squint) or one appears to fixate as the other deviates (apparent squint).

1. *Observation Made during Cover Test* (Fig. 6.4)

The next step is to **cover** the apparently fixating eye and observe what happens to the other (apparently deviating) eye. If that move to take up fixation, it confirms the presence of a manifest or true squint (heterotropia). If

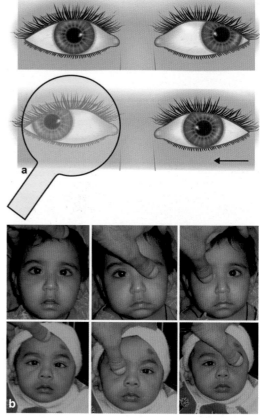

Fig. 6.4: Cover Test in the schematic diagram. (a) Observation of outward deviation of left eye, (b) Covering the straight (fixating) eye which is right eye here, causes straightening of the left eye, confirming a left exotropia. Top pictures shows pseudoesotropia and bottom pictures show true esotropia.

one had used a translucent occluder (Spielmann's one would have observed the eye behind the cover, deviating.

However, if both the eyes appear to fixate in the first instance, the examiner attempts to cover either of the eyes to observe the behaviour of the eyes. If it moves to confirm a heterotropia it would imply a true squint masked by appearance.

2. *Observations Made during Uncovering* (Fig. 6.5)

The second part: **"Uncover",** is helpful in unmasking the latent squint (heterophoria)

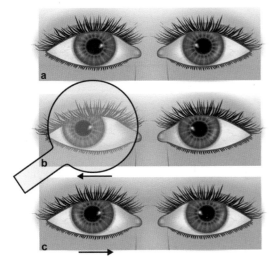

Fig. 6.5: Cover-uncover test. (a) Observation indicates no manifest deviation, (b) on covering right eye, no movement of left eye confirms that left eye was not deviating. Behind cover the right eye moves out, if there is a tendency to diverge, (c) on uncovering the right eye moves in to confirm that it had moved out behind cover. This indicates a latent exodeviation (exophoria). The speed of recovery should be noted.

which presents with both eyes appearing to fixate the target. One of the eyes is covered, which breaks the fusion, and if there is any heterophoria (tendency for squint) the eye behind cover deviates (in/out/up/down). The examiner then observes the behaviour of this eye as he removes the cover. If it remains deviated it confirms a latent squint with poor fusion **(poor recovery)** and if it recovers the examiner observes the **speed of recovery.** The speed of recovery indicates the strength of fusion and is an important prognostic sign.

Another observation can be that on uncovering the eye, the uncovered eye reassumes fixation as the other eye deviates. This indicates the presence of a squint with the "uncovered" eye being **dominant.** This also indicates that the visual acuity is unequal in the two eyes. A **free alternation of fixation** between the two eyes indicates equal vision in the two eyes. The correction of a ptosis of a hypotropic eye, when this eye fixates implies that it is a **pseudoptosis.**

Prerequisites of Cover-uncover Test

The cover-uncover test requires the following prerequisites:
- Ability of both eyes to fixate the target
- Ability of both eyes to have central fixation
- Ability of both eyes to have no gross/severe motility defect.

Thus, in the presence of one eye being blind or markedly subnormal vision or a severe restriction or limitation movement or an eccentric fixation, which will not permit the eyes to refixate, so that the cover-uncover test may be fallacious even though a squint is present.

For **infants,** who would not allow an occluder or a hand close to their face, the examiner can use **indirect occlusion test or distant cover test.** Here the fixation light or target is obstructed for one eye by an occluder at some distance away from the child.

Information from Cover-uncover Test

Thus the cover-uncover test confirms a true manifest or latent squint as also its type: Exodeviation, esodeviation or vertical deviations. It also indicates the visual dominance or the presence of amblyopia. A good cover-uncover test is the test which pays rich dividends, what remains to be done is only a quantitative measurement. A cover-uncover test needs to be done in all the nine cardinal positions of gaze, as also for near and distance fixation. With experience the examiner can detect even small angle squints leaving only the microtropia of less than 5 prism dioptre deviation.

Measurement of Deviation

Deviations can be measured by two methods: **objective** and **subjective.** Both require the co-operation of the patient, but in subjective tests the patient's subjective response is also required. The objective tests depend on the observations by the examiner of the patient's fixation pattern. Inherently the subjective tests are more precise and reveal status of the sensory system. They are not possible to be done if the patient lacks binocular vision, or the ability to comprehend the directions or express the response. Both the tests would have to be used judiciously by the examiner in order to understand the sensorimotor aspects of squint. For fixation targets colour toys or attractive figures are used (Fig. 6.6).

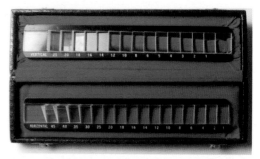

Fig. 6.7: Prismbar set: Vertical and horizontal.

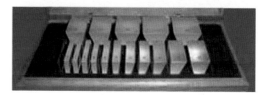

Fig. 6.8: Loose prisms

and for exodeviations they are placed base in (BI) (Fig. 6.9). A simple rule to remember is: **the apex of the prism should point towards the deviation.** Thus, in a vertical deviation,

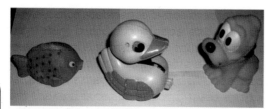

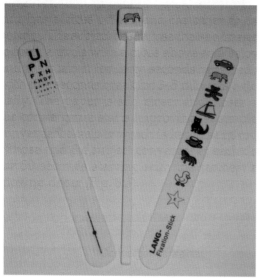

Fig. 6.6: Fixation targets for children.

Prism Bar Cover Test (PBCT)

The deviations can be measured whether subjectively or objectively by various methods.

The simplest and the best is using prisms or prism bar with the cover test and is described as the Prism Bar Cover Test (PBCT), (Figs 6.7 and 6.8). In essence it is the cover-uncover test with the addition of neutralisation of the deviation by the prisms.

For neutralising esodeviations (convergent squint) the prisms are placed base-out (BO)

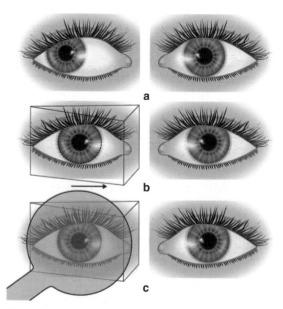

Fig. 6.9: Prism cover test. Deviation in (a), neutralised by prism (base in for exo) in (b), Cover-uncover test conducted to check the complete neutralization of deviation in (c).

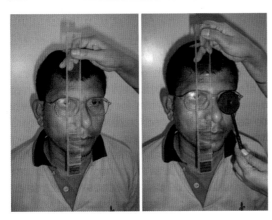

Fig. 6.9d: Prism cover test: Clinical procedure.

the prism is placed base-up in front of the right eye if there is right hypotropia and base-down in case of right hypertropia. If there is a combination of horizontal and vertical deviation, the prisms are placed horizontally in front of one eye and vertically in front of the other eye. For large deviations a loose prism of 30 or 45 prism dioptre is placed in front of one eye and an additional prism bar used in front of the other eye.

The plastic prisms are placed in the **frontal position** (Fig. 6.10) that is, parallel to the infra-orbital margin. But the glass prisms are placed in the **Prentice position** (Fig. 6.10a) that is, the posterior face of the prism is perpendicular to the line of sight.

It may be reiterated that the **fixation distance** (both for near and distance), the **fixation target** (6/9 Snellen size for accommodative control), and **proper dissociation** of the two eyes should be ensured. A hurriedly done test can be fallacious. In cases with variable deviation due to accommodative or fusional convergence, the two should be relaxed. The latter by making the subject wear occlusion for at least 4 hours (even extended up to 24 hours in cases of intermittent exotropia of simulated divergence excess type). The accommodative convergence should be controlled by making the subject wear his proper refractive correction for the

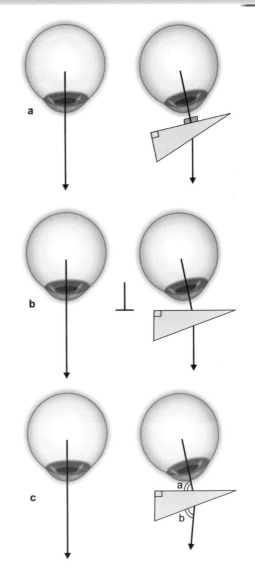

Fig. 6.10: Placement of prisms. (a) Glass prisms are calibrated for use in Prentice position, rear surface of prism perpendicular to visual axis, (b) Plastic prisms are calibrated for use in minimum deviation position (angle a = angle b) as shown in (c) but can be used in the frontal position (b) with minimal error.

test distance. For near fixation additional reading add may have to be added in cases of accommodative esotropia of convergence excess type.

It is important to understand that the deviation to be measured is to be **static**

deviation and should be free of the aforementioned **dynamic factors** of **accommodation and fusion.** It is the static angle which requires surgical correction whereas the dynamic deviation of accommodation should be corrected by glasses.

Effect of high plus or minus glasses on measuring squint deviations.

Plus lenses always measure less deviation than actual, both in esodeviation and exodeviation (base-out effect in eso and base in effect in exo).

Minus lenses always measure **more** deviation than actual, both in esodeviation and exodeviation (base in effect in eso and base-out effect in exo).

$$\frac{\Delta MD}{\Delta AD} = \frac{1 - 0.025 \times D}{1}$$

Note: MD: Measured deviation

AD: Actual deviation

D is + for convex lenses – for concave lens

For + 10 D sph

$$\frac{\Delta MD}{\Delta AD} = 1 - 0.025 \times 10 = 0.75$$

i.e. DMD = 0.75 × AD

For – 10 D sph $\frac{MD}{AD} = 1 + 0.025 \times 10 = 0.75$

i.e. MD = 1.25 × AD

Prisms should be split between the two eyes rather than being stacked over one eye for larger deviations to avoid error (Fig. 6.11).

Different Aspects of Measurement

The deviations need to be measured in various ways to determine different aspects.

1. Deviation with **distance and near fixation** to determine its nature as to:
   - Esotropia: Basic/convergence excess/divergence insufficiency.
   - Exotropia: Basic/convergence insufficiency/divergence excess.
2. Deviation **with and without glasses** (also near and with bifocals if any) to determine the accommodative element.
3. Deviation in **9 different cardinal positions of gaze** to determine any incomitance (paralytic, restrictive or spastic).
4. Deviation in **up gaze of 25°** and **down gaze of 35°** for determining AV patterns.
5. Deviations with **right and left eye fixating** alternately to determine primary and secondary deviation in case of paralytic squint.

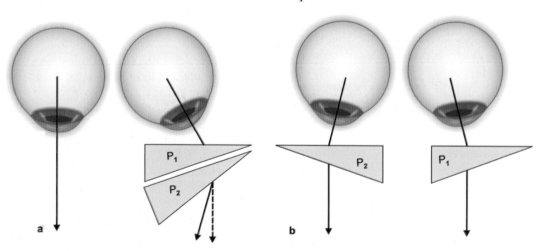

Fig. 6.11: (a) Avoid "stacking" of prisms for larger deviation, (b) Split the prismatic effect between the two eyes.

6. Deviations with **subjective method** and **objective method** to determine the type of retinal correspondence (normal or anomalous).

7. Deviations **after prolonged cover** to differentiate a true divergence excess type from a simulated divergence excess exotropia as also to determine the fully undissociated deviation.

Examination of Eyes in Nine Gaze Positions

It is important to measure the ocular deviations in different gaze positions for diagnosing motility defects. Although, except for the down gaze, one does not use 35° gaze positions physiologically, these are helpful for diagnosis. These are therefore called **diagnostic positions.** Just like the measurements in the primary position, measurements in these peripheral eight positions are also best done by prism bar cover test, with an accommodative target. Some people prefer to use **deviometers,** which are devices that can give different fixed and repeatable fixation target positions. For near measurements any Lister's perimeter or simply a vertical stand with a vertically rotatable arm around a pivot, with the free end carrying the fixation target, can be used. For distance measurements one may use multiple fixed points on the opposite wall.

Alternatively a single fixed target may be used with the head being turned to bring the eyes in the desired positions. The deviation of the head can be read on a protractor along with a scale. A **cephalodeviometer** a calibrated mirror can also be used (*see* AV phenomena) (Fig. 6.12).

Synoptophore

This is a basic orthoptic instrument based on the haploscopic principle. They have been variously called amblyoscope (major, Curpax—major types), troposcope, and synoptophore. It consists of a chin rest and forehead rest with two tubes carrying the targets seen through an angled eyepiece. The tubes are placed

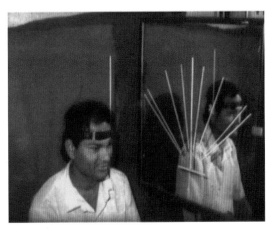

Fig. 6.12: Cephalodeviometer.

horizontally and are movable in the horizontal and vertical planes. The distance between the two tubes can also be adjusted with the subject's interpupillary distance (IPD). The targets in the tubes are illuminated slides which can be raised up or lowered and also be tilted to test for vertical and torsional deviations. All these adjustments can be read on the scales in degrees and prism dioptres. The tubes can be locked individually or both with respect to each other. The illumination of each target can be increased or decreased and flashes given if desired. Additional devices like **Haidinger brushes** can be attached. The targets are placed at a fixed distance from the eyepiece which are of +6.0 or +6.5 D, so that the targets are at optical infinity. This should theoretically not stimulate accommodation. However, in reality proximal convergence does come into play distorting the deviations. This factor has significantly reduced the applicability of the synoptophore as a reliable instrument to measure deviations, especially horizontal deviations.

Uses

In cyclovertical squint the synoptophore is a useful instrument **to measure torsion.** It is also useful for studying **accommodative convergence relationship** and for imparting several **orthoptic exercises.**

The **synoptoscope** of Curpax—major is a modification which uses semitransparent mirrors in place of opaque mirrors in front of eyes. This allows the subject to view a distant object superimposed on the targets in slide holders. The synoptometer (oculus) is a modification which allows measurement of deviations in peripheral positions with the help of mirrors.

Corneal Reflection Tests

Hirschberg's Test

The corneal reflection (first catoptric image of Purkinje) can be used to estimate the ocular deviation in a gross or semiquantitative manner. The corneal reflections, even normally are **not exactly centered,** because of angle kappa, but are **symmetrical** in the absence of a squint. In case of esodeviations the corneal reflection falls more temporally and *vice versa.* Roughly a 1 mm shift signifies a 5° deviation (earlier thought to be 7°). Thus if the reflex falls on the nasal limbus, the exodeviation is 30° (approximately 60 prism dioptres). This test can be used in infants, who are not very cooperative or in cases of eccentric fixation or nonfixation (blind eyes). This is the Hirschberg test (Fig. 6.13).

Krimsky Test

By utilising a prism bar one can quantify the deviation using the corneal reflection. This is the Krimsky test or **prism reflex test.** It is preferable to place the prism bar on the fixating eye and to neutralise the amount by observing the corneal reflex in the deviating eye (nonfixating eye) (Fig. 6.14).

Subjective Tests of Deviation

These tests utilise the subject's perception of the deviation. When there is misalignment, the subject perceives diplopia and the separation between the two images indicates the subjective deviation. This is the **diplopia principle.** Here the single "physical location" is perceived by the subject as two "perceptual

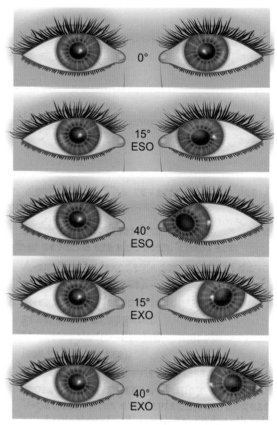

Fig. 6.13: Hirschberg's corneal reflection test for esodeviation and exodeviations. For orthotropia the corneal reflections may not always be in the centre of the pupil but are symmetrically placed

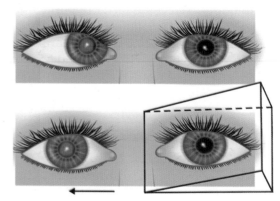

Fig. 6.14: Krimsky's corneal reflection test for neutralization of deviation by prisms in cases were cover-uncover test not possible. Prism is placed before the normal eye to see the centering of the nonfixating eye.

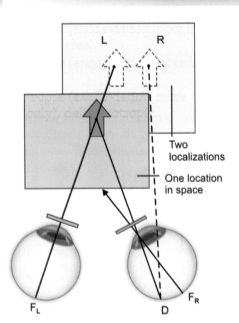

Fig. 6.15: **Diplopia testing principle.** One object seen double viewed through red-green glasses.

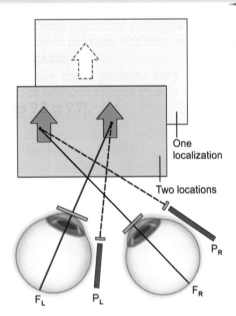

Fig. 6.16: **Haploscopic principle on Hess charting.** Two projections in space from projectors PL/ PR/ seen as one localization in space through appropriate glasses.

localizations". Diplopia testing with red-green googles is based on this principle (Fig. 6.15). Measurement of deviation on Maddox tangent scale with the help of Maddox rod is also based on it subjective tests can also be done

on the **haploscopic principle,** where two "physical locations" are used to have one "perceptual localization". The examples are synoptophore (when tested subjectively) or the Hess/Lees screen (Figs 6.16 and 6.17).

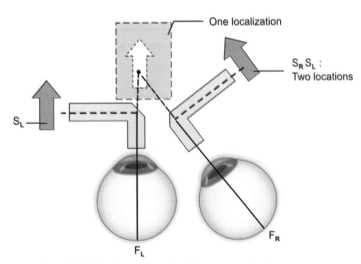

Fig. 6.17: Haploscopic principle on synoptophore.

Diplopia Testing

Red and green glasses over the right and left eye respectively, dissociate the two images and are seen double in cases of squint. Esodeviations cause uncrossed diplopia **(homonymous diplopia)** and exodeviations cause crossed diplopia **(heteronymous diplopia).** In the former the image falls on the nasal half of the retina and is projected on the temporal half of the field, and so is seen uncrossed (same side as the eye). In exodeviations the image falls on the temporal retina to produce crossed diplopia.

It is preferable to use an **illuminated slit target** and to use the slit vertically for charting horizontal deviations and to use it horizontally to chart vertical deviations. A tilt of the image is also better appreciated with a slit target. The test can be done both for near (33 cm) and distance (6 m). For distance one may utilise the Maddox tangent scale or cross, to quantify the deviation otherwise prisms for neutralisation are used.

The separation between the two images is recorded for each of the nine diagnostic gaze positions. A red filter alone can also be used but the dissociation is then not complete as with red and green glasses. This test is a very useful test for diagnosis and follow-up of incomitant squints.

Hess/Lees Screen

Here two test objects (two locations) are shown to the patient which is seen by the patient as one localization. The dissociation may be done by red-green glasses as in the Hess screen test or by a mirror septum as in the Lees screen. The Lancaster red-green test with the two Foster torches use red-green filters in the torches and red-green glasses. Polaroid dissociation can also be used in order to have a more physiological dissociation.

These haploscopic tests are very good for documentation of ocular paralysis and restrictive conditions (*see* chapter on paralytic squint).

The Hess chart has a grid pattern where each square represents 5° excursion for the fixating eye. Thus the inner square tests for 15° eye movements from the primary position. The outer square (each side is curved inwards) represents 30° excursion for the fixing eye. The outer square is usually charted to mild underactions. The Hess chart is a very good test which can document the under- or overactions of the muscles.

Measurement of Cyclodeviations

While the objective tests are difficult, the subjective tests are very good for measuring cyclodeviations. **Diplopia charting** with a slit target is used to make the patient appreciate the tilt. A horizontal slit appears to be tilted in the opposite direction to the cyclodeviation of the eye. In case of excyclodeviation of the right eye the tilt is anticlockwise and in case of incyclodeviation it will be clockwise.

By using two Maddox rods, preferably one white and the other red, the tilt is neutralised by rotating the Maddox rods in the requisite direction. The change of axis on the trial frame can be read to give the actual cyclodeviation. This is the **Double Maddox Rod Test.** A vertical prism of 5 prism dioptre can be added to create a separation between the two horizontal lines seen through the Maddox rods.

The **synoptophore** is a good instrument to measure cyclodeviations, the slides can be tilted to make the patient appreciate straightening of the torsion in the slides. The slides used should have vertical features or one can use the after image slides.

For **objective evaluation of the cyclodeviations** the indirect ophthalmoscopy and fundus photography are useful methods. These are good to semiquantify the cyclodeviations. Normally, the fovea is located between the two horizontal lines, one passing through the centre of the disc and the other cutting the lower pole of the disc tangentially. The usual location is in the middle of these two horizontal lines, that is, 0.3 disc diameters below the horizontal line through the centre of the disc. A difference of 0.25 disc diameter or more between the two eyes is considered abnormal (Fig. 6.18).

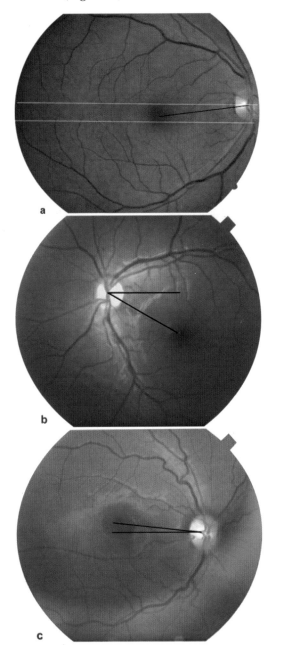

Fig. 6.18: Fundus photographs showing normal (a), extorsion (b), and intorsion (c).

Limitation of Movements

In addition to measuring the ocular deviations, it is valuable to note the limitation of movements. In restrictive squints, the limitation of movements is severe compared to the ocular deviation which is small. In contrast in the paralytic squints the two corroborate each other. Both the ductions and the versions should be noted and documented. Usually a subjective assessment is made on scale of 7 points (+3 to –3) or 9 points (+4 to –4). This is usually helpful in follow-up of cases of incomitant strabismus (Fig. 6.19).

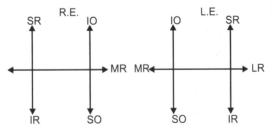

Fig. 6.19: Documentation of action of extraocular muscles: The underaction is indicated by 1–, 2–, 3– and overaction as 1+, 2+, 3+, for each extraocular muscle. Normal action is left unmarked. This grading is on a scale of 7. If a scale of 9 is chosen an additional degree 4–, and 4+ for both underaction and overaction is added.

It should be noted that due to variations in the adnexal structures, there cannot be a foolproof method of assessing such excursions. Normally, **adduction** is normal when the nasal one-third cornea crosses the lower punctum. Less than this is considered to be limited. For normal **abduction** the temporal limbus should touch the lateral canthus. **Vertical movements** are more difficult to assess due to variability of palpebral aperture. More so for the obliques.

Grading Oblique Overactions

The **overaction of the obliques** can also be indirectly assessed in the following manner.

- If the vertical deviation (hypertropia for inferior oblique) is appreciable only in sursum adduction it is **mild overaction.**
- If it is appreciable on adduction itself, it is **moderate overaction** and in case of **severe overactions** (unilateral) a hypertropia is seen in primary position itself.
- While judging the relative hypertropia of the eye in adduction we should focus on the relative hypertropia of the inferior limbus for the inferior oblique overaction rather than the coverage of the cornea.

Grading Oblique Overactions

Another useful clinical test to grade the inferior oblique overaction is by observing the angle the adducting eye makes with the horizontal line as it elevates and abducts (if overacting) on lateral version to the opposite side. It may be noted that in the absence of an oblique overaction the eye would remain in the horizontal line. For example, the inferior oblique of the right eye can be graded as follows (Fig. 6.20):

- Grade 1+: Up to 15° angle with the horizontal line (Fig. 6.20)

- Grade 2+: Up to 30° angle with the horizontal line
- Grade 3+: Up to 60° angle with the horizontal line
- Grade 4+: Up to 90° angle with the horizontal line.

Grade 1+ may not be detectable easily on lateral version and is better appreciated only in tertiary position (e.g. levoelevation for RIO).

Analogous to this grading the superior oblique also can be graded. The angle, the adducting eye makes with the horizontal line as it depresses and abducts on a lateral version is noted:

- Grade 1 + (15°)
- Grade 2 + (30°)
- Grade 3 + (60°)
- Grade 4 + (90°)

Measurement of Vergences

In actual practice the manifestation of a squint (heterotropia) only occurs if the latent tendency for squint (heterophoria) is not overcome by the fusional vergences. Thus the measurement of vergences is very important, as it determines the capability of the motor

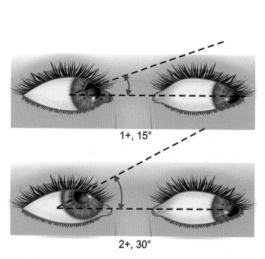

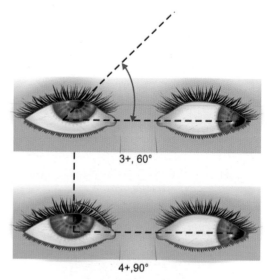

Fig. 6.20: Grading of inferior oblique overactions by the angular deviation of the eye in adduction as a lateral version is performed Grades 1+, 2+, 3+ and 4+ are shown.

system to cope with an induced misalignment of visual axes. If these vergence amplitudes are large, even a large angle squint remains latent and asymptomatic, and if they are small, even a small angle squint manifests or if still intermittent, remains symptomatic. Vergences are tested in the three planes:

- **Horizontal vergences:** Convergence and divergence
- **Vertical vergences:** Sursumvergence and deorsumvergence
- **Torsional vergences:** Incyclovergence and excyclovergence.

In principle, to measure the vergences the visual axes are misaligned artificially, and this may be done with prisms or on the synoptophore. The horizontal and vertical vergences only can be measured by prisms in this manner, as the prisms cannot induce a torsional misalignment.

Horizontal Vergences
Near Point of Convergences

The simplest way to measure the convergence is to bring a line drawn on a paper (or any other linear target) closer to the eyes, till the point, it becomes double. This determines the near point of convergence (NPC). It is important to note that the line should appear to be **double, not blurred.** The point at which it becomes blurred would determine the **near point of accommodation (NPA).** The latter is done with each eye separately (monocular) and also with both eyes together (binocular). For testing NPC in presbyopes or any refractive error, suitable glasses should be used by the subject. The point at which the line becomes double is called the **break point convergence.** If the line gradually withdrawn away, at some point the line becomes single again which is the **recovery point convergence.** The two differ from each other. The measurements are made from the bony margin of the lateral canthus. Normally, it is **8–10 cm.** NPC of 10 cm or further away is considered defective. Apart from the patient describing

the diplopia, an objective assessment is made by the examiner by seeing one of the eyes deviate out. Near point ruler, Royal Air Force binocular gauge and Livingstone gauge are instruments based on this principle.

Convergence Sustenance

A further assessment needs to be made to assess the ability of the eyes to hold the convergence at the near point. This is **convergence sustenance.** It gives a good parameter to assess the strength of fusional convergence. Normally, one should be able to hold it for 45 seconds to 1 minute, less than 30 seconds is definitely poor and indicates symptomatic exodeviation.

Measurement of Vergences with Prisms

Convergence and divergence can be measured both for distance (6 m) and near (33 cm) fixation with the help of a **prism bar** or a **rotary prism.** With the patient properly seated and made to fixate at a fixation target at distance or near as desired, the prism bar is moved with its prism strength increasing. The end point is noted as **break point,** when one eye deviates out or diplopia is reported. The prism strength is then gradually reduced till the object is seen single again, this is noted as the **recovery point.** The break point is usually more than the recovery point but within 3 to 5 dioptres. A larger difference would indicate poor recovery as in cases of intermittent exotropia who are symptomatic. **Using base out prisms the convergence amplitudes are measured and using base in prisms the divergence amplitudes are measured.** The vertical vergences are similarly measured using **prisms base up for deorsumvergence and prisms base down for sursumvergence.**

The **order of testing** the vergences should be convergence, deorsumvergence, divergence and sursumvergence. This is to avoid any artifactual changes. The normal values are as follows (Table 6.1).

Table 6.1: Fusional vergences

Vergence with prisms	Distance (6 m) in pd.	Near (33 cm) in pd.
Convergence	14–20	35–40
Divergence	5–8	15–20
Vertical vergence	2–4	2–4
Incyclovergence*	10–12°	10–12°
Excyclovergence*	10–12°	10–12°

Note: *Though cyclovergences (in degrees) are as good as above on synoptophore, the tolerance in practice is up to 4° only.*

Examination of the Sensory Status

The examination of the sensory status is as important as that of the motor status. It comprises the assessment of the binocular status of the eyes and the nature of correspondence between them. It determines the prognosis of a case of squint, whether a **functional** improvement is possible or just a **cosmetic** alignment would have to be contented with. Many of the so-called cosmetic cases may have binocular potential and surprise a surgeon postoperatively with unexpected diplopia, or have peripheral fusion and thus have a better postoperative prognosis.

The sensory status is examined with the following questions in mind:

1. Is binocularity present?
2. Is there any diplopia present, what type?
3. What is the type of correspondence?
4. Is suppression present, its extent and depth?
5. Is amblyopia present?
6. Is stereopsis present, what grade?

Binocularity and Diplopia

Presence of "binocular" diplopia indicates presence of binocularity. Diplopia should be confirmed to be **"true"** diplopia (not just blurring or elongation of an image due to astigmatism). Secondly, it should be **binocular,** that is present with both eyes open and becomes single on covering one eye. **Monocular diplopia** can be due to astig-matism, subluxated lenses, large peripheral iridectomy, corneal edema or corneal facet or in some neurological conditions. Long-standing cases of squint even of adult onset may not complain of diplopia as they learn to ignore the other image. Use of **red-green goggles** helps in dissociating the visual stimuli of the two eyes and helps in visualisation of diplopia. Similarly, other modes of dissociation of the eyes like **Bagolini's glasses** or single or **double Maddox rod test** can help.

In the absence of squint or squint without diplopia, the dissociation tests help in identifying whether binocular perception is present or not.

Type of Correspondence

The next step after establishing binocularity is to know what type of correspondence is present. A bifoveal correspondence is called Normal Retinal Correspondence (NRC). A correspondence between fovea of one eye and extrafoveal point of the other eye (deviating eye) is called anomalous retinal correspondence (ARC).

Suppression

Suppression is a sensory adaptation to squint in which only one eye functions. It may be **unilateral** or **alternating**. It may be **facultative** (only during binocular conditions) or **obligatory** (also during monocular conditions). Its **extent** (area of suppression) and **depth** (its intensity or severity) should be noted. The commonly used tests are:

1. Bagolini Striated Glasses

It is the most physiological test for dissociation of the eyes. A pair of striated glasses are used in front of each eye. A source of light is seen as a line at right angles to the striations. The axis of striations of the two eyes is kept at right angles to each other. The different responses are (Fig. 6.21):

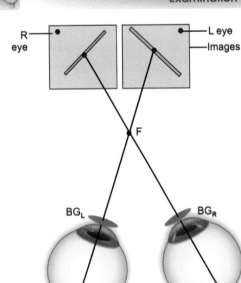

Fig. 6.21: Bagolini striated glasses test. A spot light F seen through Bagolini's striated glasses. Possible perceptions: (a) Cross response (NRC with no squint or HARC with squint), (b) Right suppression, (c) Left suppression, (d) Right central scotoma.

i. Symmetrical cross response
- In the absence of a manifest squint, a cross response indicates a normal bifoveal correspondence (NRC).
- In the presence of a manifest squint, a cross response indicates an anomalous retinal correspondence (ARC) of harmonious type (subjective angle of deviation of zero).

ii. Asymmetrical cross response or two lines cutting each other at some other point than midline, indicates an incomitant squint with normal retinal correspondence **(diplopia response).**

iii. Single line seen: If only one line is seen, it indicates suppression of the other eye **(suppression response).**

iv. **Cross response with central gap in one line** indicates a central suppression scotoma in that eye.

2. Worth Four Dot Test (WFDT)

WFDT is a simple test utilising red-green colour dissociation. It is more dissociating than the Bagolini glasses and so less physiological. The four dots (red top, white bottom, and two green horizontal) are viewed through red-green goggles (red before right eye). The following responses are seen (Fig. 6.22):

  i. **Four dots:** (a) Normal binocular response with no manifest deviation (NRC with no heterotropia).
    (b) harmonious anomalous retinal correspondence with manifest squint.

  ii. **Five dots:** Normal retinal correspondence with manifest deviation. The two vertical red dots and three green dots (inverted triangle) are separated differently depending on the type of deviation.
    – **Esodeviation:** Uncrossed pattern (red on right side).

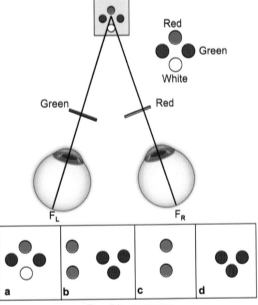

Fig. 6.22: **Worth Four Dot Test (WFDT).** Four spots seen through red (before right eye) and green glasses. Responses are: (a) Normal bifoveal or harmonious ARC, (b) NRC with squint, (c) Left suppression, (d) Right suppression.

- **Exodeviation:** Crossed pattern (red on left side).
- **Vertical squint:** Vertically displaced sets.

iii. **Three dots** seen, indicate suppression of right eye.

iv. **Two dots** seen, indicate suppression of left eye.

The test is normally done at 6 metre distance and the WFDT subtends an angle of 1.2°.

In case of central scotoma larger than this size, WFDT will not be visualised. The WFDT can be brought closer to the patient to increase the angle subtended by it.

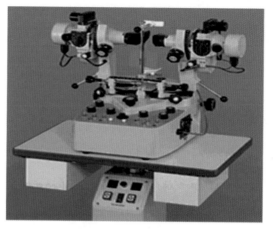

Fig. 6.23a: Synoptophore.

3. Synoptophore

The synoptophore is a versatile instrument and has special sets of slides for testing (Figs 6.23a and b):

   i. Simultaneous perception (SP) (foveal, macular, paramacular)

  ii. Fusion (foveal, macular, paramacular)

 iii. Stereopsis.

These are the three levels of binocular vision. The **SP slides** are dissimilar but overlapping the same retinal areas (soldier-gate). Presence of SP indicates basic level of binocularity. However, at times binocularity may be elicited by fusion slides and not by SP slides as fusion slides are more physiological. The **fusion slides** are almost identical in the main part with dissimilar peripheral parts to act as controls. **Stereopsis slides** are similar with some areas causing disparate stimulation. These areas are seen three dimensionally raised or deeper. Presence of stereopsis indicates good binocular single vision. However, with anomalous retinal correspondence in microtropia low grade stereopsis may present.

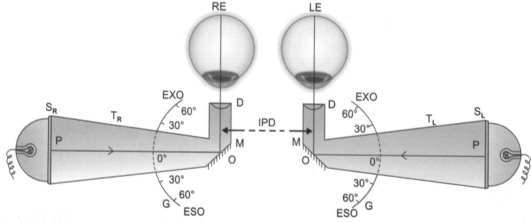

Fig. 6.23b: A schematic diagram of a synoptophore with two tubes. T_R and T_L which have the two arms such that the focal length of lens at D is DOP. The arms of the tubes can be brought closer or farther to correct IPD and each rotated around a graduated scale, G. The slides S_R and S_L can be changed, raised-lowered or even tilted (*Adapted from:* Keith-Lyle).

4. After-image Testing

This is a highly dissociating orthoptic test in which the fovea of the two eyes (or eccentric fixation point) is flashed with linear after-image horizontal in right eye and vertical in left eye since each eye is individually stimulated, only the fovea (or fixating point in eccentric fixation) are at the centre of the after-images. The responses are (Fig. 6.24):

i. **Cross response:** A symmetrical cross indicates a normal bifoveal correspondence (if eccentric fixation is excluded). This is irrespective of deviation between the two eyes. That is any eso- or exo-deviation with NRC still gives a symmetrical cross response.

ii. **Asymmetrical crossing:** In case of anomalous retinal correspondence the horizontal and vertical lines have their centres separated. The amount of

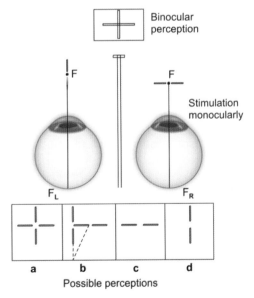

Fig. 6.24: After-image testing: After-images created in each eye monocularly centered at the fixation point of the eye (fovea). Binocular response depends on the correspondence between the two eyes: (a) NRC with or without squint = cross response, (b) ARC with squint "asymmetric cross", displacement proportional to the angle of anomaly (a),(c) left suppression, (d) right suppression.

separation is dependent on the **angle of anomaly.**

After-images are not physiological in their testing methodology and do not give the real picture always. It however does indicate the deep-rooted tendency of the sensory status.

Testing Extent of Suppression

Suppression scotoma can be charted under binocular conditions (fixating with one eye, while the field of other eye is charted). This may be done by different methods.

i. **Prisms** to displace the central object peripherally till it can be visualised in different directions.

ii. **Synoptophore:** Charting of one eye, while the other eye is used for fixation.

iii. **Lees' screen or Hess screen:** Charting of one eye while other eye fixates (through mirror in Lees', and red-green dissociation in Hess charting).

iv. **Polaroid scotometer:** Using polaroid dissociation. While one eye is fixated, the field of other eye is charted.

Different responses are observed:

i. With more dissociating tests like prisms, Lees' screen, etc. **single large coarse** scotomas are seen, these extend from fovea to the diplopia point. Jampolsky demonstrated hemiretinal scotoma in exodeviations, whereas esodeviations showed more discrete scotoma.

ii. With less dissociating tests like Aulhorn phase difference haploscope and polaroid scotometer, **two** discrete scotoma are seen. These are **foveal scotoma** about $2°$–$3°$ in size and **diplopia point scotoma.** This was seen in both esodeviation and exodeviation, but in exodeviation the foveal scotoma showed a vertical step like the hemiretinal scotoma of Jampolsky, (*see* Figs 7.3 and 8.3).

Depth of Scotoma

The depth or intensity of scotoma can be seen by using differential stimulation of the two eyes. The **graded density filter bar** of Bagolini is useful. As the denser filters are brought over the dominant eye, the relative scotoma of the amblyopic eye starts disappearing or shrinking in size.

Assessment of visual acuity, stereopsis, vernier acuity has been discussed in chapter 5, specific tests for amblyopia and ARC are described in chapter 4.

FIXATION DISPARITY

The concept of fixation disparity is important to understand the relationship of binocular vision and heterophoria. The evaluation of **fixation disparity** and the "associated" **phoria** is helpful in the clinical setting as it provides additional information on the binocular interactions, apart from being important in vision and fusion research. The phoria that is measured after disrupting fusion by coveruncover test or similar methods is **"dissociated phoria"**. Under binocular conditions there may be a misalignment of the fixation points in two eyes within the limits of the Panum's area of fusion, which is fused and is seen as one. This fusible misalignment is **fixation disparity.** This is quantified in minutes of arc.

Under binocular conditions of viewing a vertical line is shown such that the upper half is seen by right eye and the lower half by the left eye, each viewed through polaroid dissociation. If there is a misalignment reported (which may be horizontal: Eso-or exophoria), prisms are used to align the two halves. This is **"associated phoria".** The rest of the picture shown (apart from the vertical lines) is seen by the two eyes and functions as a **fusion-lock.** The associated phoria is different from the phoria seen under dissociation and is therefore, named differently (Fig. 6.25).

Fixation Disparity Curves

Under forced vergence situations, using 3, 6, 9, 12 pd. prisms base-in, base-out alternatively the fixation disparity and the associated

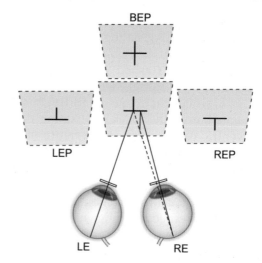

Fig. 6.25: A schematic diagram for testing fixation disparity. An exofixation disparity is shown. Dotted lines show the left eye (LEP) right eye (REP) and binocular perception (BEP). The BEP shows fusion inspite of an actual separation seen. The two eyes look through polaroid dissociation at stimuli (vertical lines) which are seen by one eye only.

phoria can be charted and plotted. These plots are called **fixation disparity curves.** There are four common types of fixation disparity curves. Individuals with type I curves are frequently asymptomatic. Those having a steep slope, greater than 0.77 minute/prism dioptre in esophoria and 1.06 minutes/prism dioptre in exophoria are usually symptomatic. Type II curve is associated with high esophoria and type III curve with high exophoria. Both these curves do not intersect the X-axis. Type IV curve is associated with unstable binocularity. The individuals with types II, III and IV are usually symptomatic. The flatter portion of the curve represents the condition of rapid adaptation to the vergence stimuli. Vision therapy may be considered to successfully flatten these curves and make the patient asymptomatic.

Forced fixation disparity curves can also be plotted using different spherical lenses (in pre-presbyopes) using lens power + 2.0 D to –3.0 D in 0.5 D or 1.0 D steps. These forced fixation disparity curves are also used to measure AC/A ratio.

The fixation disparity and associated phoria can be measured by Sheedy's disparometer, Mallet unit, Wesson's card, etc.

Disparometer

A close-up view of the fixation disparity targets on the disparometer is shown in figure. The fine reading print shown adjacent to the fixation targets provides more natural circumstances and provides a fusion lock and are visible equally by both eyes. The central fixation target for vertical associated phoria has two half split horizontal lines, each half visible by the right or left eye. For horizontal associated phoria, the split half lines are vertical.

For measuring associated phoria the adjustment knob (to move one-half line) is kept at zero. And prisms are used to correct the misalignment that is reported by the patient. Both vertical and horizontal associated phoria can be measured.

For measuring fixation disparity, the knob is shifted to set 10 minutes of exofixation disparity. If the patient reports misalignment the knob is taken to the other end till the patient reports misalignment in the reverse direction. Finally, the misalignment is decreased till the patient reports alignment. The viewing time should be limited to a few seconds.

Wesson's Card

This card has also to be viewed through polaroid glasses. It has vertical lines in the upper half (seen by one eye) and an arrow in the lower half (seen by the other eye). The rest of the card is viewed binocularly.

Suggested Reading

1. Adelstein FE and Cuppers C. Analysis of the motor situation in strabismus in Arruga A. editor. International strabismus symposium (university of Giessen, 1966) New York 1968. S. Karger AG. pp. 139–148.

2. Bagolini B. Teenica par L'esame della visione binoculare sensa introduzone di elimenti dissocianti "test del vetro striato". Boll. Ocul. 37. 195, 1958.

3. Bielschowsky A. Lectures on motor anomalies, Hanover NH 1943. (reprinted 1956) Dartmouth College Publications.

4. Burian HM. Normal and anomalous correspondence in Allen J.H. editor. Strabismus Ophthalmic symposium II St. Louis, 1958 The CV Mosby Co.

5. Capobianco NM. The subjective measurement of the near point of convergence and its significance in the diagnosis of convergence insufficiency. Am. Orthopt. J 2: 40, 1952.

6. Spielmann A. A translucent occluder to study eye position under unilateral or bilateral cover test. Am. Orthopt. J. 36: 65, 1986.

7. Urist MJ. Pseudostrabismus caused by abnormal configuration of the upper eyelid margins, Am. J. Ophthalmol. 75:455,1993.

8. Brodie SE. Photographic calibration of the Hirschberg test. Invest. Ophthalmol. Vis. Sci. 28: 736. 1987.

9. Bruckner R. Exakte strabismus diagnostik bei ½—3 jahrigen, Kindern mit einem einfachen "Durch leuch tungs test" Ophthalmologica 144. 184, 1962.

10. Veronneau—Troutman S. Prisms in the Medical and Surgical Treatment of Strabismus. CV Mosby Co. St. Louis, 1994.

6

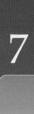

7

Esotropia

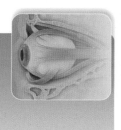

Esodeviations commonly confront a practicing ophthalmologist especially in infancy. Many a time it may be a pseudoesotropia due to prominent telecanthus or epicanthus and need reassurance. But some of these cases could be harboring a true squint or may develop one and so require a proper follow-up. True esodeviation may be incomitant or concomitant (Table 7.1). The concomitant squints could be accommodative or non-accommodative.

TYPES OF ESODEVIATIONS

- Incomitant
  a. Paralytic
     i. Neurogenic (e.g. abducens palsy, divergence palsy)
     ii. Myogenic (e.g. myasthenia)
  b. Restrictive
     i. Musculofascial (e.g. Duane's)
     ii. Other restrictive conditions (tumor, postoperative, dysthyroid, strabismus fixus).
  c. Spastic
- Concomitant
  a. Accommodative
     i. Refractive (hypermetropic)
     ii. Nonrefractive, hyperaccommodative, hypoaccommodative
  b. Partially accommodative
  c. Nonaccommodative
     i. Essential infantile
     ii. Essential acquired or late-onset

- Basic
- Convergence excess
- Divergence insufficiency
iii. Acute concomitant
iv. Microtropia
v. Cyclic esotropia
vi. Sensory esotropia
vii. Nystagmus blockage syndrome
viii. Esophoria

ESSENTIAL INFANTILE ESOTROPIA

This entity is of special importance because of its early onset that compromises the binocular vision which may be unrecoverable if not treated in time and even when that is done the results of full binocular potentials are poor. A prevalence of 0.1% of newborns highlights its importance further. While it has been called "congenital" esotropia, that seems to be incorrect and it would be proper to call it **essential "infantile" esotropia** (Fig. 7.1).

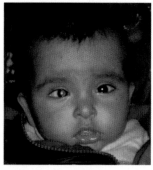

Fig. 7.1: Infantile esotropia showing bright Bruckner reflex in the squinting right eye.

In an extensive study done on 4211 newborn children, some important deductions have been made. It may be of interest to note that at birth majority of children have exotropia. True "congenital" esotropia, observed at birth is very rare, their eye alignments remain in a state of flux till about 4 months of age. The eyes undergo an orthotropization curve in that period. Therefore, it is imperative to observe these children closely in the first four months before establishing a diagnosis of esotropia. However, overdue delay may actually be detrimental in view of regaining binocular potentials. Esodeviations present after 4 months of age should be considered abnormal. The multicentric Congenital Esotropia Study has concluded that small angle esotropia less than 30 pd may be observed as some of these may spontaneously get corrected, but the larger esodeviations do not resolve and need surgical treatment.

Characteristics

- **Large angle esotropia,** usually more than 30 prism dioptres.
- **Free alternation** or **cross fixation** in alternators, and fixation preference of the normal eye in amblyopes.
- No significant refractive error **(deviation not contributed by refractive error).**
- **No neurological defect.**
- Confirmed by **4–6 months.**

- May be associated with **inferior oblique overactions** (68%), **nystagmus**(33%), or **dissociated vertical deviations**(50%). Inferior oblique overactions are associated with V-phenomenon, rarely superior oblique overactions may be associated along with A-phenomenon. DVD may not be present at the first presentation, but may appear in subsequent examinations, irrespective of surgery.
- **Asymmetric optokinetic nystagmus.** This is an asymmetry of smooth pursuit movements: tracking of objects temporal to nasal is smooth while tracking nasal to temporal is cogwheel (Fig. 7.2).

The suppression is alternating in alternators and unilateral in unilateral squints with more physiological tests like **polaroid scotometer, two point scotoma** are seen, one at the fovea and the other at the diplopia point (Fig. 7.3). With more dissociating tests a **single large scotoma** is seen.

Variants

Two common variants are the **Ciancia syndrome** and the **Lang's syndrome**.

Ciancia syndrome (Fig. 7.4) in addition to early onset esotropia has bilateral limitation of abduction with manifest-latent jerk nystagmus (fast phase in the direction of the fixing eye), increasing in abduction and decreasing in adduction. This causes a face turn towards

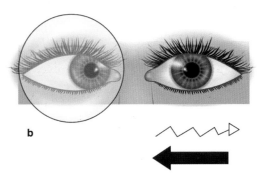

Fig. 7.2: Temporal to nasal movements are smooth in each eye but nasal to temporal movements are cogwheel. (a) Right fixation, (b) Left fixation.

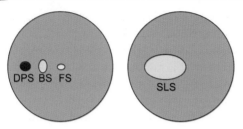

Fig. 7.3: Twin point scotoma on binocular testing of fields on polaroid scotometer in esotropia: one scotoma at fovea (FS) and the other at the diplopia point (DPS).

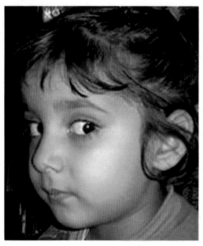

Fig 7.4: Infantile esotropia with nystagmus in abduction (IENA) or Ciancia syndrome.

the side of fixing eye, that is the fixing eye remains in adduction, as there is a null position in adduction, Even if one eye was to be enucleated, the remaining eye is held in adduction with a face turn to that side (one eyed esotropia).

Lang's syndrome is characterized by early onset esotropia with DVD, nystagmus and excyclodeviation of the non-fixing eye. This is associated with torticollis.

Differential Diagnosis

All the other cases of esotropia should be kept in mind. **Abducens or VI nerve palsy** in cases of limitation of abduction needs to be excluded as some cases of infantile esotropia show limitation of abduction due to cross fixation

or long-standing esotropia. True limitation can be confirmed by testing doll's eye movements (vestibulo-ocular reflex movements). This can be done by spinning the head or the whole infant in the opposite direction while observing the reflex eye movements. If available saccadic eye movements can be recorded or observed by inducing optokinetic nystagmus. Testing for ductions after prolonged cover of the other eye also excludes limitation due to cross fixation or inhibitional or habitual palsy. Forced duction testing confirms any restrictive limitation.

Cases of **Duane's retraction syndrome type I** is differentiated by retraction, changes in palpebral aperture and associated upshoots or downshoots on adduction.

Central nervous system anomalies in **Down's syndrome** and **Mobius syndrome, cerebral palsy** and **albinism** need to be excluded. **Accommodative esotropia** and accommodative part in a **partially accommodative esotropia** should be excluded by a full cycloplegic refraction. In cases with nystagmus it is important to exclude the **nystagmus blockage syndrome** which is characterized by an inverse relationship between the amplitude of nystagmus and the degree of esotropia.

Etiology

The etiology of infantile esotropia is not known, that is why it has the prefix **"essential"**.

Various hypotheses have been given from time to time blaming hyperopia, over-accommodation, over-convergence, subclinical paresis, maturation delay of VI N compared to III N, etc. But none of these stand to be substantiated. The etiology appears to be multifactorial, some of the factors may be heritable as evidenced by monozygotic twins showing esotropia. Some anomaly in the developmental process in the first four months seems to be responsible.

Phenomenon of Saccadic Underactions

The study of eye movements by electro-oculography has shown abnormalities in pursuit in amblyopes and also in alternating esotropia. The temporal-nasal asymmetry of optokinetic nystagmus has already been referred to earlier. Even saccades have been found to be affected in essential esotropes. The alternating esotropes showed **underaction of saccades of the covered eye (non-fixating eye)** both for adduction and abduction. When the fixation was switched to the other eye, the saccades became normal and those of the previously fixating (now-covered) eye became underacting. This is described as phenomenon of alternating saccadic underaction (Fig. 7.5). Cases of unilateral esotropia with one eye amblyopic eye have underaction of saccades of amblyopic eye when normal eye fixates but no such underaction occurs when the amblyopic eye fixates. Thus the underaction of the non-fixating eye appears to be a phenomenon, an abnormal reflex activated by dominant eye only. This underaction is different from the underaction seen in an esodeviation due to acquired paralytic squint as in lateral rectus palsy, where only saccades of lateral rectus show paresis which is same irrespective of which eye fixates (Fig. 7.5d).

Management

Once a proper diagnosis is made the management depends on the treatment of amblyopia if any. A full cycloplegic refraction with atropine 1% ointment (rice grain size) applied thrice a day for three consecutive days is desirable for the dark iris people. Other cycloplegic drugs may not fully relax the accommodation. Full hyperopic correction is desirable, in the presence of esotropia in case of doubt one should err on the side of making the child slightly myopic (his area of interest is at near fixation). In case of inability of testing visual acuity, unilateral preference of fixation or resistance of the child to allow covering one eye indicates amblyopia. Occlusion should be started. Conventional full-time, fully opaque occlusion of the dominant eye is advocated. This is done for 2 days up to 2 years of age

and subsequently up to 6 years of age the duration is increased 1 day for every year. This is alternated with one day of occlusion of the amblyopic eye, at no time is binocular viewing allowed during the treatment. Thus the patching is done for 3:1, 4:1, or 5:1 days, for a 3, 4, or 5 years old child. Above 6 years age the regime remains 6:1 for all ages. The vision is assessed monthly, but for infants it is preferred to be fortnightly. The end point is free alternation of the two eyes which is equally maintained. Recent studies have stressed the role of occlusion (alternate day, 1:1) even for the alternators prior to surgery, as it corrects the temporal-nasal bias.

Surgery: When?

Early surgery is advocated as children operated early have been restored better binocular functions. A report of a child with large esotropia documented since one week of birth and who was operated at about three months age had bifoveal fusion with 40 arc seconds stereopsis at 5½ years of age. It may be therefore recommended that a large angle esotropia (constant deviation) should be operated at the earliest, 4–6 months of age, or once the diagnosis and the deviation and associated overactions can be assessed properly. Small angle esotropia are to be carefully monitored with proper hyperopic correction till about 6 months or till the examination can be done satisfactorily.

Factors to be Considered

The surgical outcome depends on a careful and proper evaluation of associated inferior oblique (and rarely superior oblique), V-pheno-menon (or A-phenomenon), amblyopia therapy, nystagmus, DVD, etc. It may be noted that surgery in very young children is more demanding, yields more results per mm of muscle surgery, similarly larger deviations, and smaller eyeballs yields more correction. Medial recti surgery gives more effect than the lateral recti for each mm in the ratio 3:2.

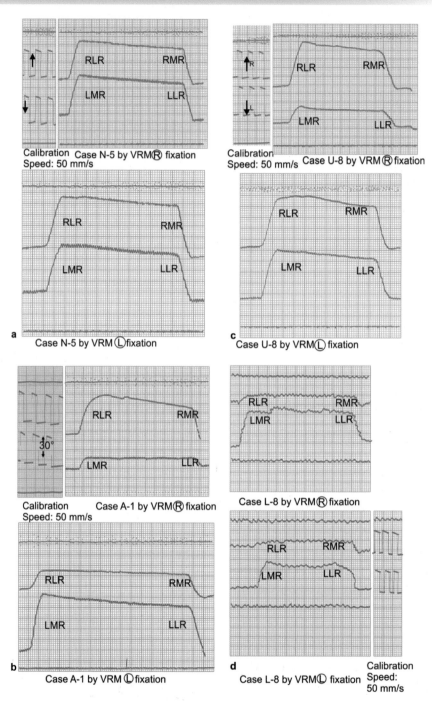

Fig. 7.5: (a) Electro-oculogram (EOG) in a normal subject showing equal saccades on either eye fixating, (b) EOG in an essential alternating esotropia showing saccadic underactions in the deviating eye, (c) EOG in a unilateral esotrope showing saccadic underaction in the deviating eye but no underaction of the dominant eye on change of fixation, (d) EOG in a left lateral rectus palsy showing underaction of saccades of left lateral rectus only.

Monocular recession-resection surgery is also more effective. Cases of eccentric fixation or uncorrected amblyopia have unpredictable results.

Surgical Guidelines

Results of surgery vary from surgeon to surgeon depending on his dissection of adjacent structures (intermuscular septum and check ligaments), and surgical technique of suturing, bites in the tendon stump left, etc. Nomograms of one surgeon are not applicable to another. Generally speaking 1 mm surgery on the medial rectus corrects 3–4.5 pd of deviation, while 1 mm of lateral rectus corrects 2–3 pd. The effect varies depending upon the various factors considered above. A minimal recession-resection procedure corrects about 15–20 pd and a maximal of 50–60 pd.

Large single muscle surgery may produce spectacular corrections in the primary position but may also produce undesirable changes in the palpebral aperture and incomitance in the lateral gazes. It is recommended that the surgery be divided between two or three recti depending on the size of the deviation. The choice of bi-medial recession vs. monocular recession-resection surgery depends on the surgeon's preference in the absence of convergence excess or divergence insufficiency or other factors.

In infants of 6 months age the posterior segment is still developing and surgery may be unpredictable. The measurements from limbus may be taken if the distance from the limbus and the recti is variable. If the conjunctival restriction is detected on FDT conjunctival recession can be planned.

Postoperative Results

Binocular vision is generally difficult to be accomplished, though early surgery helps (Figs 7.6 a and b). According to von Noorden four possible outcomes are as follows:
• **Optimal goal:** Subnormal binocular vision. Such cases have orthotropia or asymptomatic heterophoria with normal visual acuity in

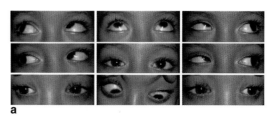
a

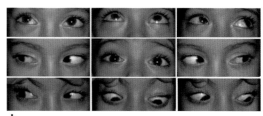
b

Fig. 7.6: Preoperative (a) and postoperative (b) of esotropia with V pattern with bilateral inferior oblique overactions.

both eyes, normal retinal correspondence, fusional amplitudes with reduced stereopsis but stability of alignment.
• **Desirable goal:** Microtropia. Such cases have very small angle squint, eso- or exo (up to 8pd) with features of microtropia: mild amblyopia, central or parafoveolar fixation with ARC with fusional amplitudes and reduced or absent stereopsis. There is some stability of alignment and no therapy other than amblyopia is desired.
• **Acceptable goal:** Small angle esotropia. Such cases have small angle (10–20 pd) eso- or exotropia, which is cosmetically acceptable, Majority of the cases have ARC, rest having suppression or amblyopia. The alignment is less stable.
• **Unacceptable goal:** Large angle strabismus. Large angle (over 20pd) eso or exotropia in the form of residual or consecutive squint, which is cosmetically unacceptable. Suppression prevails and the angle is unstable. Such cases require re-surgery or until that is done the eyes are aligned by prisms or glasses.

Role of Botulinum Injections

Botulinum injections have been used as an alternative to surgery in adults but its effect lasts for short duration. In infants the weakening effect has been claimed to be prolonged due to the immaturity of the infant's myofibrils by McNeer's studies. A paresis of the medial rectus also triggers a spread of comitance favorably aligning the eyes. More studies have not confirmed these observations so the role of Botulinum injections is limited and surgical therapy is the mainstay.

ACCOMMODATIVE ESOTROPIA

Esodeviations due to excessive convergence associated with accommodation are called accommodative esotropia (Fig. 7.7). They can be classified as:

1. **Refractive** (hyperopic)
   - Normo-accommodative (normal AC/A ratio)
   - Hyper-accommodative (high AC/A ratio)
2. **Nonrefractive**
   - Hyper-accommodative (high AC/A ratio)
   - Hypo-accommodative (normal AC/A ratio, weak accommodative mechanism)
3. **Partially accommodative** (with associated nonaccommodative esotropia with or without convergence excess)

Clinical Presentation

The most consistent feature of all these cases is a variable angle of esodeviation, which increases with the effort of accommodation.

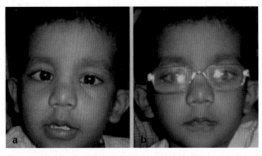

Fig. 7.7: (a) A case of accommodative esotropia without proper glasses, (b) Correction of accommodative esotropia after proper glasses.

Refractive normo-accommodative esotropia cases have an uncorrected hyperopia. In order to see clear at distance they accommodate and have esodeviation for distance fixation. Since they have a normal AC/A ratio the esodeviation is the same for distance and near fixation (within 15 pd), i.e. they lack convergence excess. Such cases respond well to their full correction of hyperopic error as determined under cycloplegia. Usually they have mild to moderate hyperopia (+2 to +6 dioptres). Very high hyperopia may not accommodate and may only have bilateral amblyopia. In addition to esotropia and amblyopia they may present with asthenopia due to constant accommodative effort.

Refractive hyper-accommodative esotropia cases have an esodeviation at distant fixation, as above, but also have a convergence excess esotropia for near fixation at 33 cm, more than 15 pd excess of that at distant fixation. They have high AC/A ratio (normal AC/A ratio is 3–5 pd/D.) Thus a +3 hyperope with a AC/A ratio of 7, will have 21 pd esotropia for distance fixation and 42 pd esotropia for near fixation at 33 cm. And even with the full correction for distance will have residual esotropia, that will be corrected with near add as bifocals.

Nonrefractive accommodative esotropia cases have no clinically significant hyperopia. They have high AC/A ratio resulting in no significant esotropia for distant fixation but more than 15 pd esotropia for near fixation, **(hyper-accommodative type).** Such cases do not accommodate for distance but only for near fixation.

Another type **hypo-accommodative** esotropia has a weak accommodative mechanism and in order to see clear they have to over-accommodate, though AC/A ratio is normal, and thus have convergence excess. They have a remote or distant near point of accommodation (NPA) and near point of convergence (NPC). This differentiates them from the hyper-accommodative type who have a normal NPA. Early presbyopes or cases under mild cycloplegic drugs can present like these cases.

Age of Onset

The accommodative esotropia cases usually present in the 2nd year of life, but some cases present as early as about 3 months of age. It may depend on the personality of the child as to whether and when he accommodates to see clear in the presence of optical blur. A variable angle of esotropia, presence of convergence excess, and the full cycloplegic error should be looked for.

Management

It depends on giving **full cycloplegic correction** to correct the esotropia. In case of doubt one may err to slightly over correct to make the child myopic rather than leave him with residual hyperopia (Figs 7.7 a and b). The frames have to be light in weight but with apertures big enough to cover the eyes in all position of gaze. Harness frames may be chosen for small infants. Monitoring for residual esodeviations should be done frequently. Children accept glasses more readily than expected, otherwise mild cycloplegic drugs like cyclopentolate drops are used for a few weeks. Contact lenses can also be used for those reluctant to wear glasses.

If convergence excess is present, **bifocal glasses** are prescribed (Fig. 7.8). The minimal plus add that corrects the convergence excess esotropia is added (Fig. 7.9). While testing accommodative targets should be used and sufficient time allowed to relax or exercise his accommodation. The lower segment should be large executive type, such that the line bisects the pupil. For small infants a higher lower segment is preferred or only the near correction may be prescribed.

If residual esotropia persists in spite of full correction and bifocals, a **non-accommodative element is indicated.** Such cases are partially

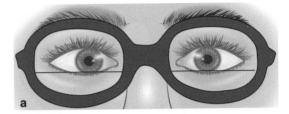

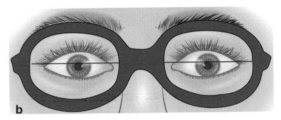

Fig. 7.8: Improper bifocals in (a) do not correct estropia, (b) proper bifocals correct esotropia.

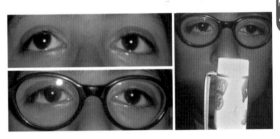

Fig. 7.9: Accommodative esotropia with convergence excess for near.

accommodative and require **surgery for the non-accommodative part** (Fig. 7.10).

AC/A ratio can be calculated by **hetrophoria and gradient methods** (Figs 7.11a and b).

Miotics can be used in place of glasses, but the latter are preferred as they have a precise correction of the refractive error. Miotics can have a variable effect at different times of the

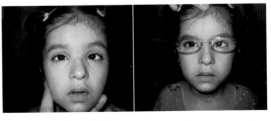

Fig. 7.10: Partially accommodative esotropia-esotropia less after glasses but still there for distance.

$$AC/A = IPD + \frac{\Delta n - \Delta d}{D}$$

Example: IPD = 5.5cm, Δn= 30 PD base out, Δd= 25 PD base out

$$AC/A = 5.5 + ((+30)-(+25))/3$$
$$= 5.5 + (30-25)/3$$
$$= 5.5 + 1.6$$
$$= 7.1^{\Delta}/D$$

Normal range: 5-7.5$^{\Delta}$/ 1 Diopter

Fig. 7.11a: AC/A ratio heterophoria method.

$$AC/A = \frac{\Delta_G - \Delta_0}{G}$$

Example: Δ_0 = 15 PD base in, Δ_G = 7 PD base in, G = -2.00Dsph

$$AC/A = (-7)-(-15)/2$$
$$= (-7 + 15)/2$$
$$= +8/2$$
$$= 4^{\Delta}/D$$

Normal range: 3 – 5$^{\Delta}$/ 1 Diopter

Fig. 7.11b: AC/A ratio gradient method.

day, and can have side effects like brow ache, nausea, abdominal cramps. The ocular side effects are iris cysts, lens opacities, angle closure glaucoma, and retinal detachment. The miotics are indicated for short term treatment till the glasses are accepted.

Echothiophate iodide 0.03% is started one drop once daily and increased to twice daily to 0.125% till desirable effect is obtained. Another miotic in use is Di-iso fluorophosphate (DFP) ointment.

For small residual deviations **prisms** can be prescribed. **Surgery** for the nonaccommodative part is medial rectus recession with or without retroequatorial myopexy (faden operation).

ACQUIRED OR LATE-ONSET NON-ACCOMMODATIVE ESOTROPIA

Cases which have esodeviations of later onset usually after infancy, but accommodative factors and no neurological cause are called **acquired essential non-accommodative) esotropia.** They may be of **basic type** (near-distant deviation same) or may have **convergence excess.** Rarely **divergence**

insufficiency may be present. They are usually considered different from the divergence palsy cases which have some neurological cause. Computed Tomography or Magnetic Resonance Imaging should be done to exclude such possibility. These are usually managed by surgery and such cases have better binocular visual potential compared to infantile esotropia.

MICROTROPIA

Ultra-small angle esodeviations which may be missed by ordinary methods of examination and usually have amblyopia of one eye with variable levels of binocularity are called microtropia.

They can be **primary** or **secondary,** the latter are residual deviations after surgery. Actually there is a spectrum of these conditions, one merging into another, with Bifoveal single vision with fixation disparity towards the normal end, through various manifestations of microtropia; to small angle esotropia at the other end.

In the so called group of microtropia we have **Park's monofixation syndrome** and **Lang's microtropia** (less than 5°).

Park's monofixation syndrome is described to have macular scotoma with good peripheral fusion with fusional amplitudes and gross stereopsis.

Lang's microtropia is described to have small angle (<5°) heterotropia with harmonious ARC with mild amblyopia and partial stereopsis. Lang further describes **three types** of microtropia, based on the fixation pattern. **Type 1** has central fixation, **type 2** has eccentric fixation without identity and **type 3** has eccentric fixation with identity. Eccentric fixation with identity implies that the angle of anomaly is the same as the eccentricity of fixation. *And once this occurs, the cover test will not pick up the tropia just as in Parks monofixation syndrome.* In types 1 and 2 the cover test will show a tropia. According to Helveston and von Noorden only Lang's type 3 is truly speaking microtropia.

The **consistent findings** of microtropia are:

1. Amblyopia (diminution of vision in one eye)
2. Anomalous retinal correspondence (ARC) (on Bagolini's or Foveo-foveal test)
3. Relative scotoma on fixation spot (as seen by 4 prism dioptre base out test or Bagolini's glasses or binocular perimetry)
4. Normal or near normal fusional amplitudes
5. Defective stereo-acuity.

And the **variable findings** are:

1. Size of deviation (5°–8°)
2. Foveal or non-foveal fixation
3. Relationship between the degree of eccentric fixation and angle of anomaly
4. Presence or absence of anisometropia
5. Positive or negative cover test.

The **diagnosis** of microtropia depends on detecting a macular scotoma by Bagolini's glasses, Four-Prism dioptre test (Fig. 7.12) or foveo-foveal test of Cuppers. Presence of amblyopia and associated refractive error should be detected. **Management** is primarily aimed to treat the amblyopia with occlusion therapy. The prognosis is good if the condition is treated in younger children.

ACUTE CONCOMITANT ESOTROPIA

Cases of concomitant esotropia which have a sudden presentation are referred as acute concomitant esotropia. These are exceptions to the usually accepted myth that diplopia is a feature of incomitant esotropia as against the concomitant esotropia. (Actually speaking, diplopia is a feature of sudden presentation of any strabismus). There are **two types** of such cases (a) Those which manifest after the fusion has been interrupted by a patch or occlusion for a short time, (b) Those which have no such interruptions to fusion but have very poor fusional control, which may be further compromised by physical or emotional stress. Three subtypes described are:

- Swan type due to occlusion
- Franceschetti type due to convergence
- Bielschowsky type due to myopia

Such cases should be investigated for any neurological lesion. The first type of cases which have otherwise good fusional control can be followed up for 6 months as they may spontaneously resolve. In case of non-resolution which is more usual in the second type, surgery is contemplated. For shorter duration prismatic neutralization may also be done for cases with small angle esotropia.

CYCLIC ESOTROPIA

Unusual cases of esotropia which have a regular cycle of presentation, usually 24–48 hours of squint alternating with similar dura-tion of no-squint are referred as cyclic esotropia. On the squint-days a large angle esotropia of about 40–50 pd appears with sensory anomalies (diplopia is rare) and deviation is usually consistent on squint days. On no-squint days binocular single vision with good fusional amplitudes are observed. No latent squint is present on no-squint days compared to intermittent squints. Such cycles last for a few months or years, before they become fully manifest squints.

Surgery as per the deviation on the squint days gives satisfactory results.

NYSTAGMUS BLOCKAGE SYNDROME

While manifest latent nystagmus and manifest nystagmus are both known to be associated with infantile esotropia (the former more often), there is a special form of nystagmus which has a dampening mechanism with eyes in adduction. Such cases have an inverse relationship between esotropia and nystagmus. Nystagmus is present when the eyes are straight and it disappears when the eyes are locked into esotropia. Such cases are Nystagmus blockage syndrome. These are distinguished from infantile esotropia with manifest latent nystagmus which lack this inverse relationship. Management of such cases is retro equatorial myopexy with or without recession of both medial recti.

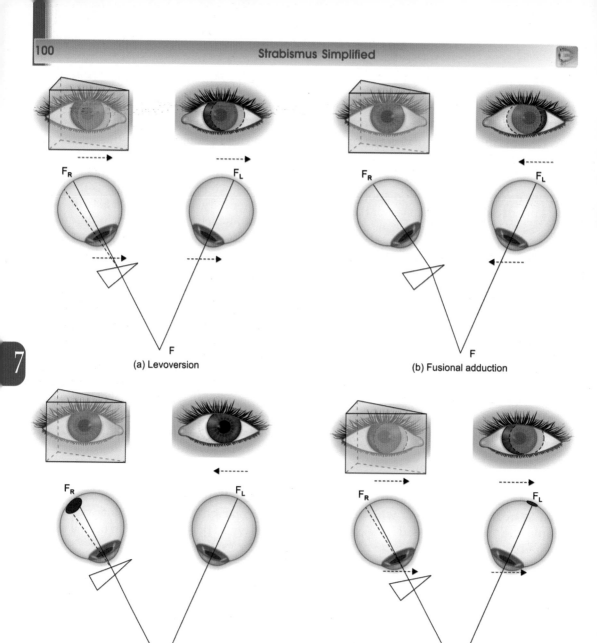

(a) Levoversion

(b) Fusional adduction

(c) No movements

(d)) Levoversion but no fusional adduction

Fig. 7.12: Four prism base out test for microtropia. (a) and (b) Depict the movements in Normals. A 4 pd B.O. in front of right eye induces a levoversion (adduction of right and abduction of left eye). This is followed by a corrective fusional adduction of left eye to refixate the left eye foveality, (c) depicts microtropia of right eye, the foveal scotoma prevents any movement, (d) depicts microtropia of left eye when the levoversion is induced by the normal eye but no corrective fusional adduction occurs as the foveal scotoma in left eye prevents this. In case of weak fusion the second movement of fusional adduction may not also occur but patient complains of diplopia.

SENSORY ESOTROPIA

Cases which have lost vision in one eye usually develop a squint over a period of time. They may develop an esotropia or exotropia depending on their convergence tonus. Generally it is observed that it is exotropia in the first year and after 8–9 years and in between it is an esotropia. In all such cases the *refractive error and accommodational status of the straight eye* needs to be evaluated before any cosmetic surgery is contemplated.

Suggested Reading

1. Helveston, EM Frank Costenbader Lecture—the origins of congenital esotropia J. Pediatr. Ophthalmol Strabismus 30:215, 1993.

2. Nixon RB, Helveston EM, Miller K. Archer SM and Ellis ED. Incidence of strabismus in neonates. Am. J. Ophthalmol. 100: 798,1985.

3. Noorden GK von. A reassessment of infantile esotropia (XLIV) Edward Jackson Memorial Lecture. Am. J. Ophthalmol. 105 : 1, 1988.

4. Noorden GK von. Current concepts of infantile esotropia (The William Bowman Lecture) Eye 2: 243, 1988.

5. Tychsen L and Lisberger SG. Visual motion processing for the initiation of smooth—pursuit eye movements in humans. J. Neurophysiol. 56: 953,1986.

6. Prakash P, Sharma P, Rao V.M., Shastry P. Polaroid Scotometer: A new device to chart suppression scotoma. J. Ped. Ophthalmol. Strabismus. 33, 181–184, 1996.

7. Jampolsky A. Characteristics of suppression in strabismus Arch. Ophthalmol. 54. 683. 1955.

8. Sharma P, Prakash P, Menon V, Gahlot DK. Saccadic underactions in concomitant convergent squint. Ind. J. Ophthalmol. 32: 461–466, 1984.

9. Jampolsky's article on occlusion.

10. McNeer KW. Tucker MG. Spencer R.E Botulinum toxin management of essential infantile esotropia in children Arch. Ophthalmol, 115: 1411, 1997.

7

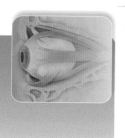

8

Exotropia

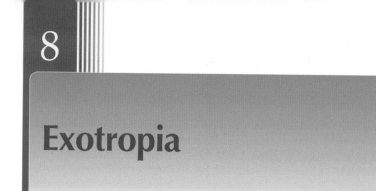

Exodeviations or divergent squint occur as a result of certain obstacles to development or maintenance of binocular vision and/or due to defective action of the medial rectus muscles. Although exophoria is almost universal, manifest exodeviations are fortunately rare due to the good fusional convergence reserves. Since essential infantile exotropia are rare unlike essential infantile esotropia, one should always exclude neurological anomalies in case of early onset exotropia (Fig. 8.1).

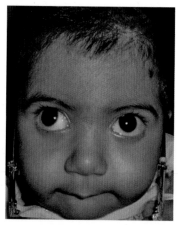

Fig. 8.1: A case of large angle exotropia.

Exodeviations can be classified as follows:

Types of Exodeviations

a. **Concomitant**

  1. Primary

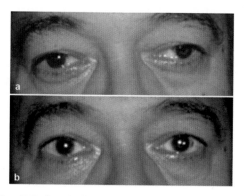

Fig. 8.2: Intermittent exotropia, (a) manifested, (b) controlled.

    • Infantile exotropia
    • Intermittent exotropia (Fig. 8.2)
  2. Secondary
    • Sensory exotropia
    • Consecutive exotropia

b. **Incomitant**

  1. Paralytic (III n., medial rectus palsy)
  2. Restrictive
  3. Musculofascial anomalies (Duane's retraction syndrome type 2)
  4. Dissociated horizontal deviation.

Duane's Classification of Exodeviations

1. **Divergence excess pattern:** Distance deviation is 15 pd larger than near deviation (Fig. 8.3).
2. **Convergence insufficiency pattern:** Near deviation is 15 pd larger than distance deviation (Fig. 8.4).

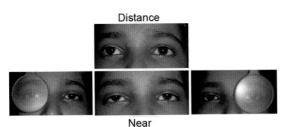

Distance

Near

Fig. 8.3: Divergence excess exotropia.

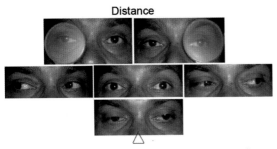

Distance

Fig. 8.4: Convergence insufficiency exotropia.

3. **Basic exodeviation:** Distance and near deviations are equal (within 10 pd).
4. **Simulated divergence excess:** A basic deviation presenting as divergence excess pattern due to part compensation of the near deviation by fusional or accommodative convergence.

Exodeviations have also been **classified on the basis of underlying fusional reserve as:**

1. Exophoria: XP
2. Intermittent exotropia: X(T)
3. Manifest exotropia: XT.

Kushner described a classification which helps in management of these cases. A comparison of Burian and Kushner's classification is shown in Fig. 8.5.

Burian	Kushner
Divergence excess	Proximal convergence,HiAC/A,4%
Simul Div XS (Occl)	Tenacious PFC, 40%
Simul Div XS (+3D)	High AC/A, 5%
Basic	Basic, 37%
Conv Insufficiency	Low AC/A, 11%
	Fusional Conv Insufficiency, 1%
	Pseudo Conv Insufficiency, <1%
	Near XT>Dist but equalize after patch

Fig. 8.5: XT Classifications—a comparison.

Clinical Presentation

Essential Infantile exotropia are primary concomitant exodeviations that lack binocularity. The term essential implies that they are not due to other causes like craniofacial abnormalities, neurological diseases, restrictive syndromes or any vision impairing ocular defects like high unilateral refractive error, cataract, corneal opacities, or macular or optic nerve diseases. Such cases are characterized by large angle (35 pd or more), alternation and early onset. They are also called congenital, infantile, or alternating exotropia. Amblyopia is a rarity and if present, usually is due to some other factor like anisometropia. *Such cases are rare, so large constant exotropia in infancy should always be investigated for neurological anomalies.*

Intermittent exotropia: These are the most common type of exotropia and are intermittent in presentation. Binocular vision is present in intermittent cases but with progression of condition one eye may be suppressed (Fig. 8.2). Such cases have fusional reserves which are partially compromised. They are usually associated with headaches, eyestrain and blurred vision especially if an effort of fusional and accommodative convergence is made to overcome the deviation. There may be occasional double vision (diplopia). Sometimes discomfort in strong light due to the manifestation of exodeviation on exposure to strong light has been loosely called photophobia, it is actually **diplopia-phobia.** Micropsia is a rare symptom of exotropia, when a patient has to use accommodative convergence to maintain BSV for distance. The image is perceived as becoming smaller and coming closer. Abnormal stereopsis for distance has been noted to be an early indicator of intermittent exotropia becoming manifest, requiring surgery.

Sensory exotropia: Exodeviations that occur secondary to poor vision in one eye due to organic causes like optic atrophy, central macular scars, dense media opacities, etc.

These may be due to disruption of fusion manifesting the ocular position of physiological rest (fusion-free position).

Consecutive exotropia: Exodeviations that occur secondary to an erstwhile esotropia either due to change in refractive status, surgery or spontaneously. These cases may have paradoxic eccentric fixation.

Incomitant squints are covered in relevant chapters.

Natural History of Intermittent Exodeviation

Untreated intermittent divergent squint (IDS) tends to increase in its frequency of manifestation to become constant divergent squint, unilateral or alternating. The latter depends on the unilateral preference of one eye or of free alternation. However, all cases of IDS do not progress and may remain stable. The extent to which an exodeviation is controlled by **fusion** depends not only on the size of the angle but also to a large extent on the general health, alertness, attention span and level of anxiety of the patient.

Factors to be Recorded for Progression

1. Loss of fusional control as evidenced by increasing frequency of the manifest phase of the strabismus.
2. Development of secondary convergence insufficiency.
3. Increase in size of basic deviation.
4. Development of suppression.

Calhounz *et al.* has described four phases of exodeviations starting as divergence excess type and progressing as above mentioned factors, as follows:

Phases of Exodeviations and Clinical Presentation

i. Exotropia at distance, orthophoria at near, Asymptomatic, goes undetected.
ii. Intermittent exotropia for distance, orthophoria/exophoria at near, Symptomatic for distance (no suppression scotoma)
iii. Exotropia at distance, exotropia or intermittent exotropia at near, Binocular vision for near, suppression scotoma develops for distance
iv. Exotropia at distance as well as near, Lack of binocularity.

Sensory Adaptations in Exotropia

Sensory adaptations in general are rare in exotropia as most of these are intermittent. Strabismic amblyopia is therefore almost non-existent and all such cases should be evaluated for some other amblyopiogenic causes or organic causes excluded. Rarely unilateral constant exodeviations do have amblyopia, otherwise alternate suppression is seen in alternating exotropia and in manifest exotropia. In very small angle exotropia of constant deviation and of early onset anomalous retinal correspondence, ARC is rarely seen. In some of IDS cases a dual binocular behaviour is observed, alternate suppression for distance (manifest exotropia) and binocular single vision for near (exophoria).

The characteristics of **suppression scotoma** vary with the test depending on its dissociation level. More dissociating tests like prisms and synoptophore produce single large scotoma from the fovea to the diplopia point with a sharp nasal cut-off (hemiretinal suppression of Jampolsky). With less dissociating tests like Polaroid scotometer or phase difference haploscope **two discrete scotoma** (Fig. 8.6) are seen: one at the fovea and the

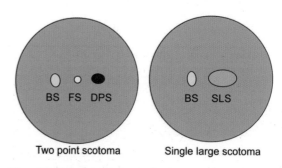

Two point scotoma   Single large scotoma

Fig. 8.6: Twin-point scotoma in exodeviation on polaroid scotometer.

other at the diplopia point. This is similar to that seen in esotropia.

Magician's Forceps Phenomenon

This is a very interesting phenomenon observed in essential or primary exotropia, having a bearing on the causation of exodeviations. Ishikawa (1978) described the **reverse phase reflex,** that is an opposite movement of the other eye when one eye (the dominant eye) was passively moved in any direction (Fig. 8.7). This reverse phase movement is dependent on the amount of passive force applied (not all-or-none) and is observed in all directions. Mitsui (1979) described a special reflex movement, on passive adduction of the dominant eye (even by slight force), the exodeviation of the other eye gets corrected or straightened.

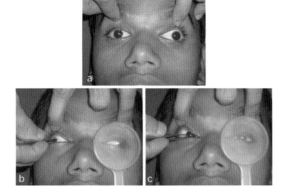

Fig. 8.7: Exotropia (a), Reverse phase reflex (b), and Magician's forceps phenomenon (c).

Moreover the exodeviation re-establishes on leaving the passive adduction. This was an "all-or-none" response and was called "Magician's forceps phenomenon" because of magical correction of exodeviation. The reflex was abolished by deep retrobulbar or procaine anesthesia of eyeball and was observed even in dark ruling out the possibility of visual fixation causing it. It is supposed to be an abnormal reflex established during the neurodevelopmental stage causing exodeviation in one eye (the slave eye). These observations have been confirmed at our centre (Garg, Menon, Prakash, 1984).

Nonsurgical Management

Intermittent exotropia presents due to poor fusional control, and the nonsurgical treatment aims to restore the control. However, it should be remembered that the **nonsurgical treatment does not actually alter the angle of exotropia.**

a. **Orthoptic treatment:** The aim is to make the patient aware of the manifest deviation and to improve his control of it.

1. **Antisuppression exercises:** The treatment is directed to diplopia recognition. Suppression scotoma is usually and initially for distance and is amenable to therapy by flashes and then the BSV is maintained by antisuppression exercises like bar-reading, or on synoptophore or Cheiroscope.

2. **Relative convergence exercises:** Binocular single vision can be strengthened by extension of the fusion amplitude and by teaching the patient relative convergence. This is a simple but effective way of treating majority of cases of intermittent exotropia as also of convergence insufficiency.

Convergence exercises: While it is true that the convergence exercises cannot affect the basic deviation and only improve the fusional control and thus decrease the manifestation of an exodeviation. *A tropia is converted to a phoria.* The lack of effect is only due to poor case selection (cases having suppression may require anti-suppression exercises prior to and along with) or improper method of exercising. *Appreciation of physiological diplopia* should be taught as the first step. Secondly training should be done to increase both the phasic and tonic control, in other words the convergence sustenance or the stamina or endurance should be exercised in addition to the fusional amplitudes. Just like any other physical exercises the results last only if the exercises are continued. Synoptophore exercises may be desirable to start with but are insufficient if not supplemented by proper home exercises.

For **home exercises,** special cards or a line on a plain paper may be made use of or a pencil tip may be used. The latter gives the name of "pencil pushups" to this regime. If convergence sustenance is not practised this may only build up biceps and not the convergence! A **simple home orthoptic trainer (SHOT)** of the author, utilising a dark circle painted on either side of a folded paper such that the circles can be superimposed and the paper slid on a foot ruler, the circle on one side has a cross on top and the other at the bottom. The subject has to fuse the two images to form a circle with a cross above and below and maintain it for forty seconds repeatedly with five seconds break for 3–5 minutes twice daily. The paper is slid closer and closer as the convergence starts improving. A simpler convergence trainer which is kept flat infront of nose and the subject converges at each dot for 50 seconds starting with the farthest at moving closer (Fig. 8.8).

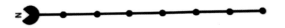

Fig. 8.8: Convergence trainer.

b. **Optical treatment:** Overcorrected concave lenses are used to stimulate convergence by inducing accommodation, thus aiding control of exotropia. This is more effective in cases of high AC/A ratio. It is at best successful as a relatively short term measure allowing surgery to be deferred to a more opportune time.

c. **Prisms:** Base-in prisms or relieving prisms can be used to compensate the strabismus in children to allow the continued use of binocular vision. It can also be used as a preoperative procedure to enforce bifoveal stimulation. Prisms are like crutches and

should be generally under-corrected to encourage the positive convergence mechanism. Lack of Fresnel prisms limits their use to about 8 pd prisms over each eye only. Even with Fresnel prisms the comfortable limit is about 15 pd prisms over each eye. The need for surgery is determined by the state of fusional control, the size of the angle and the age of the patient.

Surgery

If the nonsurgical treatment fails surgery is required.

Indications for Surgery

1. When the deviation is intermittent, that is appears and disappears on blinking or occurs only with fatigue, observation is warranted. The parents need to be told to observe how much percentage of waking hours does the child actually squint. If he does for 50% or more, surgery is advocated.

2. If the condition is progressing from Phase II to III of Calhounz, i.e. it occurs during the periods when the child is alert and lasts through blinks, or when suppression scotoma develops.

3. If diplopia is present (child covers one eye for distance viewing) or complains of "photo-phobia" or diplopia phobia, surgery is indicated.

4. If no diplopia is complained of in spite of a manifest exodeviation, a suppression is indicated. This implies that the ideal time for surgery has passed, but surgery should be still done and hoped to regain binocularity with the help of anti-suppression exercises.

5. By the time Phase IV is reached, suppression is well established and surgery may only be of cosmetic value, but some cases may develop peripheral binocular functions and some even better. Distance stereoacuity is affected earlier and should be used if possible, but atleast the near stereotests should definitely be used.

Timing of Surgery

Knapp advocated early surgery to prevent sensory changes which may become intractable later and to minimize the reinforcement of habit of squint. But Jampolsky advocated delayed surgery for accurate diagnosis and so that the child becomes cooperative for preoperative and postoperative orthoptic treatment. Also cosmetic squint would be less common and even if to occur the sequelae would be less harmful at a later age. The Newcastle score utilizes the breaking up of the exodeviation at home, and clinic both for distance and near and gives an objective value to decide the timing of surgery. The best approach is to assess the timing in each case individually as per the guidelines given above. The Newcastle score table is shown Fig. 8.9.

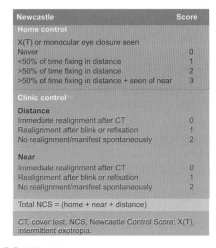

Newcastle	Score
Home control	
X(T) or monocular eye closure seen	
Never	0
<50% of time fixing in distance	1
>50% of time fixing in distance	2
>50% of time fixing in distance + seen of near	3
Clinic control	
Distance	
Immediate realignment after CT	0
Realignment after blink or refixation	1
No realignment/manifest spontaneously	2
Near	
Immediate realignment after CT	0
Realignment after blink or refixation	1
No realignment/manifest spontaneously	2
Total NCS = (home + near + distance)	
CT, cover test, NCS, Newcastle Control Score; X(T), intermittent exotropia.	

Fig. 8.9: The Newcastle score. Courtesy: *H Haggerty et al, Br J Ophthalmol 2004;88:233–235.*

Choice of Surgery

The factors which determine the choice of surgery are:
1. Comparative deviation at 33 cm, 6 m, and in the far distance (20 m).
2. The size of the AC/A ratio and determining whether the patient has a true or simulated divergence excess.
3. If there is a change of deviation on lateral versions.
4. If there is a V or A phenomenon with or without associated inferior oblique or superior oblique overaction.

The choice lies between a bilateral symmetrical surgery on the lateral recti or an unilateral recession-resection surgery on the lateral and medial recti.

Symmetrical recession of both lateral recti is indicated if there is:
- True divergence excess
- Exotropia is less on lateral versions, as amount of surgery required will be less.
- In the presence of significant V phenomenon with inferior oblique overaction when lateral recti and inferior obliques can be tackled simultaneously from the same conjunctival approach.
- In cases of V or A phenomenon (Figs 8.10a and b) without oblique overactions when vertical shifting of the horizontal recti is being planned, as it is desirable to do a vertical shifting procedure bilaterally and symmetrically.

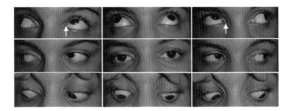

Fig. 8.10a: Exotropia with V-pattern

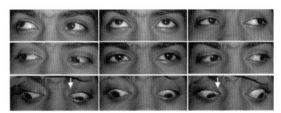

Fig. 8.10b: Exotropia with A-pattern

How much Surgery to be Done?

It is a common consideration depending on the desired postoperative result: over-correction or under-correction or an optimum correction? This depends on the age of the patient and the sensory status. In very young children, less than 5 years, one should avoid over-corrections lest esodeviations develop, which are likely to have undesirable sensory adaptations. In older children with some amount of binocularity available, a slight over-correction of 5–10 pd is beneficial in stimulating the binocular vision and to control post-surgical exo drift which is usual.

A transient diplopia for distance in place of erstwhile suppression is desirable. In pure cosmetic cases in adults, with no binocularity, one may have to take into account other factors like facial features or angle kappa as they would determine cosmesis (for further details see section on surgical management.).

Preoperative Management

- Refractive error, if any, should be optimally corrected. While myopic correction understandably favours fusion in intermittent exotropia or exophoria, hyperopic correction especially mild to moderate grade also facilitates fusion by supplying a clear visual image. In exceptional cases one may use his discretion to under or over correct the refractive error especially in residual or consecutive cases.

- Refractive error of the fixing eye assumes significance in sensory exotropia in which the other eye may have poor vision or even be blind.

- Treatment of amblyopia is important for a good functional result.

- Treatment to eliminate suppression at the divergent angle (neutralizing exodeviation) on synoptophore or with prisms can be done prior to surgery. At least the binocular status should be noted prior to surgery.

- Maximum angle of deviation should be determined. This is done by occluding one eye for 6–24 hours before PBCT in cases of variable measurements.

Postoperative Management

It is always desirable to discuss the post-operative result expected, especially if over-correction is planned. A possibility of diplopia should be forewarned. Exercises suitable to him told and a proper follow up plan explained. In case of consecutive esotropia especially in young children it should be controlled by any of the following: convex glasses and/or miotics which succeed if the AC/A ratio is high. Base-out prisms in small denominations of up to 12–14 pd, divided between the two eyes, can be used. Fresnel prisms can also be tried. In case of residual exotropia fusional vergence exercises are helpful or else base-in prisms resorted to. In case the squint cannot be overcome occlusion 1:1 till re-surgery should be instituted lest amblyopia develops in children. Thus a proper follow up is very important for a favourable outcome.

Criteria for Success

Excellent success is deemed to be achieved if the following criteria are met:
- Postoperative orthotropia or asymptomatic heterophoria for both distance and near fixation.
- Good and normal fusional vergences
- Binocular single vision with no suppression.
- Excellent awareness of physiological diplopia.
- Comfortable without asthenopic symptoms.

Suggested Reading

1. Jampolsky A. Management of exodeviations. In Strabismus. Symposium of the New Orleans Academy of Ophthalmology. St. Louis. 1962. Mosby— Year book Inc.
2. Keech RV and Stewart SA. The Surgical over correction of intermittent exotropia. J. Pediatr. Ophthalmol Strabismus. 27: 218, 1990.
3. Knapp P. Management of exotropia. In Symposium on strabismus. Transactions of the New Orleans Academy of Ophthalmology. St. Louis, 1971, Mosby — Year Book Inc.

4. Mitsui Y. Etiology and treatment of strabismus Ophthalmic Pract. 49: 1151. 1978.

5. Romano RE. Wilson M.F Robinson J.A. Worldwide surveys of current management of intermittent exotropia by M.D. Strabologists. Binoc Vision. 8: 167. 1993.

6. Scott WE and Mash AJ. The postoperative results and stability of exodeviations. Arch. Ophthalmol. 99: 1814, 1981.

7. Schlossman A. Muhnick RS and Stern K. The surgical management of intermittent exotropia in adults Ophthalmology. 90: 1166. 1983.

8. Garg R, Menon V, Prakash P: Proprioceptive reflexes in exodeviations. Ind. J. Ophthalmol 36. 168–170. 1988.

9. Prakash R, Sharma P, Rao VM, Shastry P Polaroid scotometer, a new device to chart suppression scotoma. J. Pediatr. Ophthalmol. Strabismus 33: 181–184, 1996.

8

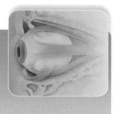

A–V Patterns

Horizontal deviations (esotropia and exotropia) which may be comitant in horizontal gazes, may not be comitant in vertical gazes, on looking up and on looking down. They are said to be **vertically incomitant comitant horizontal deviations.** In simpler terms they are described by simple alphabetic terms as **A and V patterns.** The latter is because the changes of horizontal deviation in up- and downgaze resembles the alphabets A or V.

Thus an exodeviation which becomes more divergent in upgaze and less divergent in the downgaze is said to have a **V pattern** (Fig. 9.1). An esodeviation with V pattern would be less convergent in upgaze and more convergent in downgaze. The reverse is true for **A patterns** (Fig. 9.2).

In addition to these four common patterns, other patterns are also seen. These are:

1. **A-exotropia** (exodeviation more in down gaze, less in upgaze).
2. **A-esotropia** (esodeviation less in down gaze, more in upgaze).
3. **V-exotropia** (exodeviation more in up gaze, less in downgaze).
4. **V-esotropia** (esodeviation less in upgaze, more in downgaze). It may be a pure V-pattern with exodeviation in upgaze, esodeviation in downgaze and ortho-in primary position.

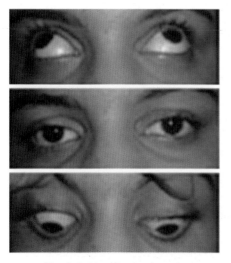

Fig. 9.1: V pattern exotropia.

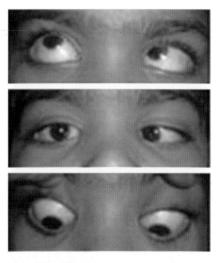

Fig. 9.2: A pattern esotropia.

5. **X-exotropia** (exodeviation more in both up and downgazes).
6. **Y-exotropia** (exodeviation more in upgaze only).
7. λ-exotropia (exodeviation more in downgaze only), delta exotropia.

8. ◆ exotropia (diamond exotropia) exodeviation only in primary position not in up and downgazes.

Clinically these patterns may be present with or without oblique muscle overactions (Figs 9.3 to 9.7).

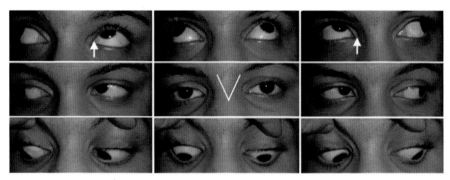

Fig. 9.3: V-exotropia with bilateral inferior oblique overactions.

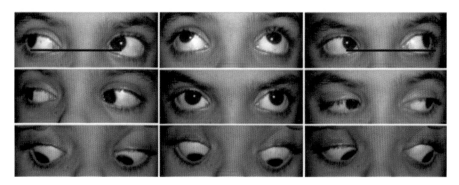

Fig. 9.4: V-exotropia without inferior oblique overactions.

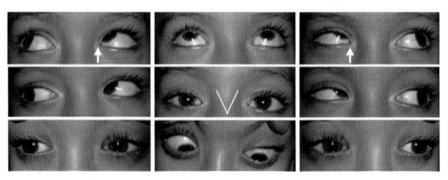

Fig. 9.5: V-esotropia with bilateral inferior oblique overactions.

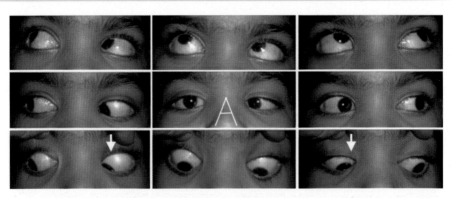

Fig. 9.6: A-esotropia with bilateral superior oblique overactions.

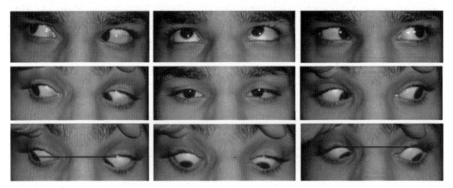

Fig. 9.7: A-esotropia without superior oblique overactions.

Prevalence

Since Urrets-Zavalia described them in 1948, A and V patterns have been commonly seen in at least one-third of esotropia and exotropia. V patterns are more common than A patterns. While esodeviations are more common in the West the exodeviations are more common in the Indian and the African races. The A-esotropia is the least type of pattern amongst the four main types, otherwise the diamond pattern is the least of all.

Etiology

From the differences in the various schools of etiology it appears none is singly correct. Multiple factors are responsible, different in different cases and more than one in some. The various factors are:

1. *Horizontal School* (Table 9.1)

Urist championed the role of horizontal recti, assuming that lateral recti are more effective in upgaze and medial recti more effective in downgaze. An overaction of lateral recti causes V-exotropia and underaction of medial recti causes A-esotropia (Figs 9.8a and b). Thus:

Table 9.1: Horizontal school

Pattern	Caused by
V-exotropia	Overaction lateral recti
V-esotropia	Overaction of medial recti
A-exotropia	Underaction of medial recti
A-esotropia	Underaction of lateral recti

Cases with A–V patterns which do not have oblique muscle overactions could be responsible because of this factor. Based on this principle Urist advocated surgery to

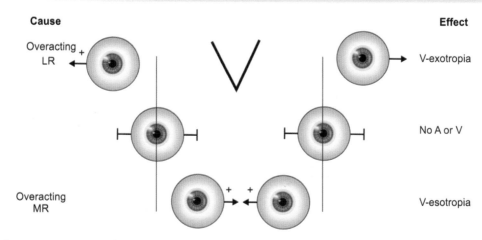

Fig. 9.8a: Horizontal school of Urist. V phenomenon caused by overacting lateral recti (V-exo) or medial recti (V-eso).

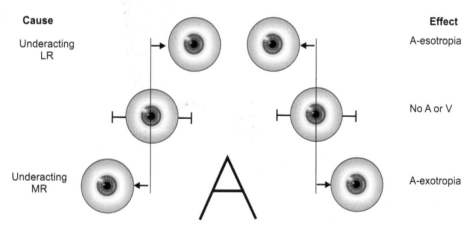

Fig. 9.8b: Horizontal school of Urist. A phenomenon caused by underacting lateral recti (A-eso) or medial recti (A-exo).

correct the specific anomaly, i.e. in case of overaction of the recti, recess them and in case of underaction resect them.

2. Vertical School

Brown stressed the role of vertical recti in the etiology of A–V patterns, the principle behind being the adducting property of vertical recti. Thus weak superior recti would result in less adducting power in upgaze causing a V phenomenon. However, it seems logical to think that the actions of vertical recti and oblique muscles are linked inseparably. Thus underacting superior recti would have underacting superior

obliques (ipsilateral antagonist of contralateral synergist). Thus it would be more appropriate to have the vertical recti and obliques as a combined factor this is the cyclovertical school (Figs 9.9a and b). The following table in brief shows the effect of these muscles (Table 9.2):

Table 9.2: Pattern and overacting muscles		
Overacting muscles	Underacting muscles	Pattern caused
Inferior oblique	Superior oblique	V pattern
Inferior rectus	Superior rectus	V pattern
Superior oblique	Inferior oblique	A pattern
Superior rectus	Inferior rectus	A pattern

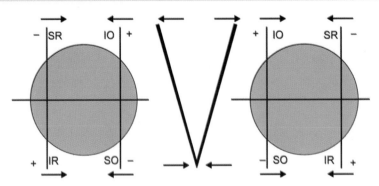

Fig. 9.9a: Cyclovertical School. V pattern caused by underacting (–) superiors (rectus and oblique), which are associated with overacting (+) Inferiors (rectus and oblique). The combination causes more abduction (less adduction) in upgaze and less abduction (more adduction) in downgaze (indicated by horizontal arrows).

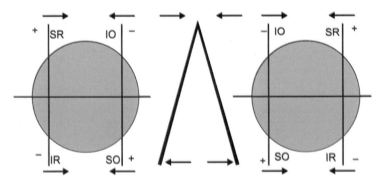

Fig. 9.9b: Cyclovertical School. A pattern caused by underacting (–) Inferiors (rectus and oblique), which are associated with overacting (+) superiors (rectus and oblique). The combination causes less abduction (more adduction) in upgaze and more abduction (less adduction) in downgaze (indicated by horizontal arrows).

Most of the A–V patterns have anomalies of oblique muscles and their respective surgery: weakening of overacting obliques and strengthening of underacting obliques does correct the respective patterns. More often it is the oblique overactions that are encountered, that is, inferior oblique over-actions in V patterns and superior oblique overactions in A patterns are seen. Rarely underactions are also seen causing these patterns. Restrictive conditions like Brown's syndrome may appear like a Y pattern but for different reasons.

3. *Structural Factors*

Variations in skull and orbital bones are known to have underaction or overaction of oblique muscles. This may be due to variation in the site of origins and insertions of the inferior or superior obliques. The trochlea acts as the functional origin of the superior oblique. The role of **sagittalization**: the oblique muscles becoming more parallel to the sagittal (anteroposterior) axis and **desagittalization**: when the oblique muscles become more parallel to the coronal plane have been stressed by Gobin. If the superior oblique is desagittalised due to the retroplacement of trochlea (as in plagiocephaly), it becomes a poorer depressor. And relatively the inferior oblique becomes a stronger elevator (Figs 9.10a and b). Similarly with a more frontally placed trochlea (as in hydrocephalus with frontal bossing), superior oblique becomes more

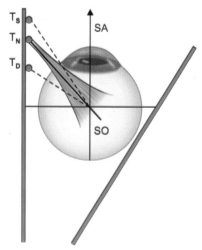

Fig. 9.10a: Sagittalization and desagittalization of superior obliques (SO) sagittal axis (SA). Trochlea (T_N = normal position) T_S: anteriorly placed trochlea = sagittalization T_D: posteriorly placed trochlea = desagittalization

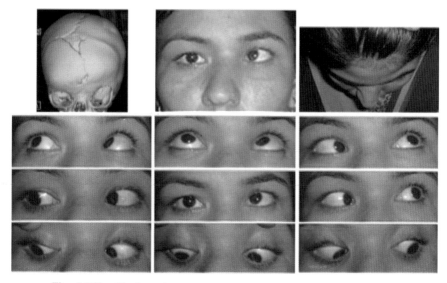

Fig. 9.10b: Plagiocephaly and desagittalization of superior oblique.

sagittalised in relation to the inferior oblique making it a stronger elevator. This relative action of the obliques can cause A and V patterns.

4. Anomalies of Muscle Insertions

Anomalies of insertions of horizontal and vertical recti or oblique muscles are also known to cause A and V patterns. Because of obliquity, horizontal, vertical, and torsional vectors are created, which create more abduction in up- or downgazes causing V or A phenomenon. In V patterns the insertions of medial recti have been reported to be higher than normal and those of lateral recti lower than normal. This will cause vertical vectors, making the horizontal vectors (for adduction or abduction), weaker or stronger in up and down positions

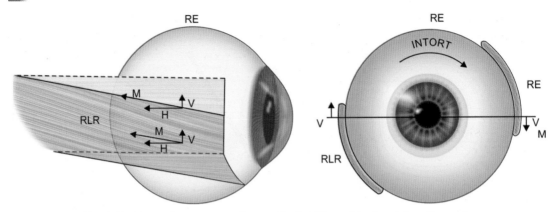

Fig. 9.11: Vector forces created on vertical shifting of horizontal recti muscles.

creating these patterns. The vertical vectors add up to form torsional vector causing extorsion of the globes in V patterns and intorsion of globes in A patterns (Fig. 9.11).

Surgery based on this principle: Vertical shifting of horizontal recti are effective in correcting A and V patterns. Slanting insertions have also been associated with A or V patterns, and these also have been used as a surgical modality.

Diagnosis

The horizontal deviations are measured in **25° upgaze** and **35° downgaze** in addition to the primary position. Sometimes it may be desirable to check in 45° downgaze position to exclude a significant A pattern. **A 15 pd difference** is taken as significant for a **V pattern** and **a 10 pd difference** is taken as significant for **A pattern.** For repeatable and reproducible measurements these positions are quantified with the help of a **scale and a protractor** on the lateral side of the head. A 35° chin-up and 25° chin-down position is used with a 6 m distance target for distance fixation measurement. For near fixation at 33 cm, either the head is similarly tilted or the target is suitably fixed. A **cephalodeviometer** has been devised using a mirror with markings drawn on it. The patient is made to wear a head band with a vertical marker, and head is suitably tilted for the required position.

The fundus should always be evaluated for the torsional changes in A–V patterns especially with oblique overactions (Figs 9.12a and b).

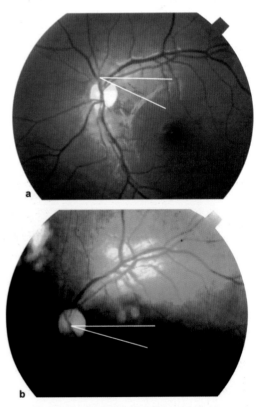

Fig. 9.12: Fundus picture of a case with V pattern with inferior oblique overaction (left eye) showing extorsion in (a), and corrected after surgery (b).

Children with V-exotropia with BSV in downgaze may have a chin-up posture and with A-esotropia with BSV in upgaze may have a chin down posture.

Treatment

The management depends on the clinical factors. If the pattern is significant and symptomatic, it needs to be operated. **All cases of esodeviation or exodeviations should be checked for A or V patterns. In case of oblique overactions being present, the obliques should be weakened** (recessed with or without anteropositioning). In case of underactions the same should be strengthened (advancement of obliques or tucking in case of superior oblique).

In the absence of oblique overactions the horizontal recti are operated (according to the horizontal school). A choice is to either weaken the lateral rectus or strengthen the medial rectus in case of exotropia. Another option is **vertical transpositioning of horizontal recti**. Thirdly, **differential (slanting) recession and resections** can be done for added effect.

The deviation in the primary position determines the amount of surgery for the horizontal recti, whereas the amount of A or V pattern and the associated overaction determines the oblique muscle surgery in case of oblique overaction or underaction or the vertical shifting of horizontal recti in the absence of oblique overactions.

Table 9.3 indicates the procedures undertaken commonly. It should be remembered that in V-esotropia esodeviation is more in downgaze so medial recti have to be weakened more in downgaze so shift them downwards **(shift the muscle in the direction you want to weaken them).** The simple rule of the thumb is: For medial recti shift them towards the apex of the A or V phenomenon that the case has the reverse in case of lateral recti.

In addition the **slanting recession** or differential recession may be undertaken to correct A or V phenomenon. Similarly **slanting resections** can also be done.

In slanting recessions the slant or differential recession determines the relative

Table 9.3: Procedure undertaken commonly	
Pattern	Surgery
1. V-esotropia with inferior overaction	• Medial rectus recession or recession-resection surgery + inferior oblique weakening
2. V-exotropia with inferior oblique overaction (Figs 9.13a and b)	• Lateral rectus recession or R-R surgery + inferior oblique weakening
3. A-esotropia with superior oblique overaction	• Medial rectus recession or R-R surgery + Superior oblique weakening
4. A-exotropia with superior oblique overaction (Figs 9.14a and b)	• Lateral rectus recession or R-R surgery + Superior oblique weakening
5. V-esotropia without overaction	• Bi-medial recession with MR down-shifted 5 mm
6. V-exotropia (no overaction)	• Bi-lateral recession with LR up-shifted 5 mm
7. A-esotropia (no overaction)	• Bi-medial recession with MR shifted up 5 mm
8. A-exotropia (no overaction)	• Bi-lateral recession with LR shifted down 5 mm
9. Pure V-pattern (exo-up, eso-down) (Figs 9.15a and b)	• Bilateral Inferior oblique weakening
10. Pure A pattern (eso-up, exo-down)	Bilateral superior oblique weakening
11. X-pattern with inferior and superior oblique overaction	Weakening of both obliques of both sides.

weakening effect. A slant of medial rectus with more recession of inferior end would correct a V-esotropia. For A-esotropia, the slant is reversed (more recession of superior end). Similarly follow for lateral recti also in cases of exotropia. V-exotropia demands more recession of upper end and A-exotropia demands more recession of lower end.

The weakening procedures for inferior oblique are graded (6, 8, 10 mm) recession for mild, moderate or severe inferior oblique overaction, for 4+ (markedly severe) over-actions the recession is combined with anteropositioning in the modified Elliot and Nankin's method (Figs 9.13a and b) (*see* chapter on surgical management). For very severe

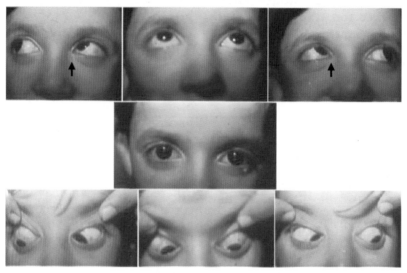

Fig. 9.13a: Pure V pattern—Exo-upgaze and Eso-downgaze.

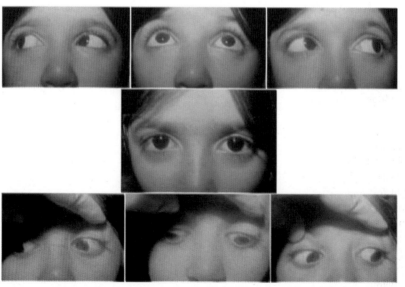

Fig. 9.13b: Pure V after inferior oblique recession and anteropositioning.

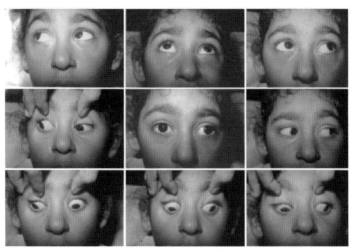

Fig. 9.14a: A pattern exotropia with bilateral superior oblique overaction.

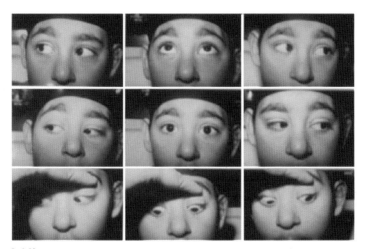

Fig. 9.14b: A pattern exotropia after posterior tenectomy of superior oblique.

overactions of IO Anterior and nasal anteropostioning (Stager's procedure) may be done. Myectomy is usually not recommended. For superior oblique overactions, graded recession or graded lengthening of superior oblique by silicon expander is recommended. Bilateral posterior tenotomy/tenectomy of superior oblique is now the first choice for mild to moderate superior oblique overactions (Figs 9.14a and b). For very severe overactions of SO translational recession of SO (Prieto Diaz procedure) may be done.

The **horizontal shifting of vertical recti** is rarely done. Nasal shifting of both superior rectus may be done in Y pattern. Nasal shifting of both inferior rectus may be done in collapsing an inverted Y or delta pattern.

Suggested Reading

1. Bagolini B. Campos E. and Chiesi C. Plagiocephaly causing superior oblique deficiency and ocular torticollis. Arch Ophthalmol. 100: 1093, 1982.
2. Boyd TAS, Leitch GT and Budd GE. A new treatment for A and V patterns in strabismus by

slanting muscle insertions: a preliminary report Can J. Ophthalmol. 6: 170, 1971.

3. Breinin GM. The physiopathology of A and V patterns. In symposium, the A and V patterns in strabismus Trans. Am. Acad: Ophthalmol. Otolaryngol. 68: 363, 1964.

4. Caldeira JA. Bilateral recession of the superior oblique in A pattern tropia. J. Pediatr. Ophthalmol. Strabismus. 15: 306, 1978.

5. Fink WH. The A and V Syndromes Am Orthopt. J. 9: 105, 1959.

6. Gobin MH. Sagittalization of the oblique muscles as possible causes for the A, V and X. phenomenon Br. J. Ophthalmol. 52: 13, 1968.

7. Knapp PA and V patterns. In Symposium on Strabismus. Transactions of the New Orleans Academy of Ophthalmology. St. Louis. 1971. Mosby—Year Book Inc.

8. Postic G. Etiopathogenic des Syndromes A et V Bull. Mem. Soc. Fr. Ophthalmol. 78: 240, 1965.

9. Urist MJ. The etiology of the so called A and V syndromes. Am J. Ophthalmol. 46: 835, 1958.

10. Ruttum M. and Noorden G.K. von. Orbital and facial anthropometry in A and V pattern strabismus. In Reinecke R.D. editor. Strabismus II New York. 1984 Grune and Stratton Inc.

11. Sharma P, Halder M and Prakash P: Effect of monocular vertical displacement of horizontal recti in AV phenomena, Ind. J. Ophthalmol. 43: 9–11, 1995.

12. Sharma P, Halder M and Prakash P. Torsional changes in surgery for A.V phenomena. Ind. J. Ophthalmol. 45:31–35, 1997.

9

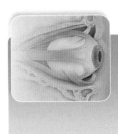

Paralytic Strabismus

Incomitant strabismus is the misalignment of the two eyes which varies in different gazes or in other words the ocular deviation is different in different gaze positions. It can be **paralytic, restrictive** or **spastic,** the last being relatively uncommon. **Paralytic strabismus** is an incomitant strabismus due to motor deficiency of one or a group of extraocular muscles. Incomplete paralysis is called **paresis** and complete deficiency is called **paralysis,** while the term **palsy** is used for both without specifying.

Intracranial course of III, IV and VI nerves should be kept in mind while dealing with paralytic strabismus (Fig. 10.1).

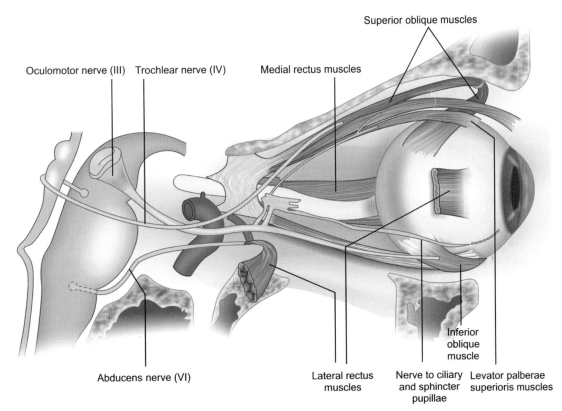

Fig. 10.1: Intracranial course of III, IV and VI nerves.

Classification

The paralysis or the motor deficiency can be

a. **Neurogenic**
  i. Supranuclear
  ii. Nuclear
  iii. Internuclear
  iv. Infranuclear
  • Fascicular (Main nerve trunk or subdivision)
    – Oculomotor nerve (III CN)
    – Trochlear nerve (IV CN)
    – Abducens nerve (VI CN)

b. **Myogenic**
  i. Nerve-muscle junction lesion (myasthenia)
  ii. Muscle
    a. **Congenital** absence, hypoplasia mal insertion or musculofascial anomalies.
    b. **Traumatic** laceration, disinsertion
    c. **Inflammatory** (myositis)
    d. **Orbito-myopathies** (dysthyroid)
    e. **Dystrophy** (CPEO)

Causes of Neurogenic Lesions

1. Congenital
2. Traumatic
3. Inflammatory
4. Neoplastic
5. Ischemic
6. Toxic
7. Demyelinating disease
8. Idiopathic

Clinical Characteristics

The paralytic strabismus is characterised by:

i. **Incomitance:** Variable ocular deviation in different position which is maximum in the field of action of the muscle (for example in a left lateral rectus palsy, esotropia is maximal in the abduction of left eye or levoversion).

ii. **Limitation of movement** of the eye in the field of action of the extraocular muscle, (in left lateral rectus palsy the abduction of left eye is deficient or limited).

iii. **Difference in primary and secondary deviation.** In all incomitant strabismus the ocular deviation measured with the two eyes fixating alternately is different (Note: Comitant strabismus is characterised by equal ocular deviation with either eye fixating) (*see* also Table 10.1). The deviation of the squinting eye with the normal eye fixing is called the **primary deviation.** And the deviation of the normal eye with the paretic (abnormal)

Differences	Paralytic	Comitant
1. Age of onset	Usually late	Usually early childhood
2. Type of onset	Sudden	Gradual, sudden manifestation
3. Precipitating events	Usually head injury systemic illness	Rarely present. Even if present no cause-effect relationship
4. Associated neurologic signs	May be present	None
5. Comitance	May develop in late stages	Usually present (except in extreme gazes)
6. Diplopia	Usually present	Absent (exceptions *see* text)
7. Headposture	Usually present	Absent (exceptions *see* text)
8. Cyclotropia	Usually present (except with horizontal muscle palsy)	Absent exception associated AV patterns or oblique overactions
9. Sensory adaptations (Suppression–amblyopia ARC)	Rare	Frequent
10. Past pointing	Present in recent cases	Absent

Table 10.1: Differences between paralytic and comitant

10

eye fixing is called the **secondary deviation.** In paralytic strabismus the secondary deviation is greater than the primary deviation. This is because the paretic eye requires more effort to straighten (come to the primary position to take up fixation) and this extra effort is passed onto the contralateral synergist, which is normal, increasing the ocular deviation. The reverse is true for spastic strabismus, i.e. the primary deviation is greater than the secondary deviation.

These are the **three main distinctive characteristics** to distinguish incomitant (paralytic) and comitant strabismus. In addition there are other characteristics which are commonly seen in paralytic squint, but are liable to change, depending on the **age of onset** and the **duration** for which the paralysis has remained. Since mostly paralytic squints occur in later age group, compared to concomitant squints which are usually of early onset, they have such characteristics. These are: **history of trauma, diplopia, past-pointing, head-posture, associated neurologic findings** or **systemic disease,** and **lack of sensory adaptations.** However, none of these may be there in a paralysis of early onset. And remember that in long-standing paralysis sensory adaptations can occur to compensate for the strabismus. At the same time concomitant strabismus, which characteristically lack the above mentioned features can have them if the concomitant strabismus has occurred in adulthood and is sudden, not allowing sensory adaptations to occur. Thus, acute concomitant strabismus or a decompensated exophoria has diplopia. Head posture is seen in some concomitant strabismus with A or V phenomenon.

One should understand that the characteristics of paralytic squint are due to the imbalance of the sensori-motor coordination which has not received a chance to get adapted because of later-onset and a shorter duration. The most characteristic findings of paralytic squint are in recent cases, while long standing cases develop features of comitance **(spread of comitance).**

Stages of Paralytic Squint

Paralytic strabismus undergoes **three** stages.
1. Paresis of the particular muscle
2. Overaction of the ipsilateral antagonist
3. Underaction of the antagonist of the contralateral synergist (Fig. 10.2).

These stages do not follow a definite rule and may take weeks to months and in some cases several years. In the **first stage** the maximal deviation is in the field of action of the paretic muscle. For example, in a case of left lateral rectus palsy, the deviation is largest in levoversion (Fig. 10.2a).

In the **second stage,** as the overaction of the ipsilateral antagonist occurs the deviation increases in the opposite field also this is described as contracture which can be confirmed by observing increased resistance to passive stretching on forced duction test. In the above example, with the left medial rectus also overacting, the duration increases in the dextroversion also (Fig. 10.2b).

In the **third stage** the underaction of the antagonist of the contralateral synergist occurs. This is known as **inhibitional palsy** (Fig. 10.2c).

In the above example, the right lateral rectus behaves like a paretic muscle. Finally the spread of comitance is complete, with the deviations being the same in all gazes and the primary and secondary deviations also becoming equal.

Cases of inhibitional palsy may confound the case as to which of the muscle is primarily paretic? This can be distinguished by doing a **patch** or **occlusion** test. If the paretic eye is occluded for some time (may be 24 hours) the inhibitional palsy disappears and the ductions in that direction improve (Fig. 10.3).

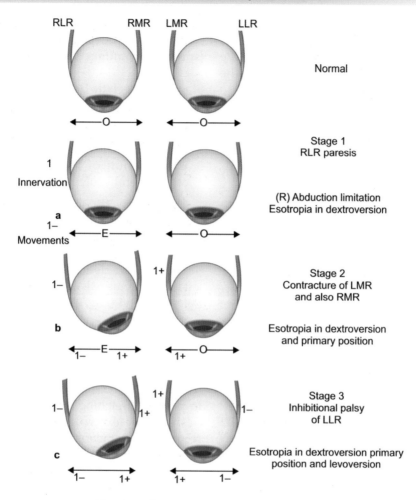

RLR   RMR   LMR   LLR

Normal

Stage 1
RLR paresis

1
Innervation

(R) Abduction limitation
Esotropia in dextroversion

a
1−
Movements

Stage 2
Contracture of LMR
and also RMR

Esotropia in dextroversion
and primary position

b

Stage 3
Inhibitional palsy
of LLR

Esotropia in dextroversion primary
position and levoversion

c

Fig. 10.2: Stages of paralytic squint (a to c).

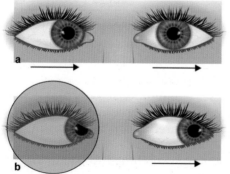

Fig. 10.3: Inhibitional palsy of left lateral rectus in a case of right lateral rectus palsy in (a), improves, abduction fully when right eye is patched (b).

Examination of a Paralytic Case

After taking the relevant history of the age of onset, type of onset, the precipitating event which may be a fever or a head injury, or other associated neurologic signs should be noted. These could be indicative of an intracranial space occupying lesion or other neurological diseases which may have to be attended to in an expedient manner.

Past pointing: Presence of past pointing indicates a recent onset. It can be tested by asking the patient to point with his finger the object viewed by the paretic eye (hand-eye

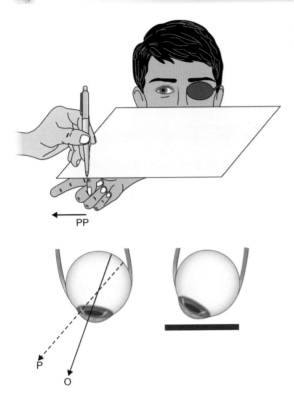

Fig. 10.4: Past pointing in right lateral rectus palsy. Paretic RLR requires more innervation to fixate an object in dextroversion causing past pointing. O is the object and P the perceived point.

coordination) with a septum not allowing him to have a visual feedback (Fig. 10.4) to correct the disturbed coordination between the eyes and the hand, due to a paresis. In the presence of paresis extra innervation is required for a movement in the direction of field of action of the paretic muscle which is perceived by the brain as if the object is located farther than it is, giving extra innervation to the hand for pointing. This causes past pointing.

Measurement of Deviation

Ocular deviation can be measured by objective method (Cover Test) or by subjective method (patient's response) using a Maddox rod or any other method to dissociate the two eyes. **Diplopia charting** is a method in which the

subjective deviation is recorded by asking the subject to quantify the separation between the double images which are dissociated by red green glasses. This is repeated in all the 9-diagnostic positions. In paralytic strabismus the separation is maximal in the field of action of the paretic muscle. Using a slit, horizontal for vertical strabismus and vertical for horizontal strabismus, one can also know the **subjective cyclotropia. Three points to be remembered are:**

1. Maximum separation is in the quadrant in which the muscle acts most (field of action).
2. The image that appears farthest, belongs to the deviating eye.
3. The image is displaced in the direction of action of the paralysed muscle. For example, in case of superior rectus the image is shifted up and inwards and tilted inwards (intorsion) (Figs 10.5a to c).

Hess/Lees' Charting

Another way of documenting the ocular deviation subjectively is the **Hess charting.** This uses red-green color dissociation, with the eye with the **red** filter **fixating,** as the projection of the other eye with the **green** filter is **charted**. This test charts the excursion of the 'other eye' (green filter) with the normal excursion of the 'fixating eye' red filter.

The fixating eye determines the innervational input and so the excursion of the other eye, if the muscle is underacting, would move less (smaller squares) and more in case of overactions. Cyclodeviations when present are seen as tilting of the squares of the eyes. **Lees charting** method utilises the dissociation by a mirror-septum (Figs 10.6a to c).

The Foster torches are two flash lights with red-green filters, with the patient wearing red-green goggles, so that one eye sees one image only and the other eye sees the other. By utilizing polaroid filters in place of red-green filters, the author has used the Foster torches with polaroid dissociation in charting scotomas under binocular conditions. But the

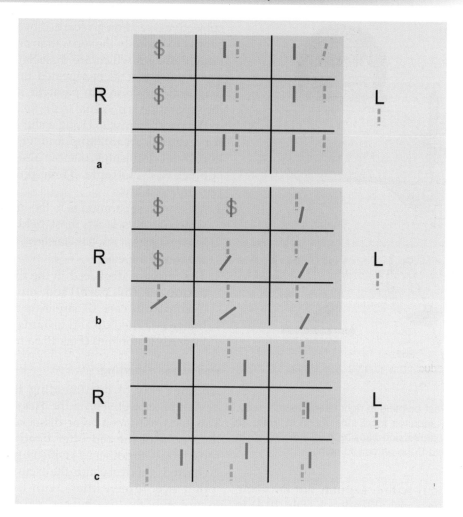

Fig. 10.5: Diplopia charting.

(a) Left lateral rectus palsy
- Binocular single vision in dextroversion.
- Horizontal diplopia in primary position and levoversion (uncrossed diplopia).
- Maximum separation in levoversion.
- Image of left eye (paretic eye) is seen more peripheral.

(b) Right superior oblique palsy
- Binocular single vision in dextroelevation, dextroversion and straight upgaze.
- Vertical deviation and tilting of right image (intorted image), in other gazes.
- Maximum vertical deviation in levodepression maximum intorted right image in dextro-depression.

(c) Left third nerve palsy involving
- Left medial rectus (partly recovered) superior rectus, inferior rectus and inferior oblique.
- The horizontal separation is maximum in the gaze of dextroversion (medial rectus).
- The vertical separation increases both in up- and downgazes (may vary depending on relative involvement of superior-inferior rectus and inferior oblique). There may not be any diplopia-free gaze or only in levoversion.

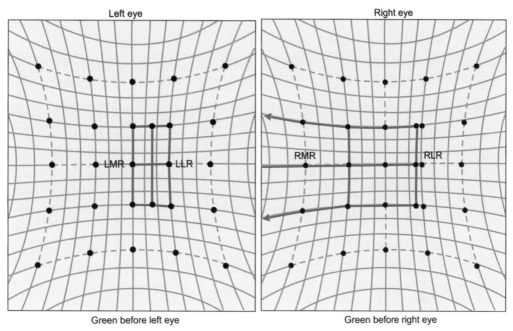

Fig. 10.6a: Left lateral rectus palsy. The horizontal excursion of left lateral rectus is markedly reduced while left adduction is normal or may be increased in some cases. The excursion of right medial rectus is markedly increased shown by arrows.

10

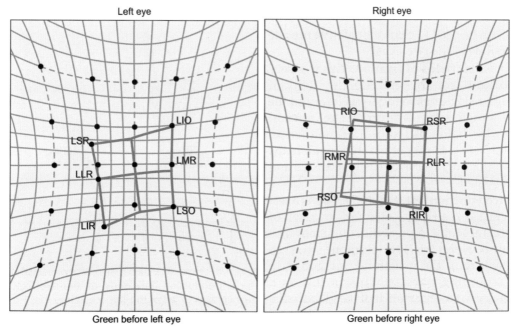

Fig. 10.6b: Right superior oblique palsy. The excursion of right superior oblique is reduced while right inferior oblique shows overaction. The whole square is extorted. A similar overaction of contralateral synergists causes extorsion of other eye square also.

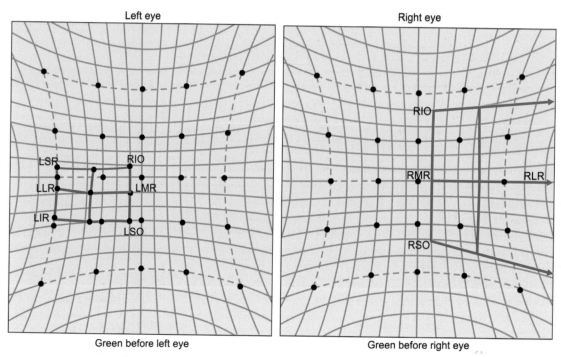

Left eye — Green before left eye

Right eye — Green before right eye

Fig. 10.6c: **Left third nerve palsy.** This case has partly recovered medial rectus so adduction is not so deficient, but overall all the muscles of left eye show reduced excursions resulting in a very small square. The overactions are seen in the contralateral synergists.

same can be used to chart the **relative muscle excursions** of the two eyes.

Binocular fields of fixation: This is a very important test to evaluate the field of binocular single vision (diplopia free) and the area which sees diplopia. The normal binocular fields of fixation are shown in Figs 10.5a to c. In case of paralytic squints the follow-up progress can be easily recorded and documented.

Forced duction test (Fig. 10.7): This is a test to detect a **restrictive** element in cases of incomitant squint. A paralytic squint may also develop a restrictive element due to **contracture** of the ipsilateral antagonist in long standing paresis. This is felt as a resistance to passive stretch of the globe in the direction opposite to that in which mechanical restriction is suspected. Sometimes **a reverse leash** effect can be seen, when there is a restrictive element on the same side as the

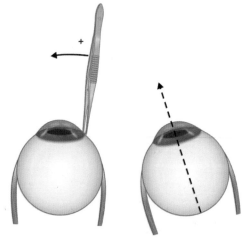

Fig. 10.7: Forced duction test in left eye held at limbus for left abduction deficiency, as the eye fixates in levoversion to relax the left medial rectus. Passive movement is free if LMR is not tight.

limitation of movement. This occurs when there is a retroequatorial adhesion.

Method of FDT

After anesthetizing the eye with topical 1% Proparacaine drops, the patient lies in supine position. The lids are retracted with speculum. The patient is asked to look in the direction of action of the muscle being tested (this relaxes the antagonist). The eye is held at the limbus with Fixation forceps or Pierse-Hoskin's forceps without pushing the globe posteriorly. It is rotated in the direction of action of muscle with the forceps. If this movement is allowed freely, the FDT is said to be negative. If it is restricted it is known as FDT-positive. For that movement, the other movements are also checked and compared. A posterior push on the globe will give a falsely negative FDT for recti muscles. However, while testing of oblique muscles a posterior push is desired to exaggerate the tautness of obliques (*see* Chapter 15).

Active force generation test (Fig 10.8): Another useful test to determine and quantify the ability of the muscle to contract is the active force generation test (AFGT). This is very useful to distinguish a restrictive squint

from a paralytic squint in which secondary restriction has developed. After holding the globe with a fixation forcep, the subject is asked to look in the direction in the field of action of the muscle being tested. If there is a normal 'tug' felt, it indicates the muscle is normal but incapable of a movement because of the restrictive element. If the 'tug' is weak, it indicates a paretic muscle which also has restriction of its antagonist. Special Scott's forceps have been devised, or otherwise transducers can be used, to actually quantify the muscle force.

Measurement of intraocular pressure (Fig. 10.9) in various positions of gaze, has also been known to indicate restrictive element. When the muscle is acting against resistance more force has to be generated this along with the restrictive (tight) muscle presses on the globe increasing the intraocular pressure.

Saccadic velocity recording (Fig. 7.5d): Using the principle of eye working as a dipole with the corneal end being **positive** and the retinal end being **negative**, the movement of eyes to and from the medial or lateral canthi

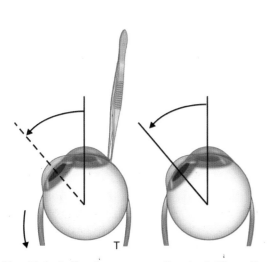

Fig. 10.8: Active force generation test. The active tug felt in the forceps holding at the limbus when left abduction is actively attempted against a tight medial rectus which causes restriction of abduction.

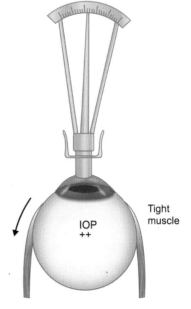

Fig. 10.9: Active contraction of the antagonist of a tight muscle causes intraocular pressure to rise.

can be recorded by sensitive electrodes at these canthi. This is the principle of electro-oculography (EOG). The eyes are capable of making saccades or fast eye movements which have a velocity of 200°/sec to 700°/sec. In case of paresis the excursions of the paretic muscles are significantly slow in velocity, and also have smaller amplitudes. In contrast, the restrictive squints have normal saccadic velocity till the restriction comes into effect, when the excursion stops abruptly. In cases of myasthenia gravis the slow saccadic velocity recorded is seen to become normal (or even overshoot) after the intravenous injection to edrophonium (Tensilon). Clinically the saccades can be seen as *quick* refixations of normal muscles compared to *slow drifts* of paralytic muscles on being asked to fixate on objects from right to left and back.

Electromyography (EMG)

Recording of muscle potentials by unipolar or bipolar leads in the extraocular muscles can distinguish myasthenia and myopathy from a neurogenic palsy. However, their role in diagnosis of paralytic squint is limited. But now with the botulinum toxin injections, they are required in the management of paralytic squints.

Restrictive Squints

Incomitant squints which are due to a restrictive element, usually in the opposite direction, are called restrictive squints. They have to be distinguished from paralytic squints, as they both present with **limitation of movement.** The two can be distinguished clinically by observing the **relationship between limitation of movement and the ocular deviation.** In case of paralytic squint both are affected in a proportional manner, i.e. more the limitation of movement, more is the ocular deviation in the primary position. In restrictive squints the limitation of movement is markedly affected whereas the ocular deviation in primary position (PP) is

not proportionally affected. A minimal deviation in the PP may be seen in a case which has total abduction or adduction deficiency, in case of restrictive squint. This can be further confirmed on FDT and AFGT.

TYPES OF PARALYTIC STRABISMUS

As outlined earlier paralytic strabismus may be involving the group of muscles supplied by the three cranial nerves: oculomotor, trochlear, and abducens. The last two nerves supply only one extraocular muscle each. Rarely individual EOM may be paretic.

Oculomotor Nerve Paralysis (III CN)

The paralysis of III CN can be distinguished as:
- Nuclear
- Infranuclear
- Fascicular
  - Complete nerve trunk (intracranial)
  - Superior or inferior division (intraorbital)

It may be **total** or **partial.** It should be remembered that III CN supplies the following muscles causing the respective functional deficits.

a. Extraocular

1. Levator palpebrae superioris—Ptosis
2. Superior rectus—Elevation weakness (more in abduction)
3. Inferior rectus—Depression weakness (more in abduction)
4. Inferior oblique—Elevation weakness (more in adduction)
5. Medial rectus—Adduction weakness

b. Intraocular

1. Ciliary body muscle—Accommodational paresis
2. Sphincter pupillae—Mydriasis.

In a total III CN palsy, all the above functional deficits are seen (Fig 10.10). However, at times incomplete involvement of all muscle subgroups is also observed. It is also possible that some of the functions have started

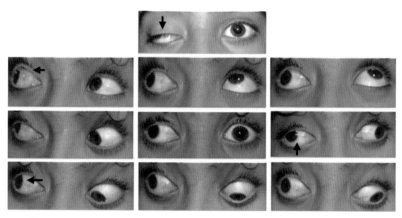

Fig. 10.10: A case of oculomotor (III) nerve palsy of right eye. Note ptosis and deficient adduction, elevation, depression in right eye.

recovering due to **regeneration.** However, in regenerations, **aberrant regenerations** (abnormal wiring) are the rule except in ischemic mononeuropathy.

Aberrant regenerations (Figs 10.11a and b) occur due to the nerve fibres subserving to one muscle group get connected to some other muscle group. Remembering that III N supplies

10

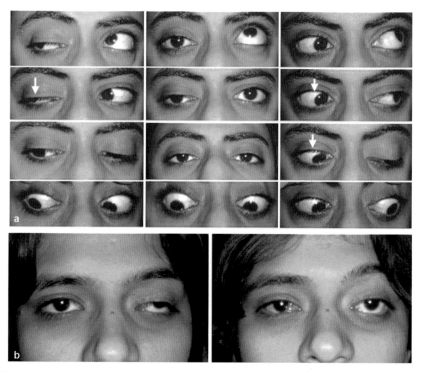

Fig. 10.11: Aberrant regeneration in oculomotor nerve palsy. (a) Pseudo-von Graefe sign: Lid retraction of right eye on attempted downgaze, (b) using aberrant regeneration to lift the left lid by normal right eye surgery.

7 muscle groups, this miswiring is not surprising after a transection is followed by regeneration. Thus the superior rectus fibres may get connected to medial rectus resulting in adduction when elevation is intended, or the inferior rectus fibres get connected to levator palpebrae superioris causing a lid retraction in downgaze (pseudo-von Graefe sign).

It is very common in aberrant regenerations to have a **tonic pupil** (Adie's pupil), in which the pupil constricts in a slow and sustained manner on light stimulation, compared to a normal brisk response. This is due to the nerve fibres for ciliary muscle getting connected to the sphincter pupillae the relative ratio being 20:1 (Table 10.2).

Ischemic mononeuropathy due to diabetes, hypertension, etc. is pupil sparing III nerve paresis which recovers almost fully in 2–3 months.

Nuclear III CN Palsy

A complete nuclear III CN may be distinguished from a complete fascicular III CN only by associated neurologic features. But incomplete lesions involving only some **subnucleus** of III CN can give a different picture. The characteristic features of nuclear III CN palsy (Fig. 10.12) are:

1. Ptosis, if present, is always bilateral.
2. Mydriasis and cycloplegia, if present, is always bilateral.
3. Contralateral superior rectus paresis or bilateral superior rectus paresis is seen.
4. Incomplete involvement of different subnuclei.

The reasons for this is a common/single median nucleus for both LPS and parasympathetic supply, and the superior rectus has a contralateral supply. But since the contralateral nerve traverses the other side subnucleus, one may encounter bilateral superior paresis.

Causes of nuclear III CN can be ischemic infarcts, degenerations, space occupying lesions or infective granulomas.

Palsy of Individual Extraocular Muscles of III CN

   i. **Superior rectus** muscle palsy presents with **weak elevation in abduction.** It is usually associated with ptosis of the same side. It is common to see congenital ptosis (complicated) to have an associated superior rectus paresis. It is usually congenital and has **poor Bell's phenomenon** (failure of the eyes to roll up and out on forced closure of lids). Head tilt may occur but is not as classical

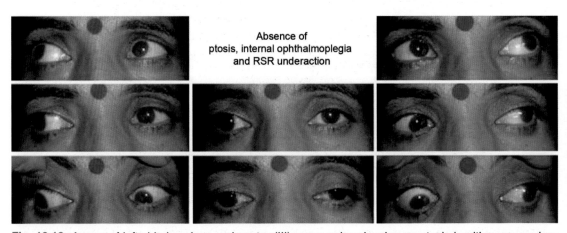

Absence of ptosis, internal ophthalmoplegia and RSR underaction

Fig. 10.12: A case of left sided nuclear oculomotor (III) nerve palsy showing no ptosis in either eye and no pupillary involvement. Contralateral elevation is affected.

Table 10.2: Pupillary involvement in oculomotor nerve palsy

Feature	Remarks
1. Pupil sparing	• Usually in ischemic mononeuropathy due to diabetes mellitus, hypertension, arteriosclerosis, coronary artery disease, hyper cholesterolemia. 90% of compressive lesions have pupillary involvement. 32% of ischemic lesion can involve pupils, but anisocoria is never more than 2.5 mm, even if pupil involved.
2. Pupil more miosed	• May be associated Horner's syndrome as in some cavernous sinus lesions or • May be an irritative lesion of oculomotor nerve. • In uncal herniation syndrome in comatosed patients the initial miosis is followed by ipsilateral pupillary paralysis with contralateral pupillary constriction. Finally bilateral pupillary paralysis may occur.
3. Isolated pupillary paralysis	• Botulism, diphtheria may have pupillary and accommodational paresis, without involvement of other extraocular muscles.

as cases of superior oblique palsy and is not dependable. A hypotropia occurs in the primary position. If the patient fixates with the normal eye, a **pseudoptosis** may be seen due to the hypotropic position of the globe. This improves on the hypotropic eye taking up fixation as against a true ptosis.

An elevator underaction if long-standing can be seen even in adduction, mimicking a double elevator palsy, this may also be secondary to an inferior rectus contracture. Double elevator palsy and other acquired causes of elevator underaction like blow out fracture, dysthyroid orbitomyopathy should be considered in differential diagnosis.

ii. **Medial rectus muscle** palsy as an isolated involvement is very rare, and presents as adduction weakness with exotropia in primary position. Some cases may have abduction nystagmus of the contralateral eye on attempts of adduction of paretic eye. **Internuclear ophthalmoplegia** may also present with ipsilateral adduction deficiency with contralateral abduction nystagmus, but it has a **normal convergence,** in spite of adduction weakness. In true MR paresis convergence is also affected.

Another related condition is **synergistic divergence** in which simultaneous abduction of both eyes occur on attempted abduction of one eye.

Dissociated horizontal deviations present with exodeviation on cover with a slow esotonic drift and redressal movement.

Causes of isolated MR underaction may be due to orbital restrictive conditions. Slipped MR muscle after a pterygium surgery has also been observed. Duane's retraction syndrome type II should be distinguished.

iii. **Inferior rectus muscle** palsy as a congenital case is exceptional. But recently several cases of acquired inferior rectus palsy have cropped up after cataract surgery. These are attributed to the injury caused by retrobulbar or peribulbar injections. The local anesthetic, Bupivacain is known to be myotoxic. Orbital trauma is also commonly associated with inferior rectus underactions.

iv. **Inferior oblique muscle palsy** is a very rare involvement and presents with deficient elevation in adduction with associated overaction of ipsilateral superior oblique. Incyclotropia is usually present. Bielschowsky's head tilt on tilting the head towards the opposite side is positive. Distinction should be made from Brown's superior oblique sheath syndrome which has a tight superior oblique on FDT and does not have an overaction of superior oblique overaction.

Associated trochlear nerve palsy with oculomotor nerve palsy: It is important to detect a paralytic trochlear nerve in the presence of an oculomotor nerve. Depression in adduction cannot be evaluated as the eye cannot be adducted. In such cases one should observe the intorsion of the globe on attempted depression. For this a limbal vessel on medial

limbus is noted as the intorsion is maximum here (*see* Fig 2.18). If intorsion is detected, the trochlear nerve is normal. Sometimes bilateral trochlear nerve with oculomotor nerve may be involved. This presents AV-pattern on upgaze (Figs 10.13a and b)

Trochlear Nerve Paralysis (IV CN)

Trochear nerve (IV CN) palsy is a common ocular motility defect. Usually it is congenital in nature but it is also common to see post-traumatic cases after road traffic accidents suffering trochlear nerve (unilateral or bilateral palsy. It presents with deficiency of

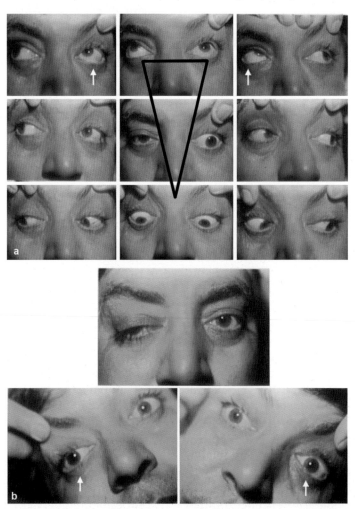

Fig. 10.13: (a) Right third and associated fourth nerve palsy, and (b) showing bilateral positive head tilt test.

depression in adduction of the involved eye. In **mild** forms the hypotropia is only seen in the tertiary position: deorsum-adduction (down and adduction). In **moderate** forms it is seen in adduction (without depression) and in **severe** forms the hypertropia is seen in primary position also. In **long-standing cases** ipsilateral inferior oblique overaction is seen and in later inhibitional palsy of the contralateral superior rectus is seen. In that stage it may be difficult to distinguish as to which paresis is primary. In such late stages spread of comitance may make the hypertropia equal in all the gazes. Some cases may present as **double depressor palsy** with more involvement of the superior oblique.

The **congenital trochlear palsy** characteristically presents with head tilt towards the opposite shoulder (Fig. 10.14). This is to correct the excyclotropia which the eye suffers due to the dysfunction of superior oblique (an intorter).

Excyclotropia can be **subjectively** tested by:
i. Double Maddox Rod (DMR)
ii. Synoptophore with torsion slides (slides with vertical elements)
iii. Field charting (noting the vertical displacement of the blind spot).

Objectively the excyclotropia can be seen on **fundus examination** with indirect ophthalmoscopy (noting the relative displacement of the fovea and the optic disk).

Unilateral superior oblique palsy may cause excyclotropia of about 7° and bilateral cases usually have excyclotropia of 10–15°. Usually excyclotropia of 4° or more are symptomatic (if not assuming head posture).

Superior oblique palsy suspect bilateral palsy if
- SO palsy following closed head trauma
- Subjective complaints of torsion
- Objective torsion more than 10 degrees
- Alternating hypertropia on alt head tilt
- V-pattern heterotropia (eso)
- Chin down head posture

10

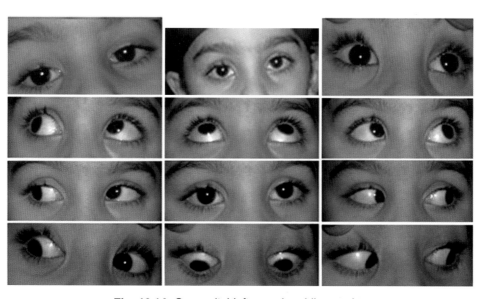

Fig. 10.14: Congenital left superior oblique palsy.

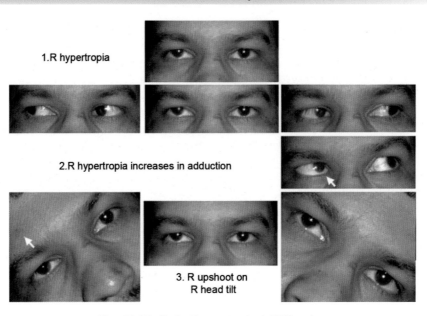

1.R hypertropia

2.R hypertropia increases in adduction

3. R upshoot on R head tilt

Fig. 10.15: Parks three step test-RSO palsy

The **head tilt test** (Fig. 10.15) Bielschowsky's test is very helpful in diagnosing superior oblique palsy. A head tilt towards the **same** side causes an upshoot of the involved eye. This is due to the extra effort of the ipsilateral superior rectus (the other intorter) to compensate for the head tilt and its elevation not being neutralised by the superior oblique (intorter but depressor).

Knapp's Classification of Trochlear Palsy

See in management of fourth nerve palsy (Table 10.3).

Abducens Nerve Palsy (VI CN)

The most common paralytic squint, especially in adults following head injury or as a non-localizing sign of raised intracranial pressure. Diabetic mononeuropathy also commonly presents as lateral rectus palsy. It has abduction limitation with convergent squint. Head posture is characteristically a **face turn** to the same side. The cases of Duane's retraction syndrome type I, infantile esotropia should be distinguished (Fig. 10.16).

Table 10.3: Management of fourth nerve palsy	
Class Maximum involvement of gaze*	*Management*
1. Levoelevation	RIO recession
2. Levodepression	RSO tucking LIR recession or modified Harada-Ito
3. All levoversion poistions	Hypertropia <25 pd R10 Recession Hypertropia >25 pd R10 Recession + RSO tuck
4. All downgaze positions and levopositions	As in class 3 + LIR recession/RSR recession
5. All downgaze positions	RSO tuck + LIR recession
6. Bilateral with V-pattern	Bilateral IO weakening or Modified Harada Ito
7. All downgazes primary position	Explore trochlea and levoversion

Note: *In the table the involvement is shown with right superior oblique palsy taken as example.

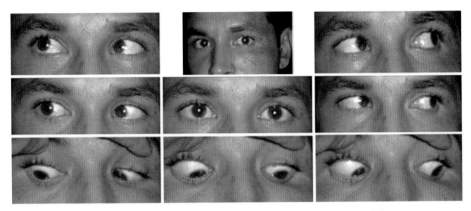

Fig. 10.16: A right lateral rectus palsy with face turn to right.

Mobius syndrome has bilateral VI and VII palsy along with other cranial nerves from the brainstem. Facial diplegia and microglossia are associated giving an expressionless face. Such cases should be investigated to exclude neurological cases of abducens paralysis (Fig. 10.17).

Skew Deviation

An episodic see-saw like presentation with alternate elevation–depression of the two eyes with rotary nystagmus, is seen in brainstem and cerebellar diseases. Disturbance of tonic-otolith organs is also implicated.

Double Elevator Palsy

Paralysis of superior rectus and inferior oblique of one eye is called **double elevator palsy** (DEP) or **monocular elevation deficit** (MED). It may occur as a congenital condition or as an acquired neurological condition described as **supranuclear paresis of**

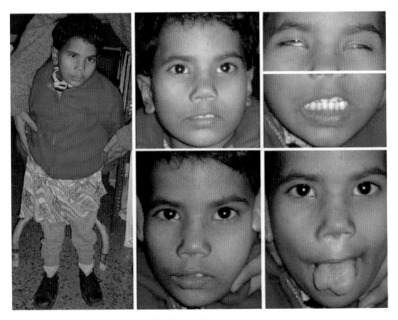

Fig. 10.17: Mobius syndrome.

monocular elevation. The latter was attributed to a unilateral lesion of the pretectum. It has no ptosis and no hypotropia in the primary position and downgaze. Hypotropia and resultant diplopia is seen in upgaze only. The Bell's phenomenon (rolling upward and outwards of the eyeball on forced lid closure) is normal. Reflex upward movements are also present on doll's eye movements.

Congenital DEP may have a similar etiology, with a postulation of supranuclear monocular vertical gaze centres. But some of the cases may be a "spill-over" superior rectus palsy (the main elevator) with secondary contracture of the inferior rectus.

Usually **true ptosis** is present along with the hypotropia in the primary position which causes an additional **pseudoptosis**. Clinically **three types** of DEP have been identified:

    i. Prominent inferior rectus restriction with FDT positive for elevation. Superior rectus saccades are normal.

    ii. Elevator paresis with reduced superior rectus saccades. FDT for elevation is negative.

    iii. Combination of both.

Acquired DEP may occur due to trauma (blow out fracture), dysthyroid orbitopathy, postretinal detachment or strabismus surgery. All such cases have positive FDT on elevation indicating a tight inferior rectus.

Double Depressor Palsy

Paralysis of both superior oblique and inferior rectus is uncommon. However, some cases of superior oblique palsy may present as one, with the underaction of superior oblique being more than that of inferior rectus. Acquired causes of restrictive underaction of depression should be distinguished.

Supranuclear Gaze Palsy

Paralysis of binocular gaze or spastic conjugate deviations can occur in different version movements. Horizontal gaze palsy are located in the Pontine Gaze centre in the paramedian pontine reticular formation,PPRF and result in equal and simultaneous underaction of both the yoke muscles involved in the horizontal version (medial rectus of one eye and lateral rectus of the other). Vertical gaze palsy are commonly located in the pretectum in the mesencephalic recticular formation (MRF). As in Parinaud's syndrome all elevators or all depressors of both eyes are involved.

Gaze palsy, as a rule being binocular and symmetrical, do not have a relative ocular deviation and so have no diplopia.

Internuclear ophthalmoplegia (Fig. 10.18) is different and is due to lesions of the median longitudinal fasciculus (commonly due to multiple sclerosis or ischemic infarction) and is characterised by ipsilateral adduction deficiency with contralateral abduction nystagmus with *intact convergence*.

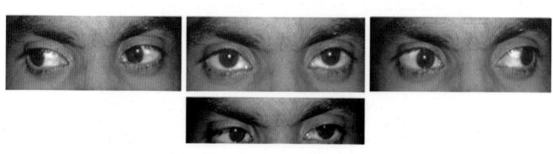

Fig. 10.18: Right inter nuclear ophthalmoplegia, INO.

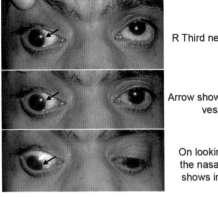

R Third nerve palsy

Arrow shows a nasal vessel

On looking down the nasal vessel shows intorsion

Fig. 10.19: Identifying fourth nerve function in the presence of a third nerve palsy.

Management of Paralytic Squint

All cases of paralytic squint should be evaluated to localise any **neurological lesion (never miss a fundus examination to look for papilledema or optic atrophy)** or other systemic causes like **hypertension, diabetes, cardiovascular anomalies,** or **lipid distur-bances.** If these are ruled out the cases should be followed up at 6 weekly intervals till about 6 months or two consecutive 6-weekly follow-ups reveal no change in motility (improvement or worsening).

Paralytic workup with the help of diplopia charting, Hess charting, recording of deviations in nine gazes are helpful in follow-up. The **nonsurgical management** can be tried during the period of follow-up to avoid diplopia by using **occlusion** or **prisms.** Prisms are helpful in providing binocular vision as also reducing the chances of development of contracture, but are useful only in small angle squints. The small angle cyclotropia is usually compensated by a head tilt.

Botulinum toxin has been used successfully in paralytic squints, whereby the ipsilateral antagonist is paralysed by chemodenervation. The effect lasts for about 2–3 months. If necessary the injection can be repeated if the original paralysis has not recovered till then.

Surgical therapy is mainly aimed to weaken the antagonist, usually ipsilateral and sometimes also the contralateral antagonist, in addition to strengthening the paralysed muscle. More than normally suggested surgical amounts are required in such cases. A severe VI CN palsy may require 8–9 mm of medial rectus recession with about 10 mm of lateral rectus resection. The amount also varies depending on which eye habitually fixates (secondary deviation or primary deviation needs to be corrected).

Another surgical principle is to **restrain the contralateral antagonist** by performing retroequatorial myopexy, this may improve the action of paralysed muscle.

In cases of contracture of the antagonist, sufficient recession is done to make the FDT negative. If still the paralysis persists, **transposition** of the available muscles can be utilised to aid the action of paralytic muscle. A **Hummelshiem's procedure** utilises the temporal halves of the vertical muscles to improve abduction in VI CN palsy (Figs 10.20a and b). **Jensen's procedure** utilizes the binding of the temporal halves of the vertical recti with the upper and lower halves of the lateral rectus by non absorbable sutures. However, it has an inherent disadvantage, as the vector forces of the vertical recti are lost as they are transmitted through a paralysed muscle.

Management of Third Nerve Palsy

Cases of III CN palsy are particularly difficult to manage because it supplies most of the EOM, except superior oblique and lateral rectus. Moreover, aberrant regenerations alter the clinical picture. Each case of III CN has to be considered on an individual basis and managed accordingly.

The most one may aim to achieve in paralytic squints is to give a diplopia-free ocular position in primary position and downgaze. The latter should never be compromised for the upgaze.

10

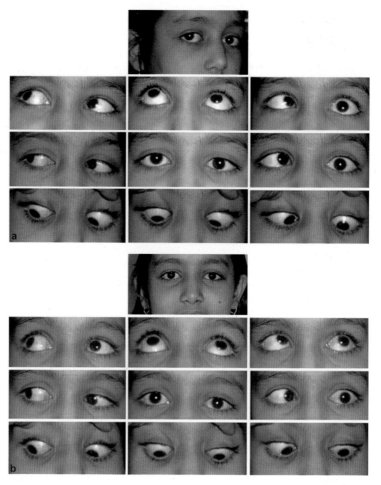

Fig. 10.20: Left VI N palsy preoperative (a) and postoperative partial VRT (b).

The available muscles have to be noted and the plan made so as to give alignment in the two important positions: **downgaze** and **primary position.**

If the MR still has some tone, supramaximal recession of 12–18 mm of lateral rectus with 8–9 mm resection of the medial rectus may correct the horizontal deviation (Figs 10.22a and b). If not then the **transpositioning** of the vertical recti can be done, provided they have normal tone. In case **superior oblique** is overacting causing hypotropia, it is disinserted.

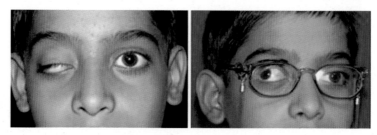

Fig. 10.21: Use of crutch glasses.

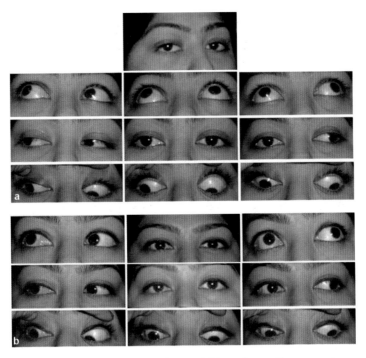

Fig. 10.22: Right III N palsy. (a) Preoperative and (b) postoperative recession and resection.

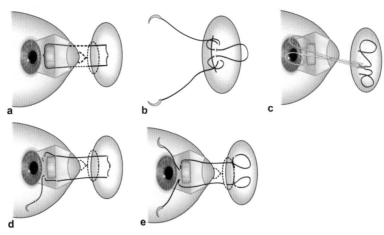

Fig. 10.23: Periosteal anchoring of globe: (a to e) surgical steps.

Some surgeons have shortened it by about 12 mm and reinserted close to the medial rectus for assisting the adduction. However, this may cause severe restriction of depression in downgaze and so not a desirable procedure.

Periosteal flaps have been raised on the medial orbital wall to fix the globe medially. The author has described **Periosteal anchoring** (Figs 10.23 and 10.24a and b) of the globe to the medial periosteal wall with nonabsorbable

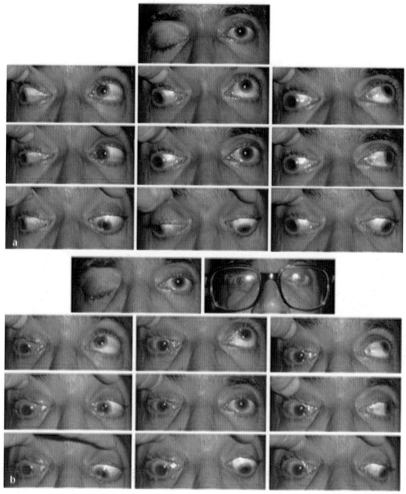

Fig. 10.24: Third nerve palsy: Medial periosteal anchoring of globe (a) Preoperative and (b) postoperative.

5–0 mersilene/Ethibond sutures. This was initially described using the Skin approach for Dacryocystorhinostomy, DCR, later the retrocaruncular approach was also used. Lately the choice procedure for such cases is **Periosteal anchoring of the lateral rectus** to the lateral periosteum by non-absorbable 5–0 Ethibond sutures and resecting the medial rectus by 8–9 mm for globe alignment in the primary position (Figs 25a and b). Use of Intramuscular **injection of Bupivacain** into the paretic MR as advocated by Alan Scott to strengthen it is under investigation.

For small accompanied vertical deviations the horizontal recti are shifted. Faden recession on contralateral vertical recti also is helpful to correct the vertical misalignment in primary position or downgaze.

Management of Fourth Nerve Palsy

The management has been systematised by Knapp's classification, modified by von Noorden (1986), as shown in Table 10.3. Inferior oblique weakening is the most common procedure for superior oblique palsy (Figs 10.26 and 10.27a and b).

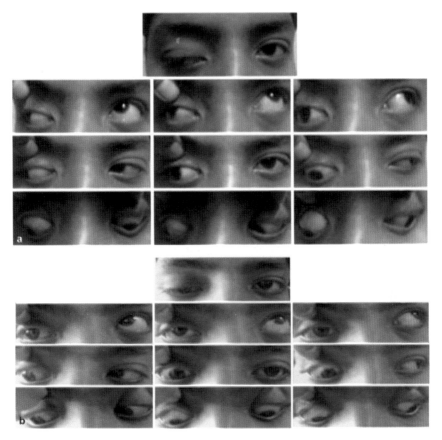

Fig. 10.25: Periosteal anchoring of lateral rectus in III nerve palsy. (a) Preoperative and (b) postoperative.

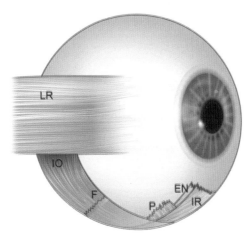

Fig. 10.26: Inferior oblique weakening: Different procedures. LR: Lateral rectus, IO: Inferior oblique, F: Fink, P: Parks, EN: Modified Elliot and Nankin, IR: Inferior rectus.

It may be further noted in the management of trochlear nerve palsy that if there is only extorsion in the downgaze with hypertropia only in the ipsilateral superior oblique quadrant, strengthening procedures like **modified Harada-Ito procedures** work well.

Tucking of the Superior obliques is done only if they show laxity on exaggerated FDT, this is usually seen in Congenital SO palsy. It is done with intraoperative adjustment such that it creates just a minimal acquired Brown syndrome to be effective (Figs 10.28a and b).

In case of class 3 and 4 the choice of surgery between **ipsilateral superior rectus recession** against **contralateral inferior rectus recession** is based on a forced duction test of the paretic eye. If FDT indicates a tight superior rectus, it

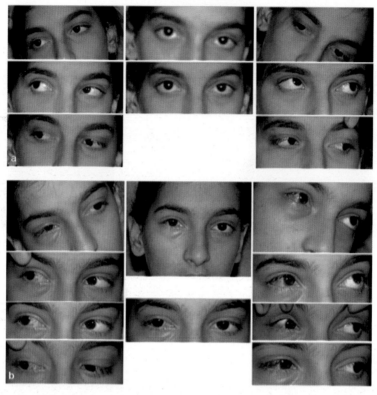

Fig. 10.27: Superior oblique palsy. (a) Preoperative and (b) after IO recession and anteropositioning.

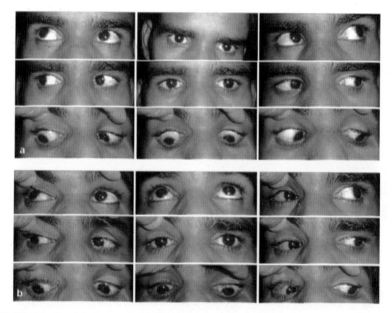

Fig. 10.28: Acquired R S O palsy without IOOA. (a) Preoperative and (b) after SO tuck.

is recessed, otherwise contralateral inferior rectus is recessed.

Double Elevator Palsy

The management of DEP is also considered in a systematic manner. A FDT should be done to exclude a tight inferior rectus, which calls for recession of ipsilateral inferior rectus. This is also indicated if a significant hypotropia in primary position is present.

If the inferior rectus is shown to be free, and hypotropia seen only in upgaze, the contralateral superior rectus and inferior oblique are weakened. The preferred alternative is to perform a Knapp's procedure, transposition of both medial and lateral rectus of ipsilateral eye close to the superior rectus. An associated horizontal deviation can be corrected by incorporating the recession and/or resection of the concerned horizontal rectus in addition to the vertical shifting.

MYASTHENIA AND MYOPATHIES

Incomitant strabismus with limited ductions, may be myogenic in nature. It may involve the muscles (myopathy) or the neuromuscular junctions (myasthenia).

Myasthenia

Myasthenia presents with ptosis and or ophthalmoplegia which tends to fluctuate, improve after rest or sleep and worsen with fatigue, exposure to bright light or during eye examination. In addition there may be difficulty in speech (dysarthria), swallowing, breathing or even fatigue of limbs.

It is an autoimmune disorder and may occur spontaneously or after major illnesses, surgical procedures or during pregnancy and postpartum period and in patients of dysthyroid disease or collagen vascular disease, and due to certain drugs.

Pathogenesis

Antibody-receptor interactions block neuromuscular transmission and subsequently destroy the receptor complex. The susceptibility of extraocular muscles is due to the retention of the embryonic acetylcholine receptor isoform by epsilon subunit. The multiply-innervated extraocular muscle (EOM) fibres are specifically targetted. EOM also have an early involvement because of their high activation rate.

Diagnosis

In addition to a history, the following tests are helpful in diagnosis.

* **Icepack test:** Ice cubes in a plastic wrap are applied onto the lids for 5 minutes which improves the ptosis in myasthenia (Fig. 10.29)
* **Tensilon test:** IV Edrophonium 1–2 mg is given as a test dose to watch for any idiosyncratic response, if no response is seen by 60 sec inject the rest 8–9 mg (0.15 mg/kg in children, up to 10 mg in

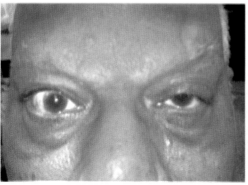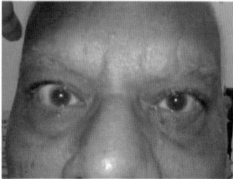

Fig. 10.29: Myasthenia with left ptosis before and after icepack test.

adults). The improvement in ptosis and diplopia is noted and preferably documented (videophotography). 0.5–1 mg atropine IV may be used when disturbing symptoms like sweating, cramps, vomiting or salivation occur. It may also be given prophylactically, 5 minutes prior. Older patients and those at risk should have an I.V. lifeline with standby cardiac monitoring.

- **Neostigmine** has a longer duration and is useful in children and patients with minimal ocular manifestations. In adults 1.5 mg neostigmine is given IM (deltoid muscle) 20 min after 0.6 mg atropine. Peak effect is seen in 30 min. This allows sufficient time to do diplopia charting, Hess/Lees charting and 9-gaze eye movement study.

- **Sleep test** improvement of ptosis and ocular motility measurements after 30 minutes of rest in a quiet dark room is a very confirmatory test.

- **Curare test and regional curare** test after injecting d-tubocurarine in the arm to increase the effect of paralysis.

- **Electromyography** especially single fibre EMG is a highly sensitive test in which decremental response (more than 10%) is seen on repetitive nerve stimulation.

- **Anti-acetyl choline** receptor anti-body assay are diagnostic (98–99%).

- **Muscle biopsy** (motor point) with binding of radiolabeled **alpha bungarotoxin** is the most sensitive and specific.

A mediastinal Roentgenogram and **MRI** to confirm thymoma is helpful in deciding the management, as **thymectomy** is very successful.

Treatment

Medical treatment depends on pyridostigmine 60 mg tablets or 180 mg SR tablets, started with 30 mg orally thrice daily and increased till response. IM injection of pyridostigmine or neostigmine can also be used.

Cases which do not respond with anticholinesterase therapy, particular ocular myasthenics require corticosteroids and sometimes immunosuppressive agents like azathioprine and cyclosporin. Plasmapheresis and intravenous gamma globulins have also been tried.

Myopathies

Ocular myopathy is a condition which has been referred as **chronic progressive external ophthalmoplegia** (CPEO). It is a disease of unknown etiology and has no neurologic involvement. Some patients may develop a progressive generalised muscular disorder. Association of ocular myopathy with tapetoretinal degeneration, various degrees of heart block has been reported as **CPEO-plus or Kearns-Sayre syndrome** (Fig. 10.30).

It starts as ptosis which is bilateral, symmetrical and progressive gradually involving the ocular motility. Due to the bilateral symmetrical involvement diplopia is not complained off (also due to the slow chronic progression). Cosmetic squint surgery may be done along with crutch glasses for ptosis.

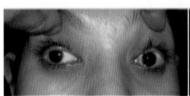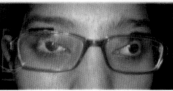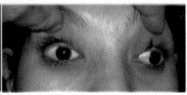

Fig. 10.30: Myopathy, CPEO.

Suggested Reading

1. Baker RS and Steed MM. Restoration of function in paralytic strabismus: alternative methods of therapy. Binoc. Vision 5: 203. 1990.
2. Ellis FD and Helveston EM editors Superior Oblique palsy. Int. Ophthalmol. Clin. 16:127, 1976.
3. Duke-Elder S and Wybar K. System of Ophthalmology vol. 6. Ocular motility and strabismus. St. Louis. 1973. Mosby—Year Book Inc.
4. Helveston EM, Krach D, Plager DA and Ellis FD: A new classification of superior oblique palsy based on congenital variations in the tendon. Ophthalmology 99:1609,1992.
5. Knapp P and Moore S. Diagnosis and Surgical options in superior oblique surgery. Int. Ophthalmol. Clin. 16:137,1976.
6. Metz HS: Saccadic velocity measurements in strabismus. Trans. Am. Ophthalmol. Soc. 81: 630,1983.
7. Metz HS, Scott WE, Madson E, and Scott AB. Saccadic velocities and active force studies in blowout fractures of the orbit. Am J. Ophthalmol. 78:665,1974.
8. Noorden GK von. Awaya S and Romano PE. Past-pointing in paralytic strabismus. Am. J. Ophthalmol. 71:27,1971.
9. Noorden GK von, Murray E, Wong SY. Superior oblique paralysis. A review of 270 cases. Arch. Ophthalmol. 104:1771. 1986.
10. Rosenbaum A and Metz HS. Diagnosis of lost or slipped muscles by saccadic velocity measurements Am. J. Ophthalmol, 77:215,1974.
11. Rush JA and Younge BR. Paralysis of cranial nerves III, IV and VI : Causes and prognosis in 1000 cases. ArcK Ophthalmol. 99:76,1981.
12. Scott AB. Miller JM and Collins CC. Eye muscle prosthesis. J. Pediatr. Ophthalmol. Strabismus. 29:216,1992.
13. Sharma P, Gogoi M, Kedar S, Bhola R. "Periosteal anchoring in third nerve palsy: a new technique.": Jour Amer Assoc of Pediatr Ophthalmology and Strabismus, J AAPOS, 2006;10:324–327
14. Saxena R, Sinha A, Sharma P, Pathak H, Menon V, Sethi H. Precaruncular periosteal anchor of medial rectus, a new technique in the management of complete external third nerve palsy. Orbit; 2006:25(3):205–8.
15. Saxena R, Sinha A, Sharma P, Phuljhele S, Menon V.. Precaruncular approach for medial orbital wall periosteal anchoring of the globe in oculomotor nerve palsy. J AAPOS. 2009 Dec;13(6):578–82.

10

Restrictive Strabismus

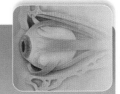

Restrictive strabismus is a form of incomitant strabismus characterised by limitation of movement which is out of proportion to the ocular deviation in the primary position. They have a **mechanical** or **innervational restrictive element** which can be confirmed by resistance to passive stretching on forced duction test (FDT).

Musculofascial innervational anomalies, a common example of which is Duane's retraction syndrome, are congenital forms of restrictive syndromes. Other examples are Brown's superior oblique sheath syndrome, congenital muscle fibrosis and strabismus fixus.

Acquired causes of restrictive strabismus are dysthyroid orbitomyopathy, pseudotumor, myopic myositis, parasitic cysts (cysticercus), and other orbital tumours and fibrosis secondary to orbital trauma and orbital surgery.

DUANE'S RETRACTION SYNDROME

Initially described by Stilling and Turk and popularised by Duane, its complete name should be Stilling-Turk-Duane syndrome but is commonly known as Duane's retraction syndrome. It is **characterised** by
- Limitation of abduction and/or adduction,
- With narrowing of palpebral aperture,
- Retraction of globe and variable upshoot and/or downshoot of globe on attempted adduction (Figs 11.1 and 11.2).

Three subtypes have been differentiated on the basis of electromyography by Huber, as shown in Table 11.1.

Pathology

The basic pathology is **abnormal and paradoxic innervational impulses to the horizontal recti on abduction and adduction.** Due to lack of innervation on

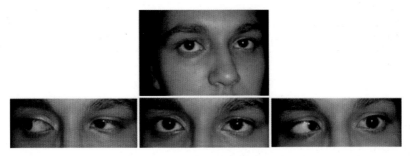

Fig. 11.1: A left sided Duane's retraction syndrome. Note slight exotropia in primary position, despite abduction limitation. On attempted adduction the left eye retracts and down shoots along with narrower palpebral aperture.

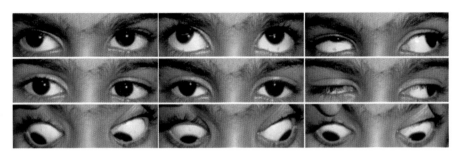

Fig. 11.2: A right side Duane's retraction syndrome with a very slight exotropia. Limitation of abduction and retraction of eyeball and narrowing of palpebral aperture on attempted adduction of right eye should be noted.

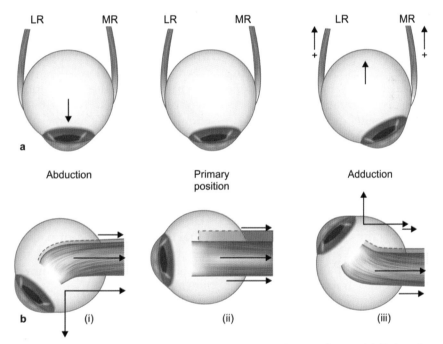

Fig. 11.3: Pathomechanism of eye movements in Duane's retraction syndrome. (a) Relaxation of both LR and MR in abduction results in a relative protrusion of eyeball and co-contraction of both LR and MR in adduction causes retraction of eyeball, (b) co-contraction of eyeball with straight eye causes retraction (i) but if the globe is down, it further downshoots (ii) and if up, it further upshoots (iii) just like a horse head on tightening the reins.

abduction causes limitation of abduction along with relaxation of both LR and MR causing slight atonic protrusion of globe with widening of palpebral aperture. During adduction the LR should relax (Sherrington's law) as the MR normally gets its innervation, but in DRS the LR gets innervated in addition to the MR, not allowing adduction, or if permitted with resistance, it causes retraction of the globe with narrowing of the palpebral aperture (due to lack of support of globe). Co-contraction of the horizontal recti with slippage of globe under a tight LR, may cause upshoot or downshoot, depending on the relative position to the globe in reference to the muscles. This is the pathomechanism for the classical form of **DRS type I** (Fig. 11.3).

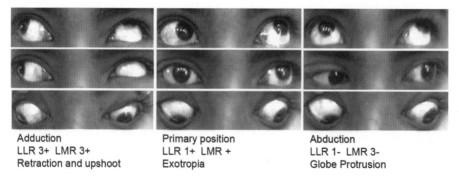

Adduction	Primary position	Abduction
LLR 3+ LMR 3+	LLR 1+ LMR +	LLR 1- LMR 3-
Retraction and upshoot	Exotropia	Globe Protrusion

Fig. 11.4: Pathomechanism of findings in exotropic DRS type II.

In **type II** the LR receives its innervation of abduction permitting abduction (unless the MR has mechanical restriction) but during adduction it still receives innervation as the MR rightly gets its innervation leading to co-contraction. The results of co-contraction on adduction are similar as in type I (Fig. 11.4).

In **type III** the paradoxic innervation is present for both LR and MR during both abduction and adduction, causing a constant retraction of the globe even in primary position. As the paradoxic innervation along with fibrosis of the MR causes severe retraction of globe, narrowing of palpebral aperture, and marked upshoot and down-shoot of globe occur. Clinically the different cases are described as **Eso DRS, Exo DRS**, or **Ortho DRS** depending on the deviation in the primary position.

Though most cases have paradoxic innervation as the anomaly, some have mechanical fibrosis of the muscle or the adjacent fascia, justifying the terminology: **Musculofascial–innervational anomaly.** The recent high definition MRI findings showing abnormalities in the innervation and muscle hypoplasia indicate that it may be a part of Cranial Congenital Dysinnervation Disorder.

Variants

There are some **variants** to the classic picture with retraction being minimal or even absent **(Duane's retraction syndrome sine retraction),** narrowing of palpebral aperture may be minimal or absent on adduction.

There may be **abnormal innervation** to the levator palpebrae superioris (causing active retraction and widening of palpebral aperture); to the inferior oblique (casuing V-phenomenon with hypertropia in primary position); to the superior oblique (causing a phenomenon with hypotropia in primary position) and; to the vertical recti causing

Table 11.1: Duane's retraction syndrome		
Types	Innervation	Clinical presentation
I	• On abduction–LR innervation absent	• Abduction limited
	• On adduction–LR innervation present	• Adduction limited due to resistance with retraction
II	• On abduction–LR innervation present	Abduction may be normal
	• On adduction–LR innervation present	Adduction limited with retraction
III	• On abduction–LR + MR innervation present	Limited abduction with retraction
	• On adduction–LR + MR innervation present	Limited adduction with retraction

11

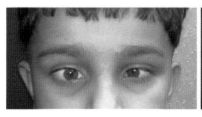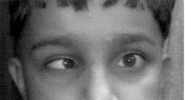

Fig. 11.5: Bilateral Eso DRS.

hypertropia or hypotropia in primary position.

Diagnosis

The most important clinical features are the paradoxic innervation causing limitation that is out of proportion to the ocular deviation, or even a **paradoxic deviation.** In type I with limitation of abduction one should expect esotropia, which is usually so but some cases may have an exotropia (paradoxic). Similarly in type II, usually exotropia is present but paradoxic esotropia is possible. **Bilaterality** (Fig. 11.5) is seen in 20% cases and of the unilateral cases **left eye** preponderance is seen in 75% cases. **Sex** probably has no correlation.

Differential Diagnosis

Cases of **orbital restrictive syndromes** should be distinguished as also long standing cases of **lateral rectus palsy or infantile esotropia** with cross-fixation. In paralytic squints with recovery of lateral rectus after the contracture of medial rectus, a retraction of globe can

occur, **but in abduction.** Similarly a **recovered III CN** palsy can have retraction in adduction but limitation of abduction is not a feature. A case of **MR entrapment** after fracture of medial orbital wall with retraction of globe increasing on attempted abduction is described as **'Pseudo-Duane's Syndrome'.** Forced Duction Testing can be fallacious in cases of innervational restriction if done on relaxed muscles (positive during active innervational effort).

Associations

Several ocular and systemic associations have been noted and they lend credence to the theory of an embryogenic defect during the development of branchial arches around 7 weeks of gestation. The development of III, IV, VI nerves occurs around 4–10 weeks. Three common syndromes associated with DRS are:

Goldenhar's syndome (oculo-auriculo-vertebral dysplasia): Epibulbar dermoids preauricular tags, blind ended fistulas and vertebral anomalies (Figs 11.6).

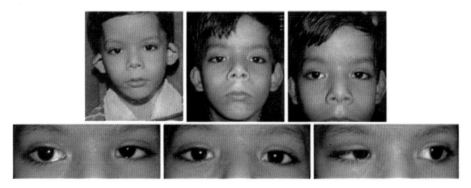

Fig. 11.6: Bilateral orthotropic DRS with abnormal pinna.

Klippel-Feil anomaly: Cervical fusion, short neck low posterior hairline with pseudopterygia.

Wildervanck syndrome: Features of Klippel-Feil with perceptive deafness.

In addition **other anomalies** listed are: iris dysplasia, pupillary anomalies, heterochromia, cataracts, persistent hyaloid arteries, choroidal colobomas, distichiasis, microphthalmos, crocodile tears (gusto lacrimal reflex), etc. Among the **systemic associations** are: cervical spinal bifida, cleft palate, facial anomalies, perceptive deafness, malformations of external ear, and anomalies of the hands and feet.

Management of DRS

In the management of DRS the following **considerations** are made:

1. Cosmetic appearance due to **deviation** of eyeball

2. Cosmetic disfigurement due to adoption of **head posture,** which gives functional binocularity.

3. **Retraction** of the eyeball and **narrowing** of **palpebral aperture** causing cosmetic disfigurement.

4. **Limitation** of movement.

If binocular vision is present with cosmetically acceptable head posture and cosmetically acceptable ocular appearance, no surgery is indicated, just for improving the limitation of abduction. The latter is the most difficult to correct. In cases where the deviation is marked and significant head posture is present or the palpebral appearance is disfiguring or severe up-shoot down-shoot are present, surgery is indicated. Prognosis for lateral rectus motility should be explained in clear terms, which is unlikely to improve (Figs 11.7 and 11.8). The **choice of surgery** is:

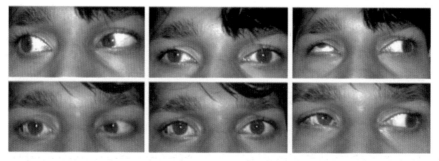

Fig. 11.7: Right exotropic DRS preoperative (top) and postoperative (bottom) after right LR periosteal fixation.

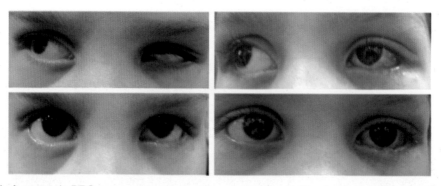

Fig. 11.8: Left esotropic DRS preoperative (top) and postoperative (bottom) after left MR and LR differential recession.

- Mild DRS with esotropia: Medial rectus recession.
- Moderate-to-severe DRS with exotropia with/without upshoot or downshoot: Ipsilateral recession of both LR and MR of differential amounts to correct deviation.
- Associated V-phenomenon with inferior oblique overaction with upshoot: Horizontal recti plus inferior oblique recession.
- Associated A-phenomenon with superior oblique overaction with downshoot: Recession of ipsilateral horizontal recti plus superior oblique weakening.

It should be emphasised that **resection of the horizontal recti of the same eye should never be attempted** even to correct the ocular deviation. It may be undertaken only in the contralateral normal eye for the latter indication. MR resection is also done for Synergistic divergence after doing periosteal fixation of LR. Recession and **retroequatorial myopexy** of the contralateral synergist can also be undertaken to correct face turn and may improve the limitation of abduction of the involved eye. **Y-splitting** of lateral recti has been tried by some workers for upshoot-downshoot. But the author recommends recession of LR and MR as effective for relieving co-contractions, and tackling obliques when indicated. Transposition of vertical recti to aid abduction are partially successful in improving abduction but usually aggravate the retraction problem and are thus avoided. Recently for Exo DRS cases the paradoxically innervated LR is disinserted and fixed to the lateral periosteum and partial Vertical Rectus transpositioning done to improve abduction.

BROWN'S SUPERIOR OBLIQUE SHEATH SYNDROME

Brown described congenitally tight superior oblique sheath syndrome with the characteristic features as:
- Absence of elevation in adduction.

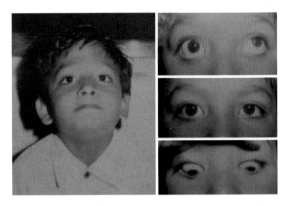

Fig. 11.9: Brown's syndrome—clinical presentation showing chin up and limited elevation.

- Unaffected elevation in primary position and abduction.
- Normal or minimal overaction of the ipsilateral superior oblique.
- Positive forced duction test (restricted elevation in adduction).
- Positive exaggerated FDT for superior oblique.
- Frequent depression of eye in adduction.
- Divergence (Y pattern) in upgaze.

Eustis, O'Reilly and Crawford have graded the Brown's syndrome as:

Mild: Restricted elevation in adduction but no downshoot, or hypotropia in primary position.

Moderate: Restricted elevation in adduction with downshoot but no hypotropia in primary position.

Severe: Restricted elevation and down-shoot in adduction with hypotropia primary position.

Jampolsky has differentiated cases with superior oblique overaction (Fig. 11.10) as **'Brown-Plus'.**

Acquired forms of Brown's syndrome have been described after **trauma** or infections of the trochlear area or after inferior oblique incarceration following **blow out fracture** and after **superior oblique tucking** surgery. The cases of Brown's syndrome and Brown-plus

11

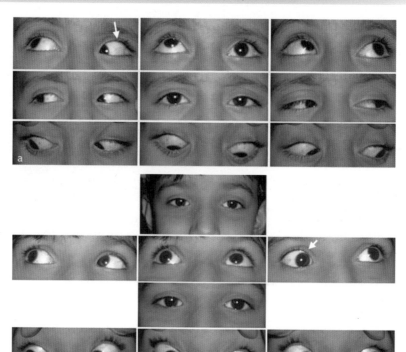

Fig. 11.10: Brown syndrome right eye. (a) preoperative and (b) postoperative after right superior oblique weakened by silicon expander.

should be differentiated from **inferior oblique palsy** (lacks Vpattern on upgaze and has overaction of superior oblique). The **Canine tooth syndrome,** caused by dog bites, with extensive scarring restricting both elevation and depression in adduction is a form of superior oblique palsy with acquired Brown's syndrome.

Management

Cases of Brown's syndrome (without superior oblique overactions) have had unsatisfactory surgical results. Complete dissection of the superior oblique sheath or complete tenectomy of SO have been tried. Some surgeons prefer to do simultaneous inferior oblique weakening. Wright has advocated superior oblique lengthening by silicon expander. These may actually be more relevant in cases with superior oblique overaction (Brown-plus). Other weakening or

lengthening procedures like chicken suture in nasal of tendon or **loop** at the insertion site are also tried. Most cases which are cosmetically acceptable and have binocularity in primary position (Grade 1 and 2 of Eustis) need not be operated.

Strabismus Fixus

Strabismus fixus convergens is a rare condition with the eyes firmly fixed in extreme adduction (Fig. 11.11). Forced duction test confirms their immobility. Rarely strabismus fixus divergens, eyes fixed in exodeviation are also seen. Usually cases are congenital in which lateral rectus palsy with medial rectus fibrosis have been described. Acquired cases with myopic myositis and amyloidosis of the lateral recti have been reported by the author.

Supramaximal recession of the medial recti with silicon expanders have been found to be of considerable functional and cosmetic

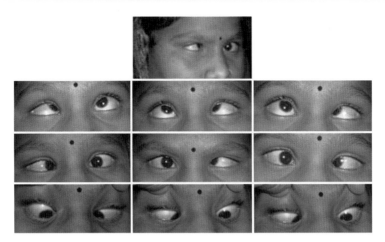

Fig. 11.11: Strabismus fixus convergens: bilateral.

benefit. In case of tight MR, otherwise reasonable results are obtained with loop myopexy of the LR and SR with non-absorbable suture or silicon sling to the sclera in the superotemporal part. This is because of the nasal slippage of the SR and inferior slippage of LR in such cases as seen on MRI (Fig. 11.12).

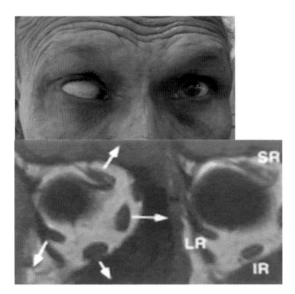

Fig. 11.12: Strabismus fixus with nasalization of superior rectus and lateral rectus. Surgical planning requires loop myopexy of right superior and lateral rectus temporally.

Congenital Fibrosis of Extraocular Muscles (CFEOM)

Brown described this condition as congenital generalised fibrosis syndrome. Autosomal recessive and also autosomal dominant pattern of transmission is described (Fig. 11.13)

Characteristics

- Fibrosis of extraocular muscles, Tenon's capsule with adhesions between muscles, Tenon's and the globe.
- Inelasticity and fragility of the conjunctiva.
- Ptosis with chin elevation.
- Absence of elevation with downward fixation of eyes.
- Perverted convergence on attempted upgaze and divergence on downgaze.
- Family history.

Associations

Ocular conditions associated are: Marcus-Gunn jaw wrinking phenomenon, choroidal coloboma, pendular nystagmus and optic nerve hypoplasia.

Systemic associations are: Ventricular septal defect, talipes equino valgus, unilateral facial palsy and facial asymmetry.

Acquired causes of restrictions should be excluded.

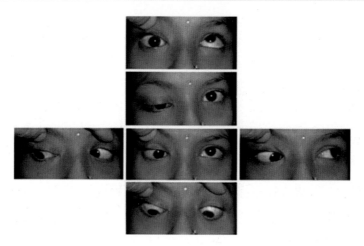

Fig. 11.13: CFEOM.

Management

Supra-maximal recession of inferior recti (6–8 mm) with frontalis sling (or crutch glasses) for ptosis is done. Associated Superior Oblique overactions and Exodeviations are corrected surgically. Perverted convergence are difficult to correct (Fig. 11.14).

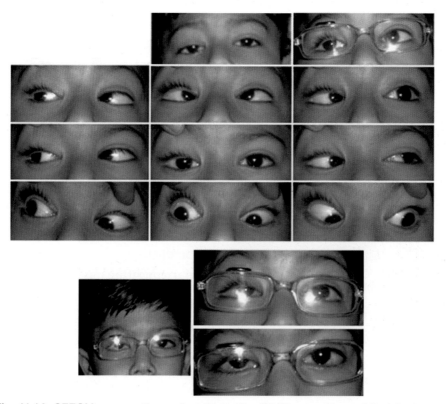

Fig. 11.14: CFEOM preoperative and postoperative-Bil IR recession and Crutch glasses.

Adherence Syndromes

Post-traumatic and post-detachment surgery cases commonly present with extensive fibrosis especially between lateral rectus, inferior oblique and inferior rectus. Prolapse of fat and fibrofatty adhesion make a lethal combination. Such cases are best avoided by careful extraocular surgery in proper tissues planes. These can be confirmed by FDT. Restriction can also be caused by buckles, encirclages, setons or fibrous adhesion with these structures.

Management requires exploration with an individualised surgical approach. Use of local application of Mitomycin C: 0.02% solution for 3–4 minutes intraoperatively is useful.

Dysthyroid Orbitomyopathy

Restrictive limitation of ocular movement is a feature of dysthyroid eye disease. It has been called as exophthalmic ophthalmoplegia, endocrine ophthalmic ophthalmoplegia, endocrine ophthalmopathy or myopathy dysthyroid myositis or myopathy, exophthalmic goitre or infiltrative ophthalmopathy.

It is characterised by lid retraction, prominence or eyeball with limitation of movement in more than one direction especially elevation, depression, abduction (Fig. 11.15). Associated conjunctival hyperemia and chemosis may be seen. Convergence insufficiency is usually present, even in milder cases. Other signs of Graves disease may be seen. There is no relationship with the levels of T3, T4, TSH, or the patient being euthyroid, hyperthyroid or hypothyroid, during activity of eye problems. (But these should be evaluated.)

The involvement is unilateral or asymmetric, if bilateral. Ultrasonography can measure the thickened extraocular muscles (EOM). But most characteristic feature is on computed tomography which shows **fusiform enlargement of the proximal part of extraocular muscles**. It is this that causes axial proptosis and threatens vision due to compressive optic neuropathy (Fig. 11.16).

Pathogenesis

Dysthyroid orbitomyopathy is an autoimmune disorder. An autoantigen is coexpressed in the thyroid gland and the orbital fibroblasts. This is recognised by the circulating T-cell lymphocytes activating the T cells (CD4 cells) triggering an immune response. The activated T-cells secrete various cytokines, interferon, gamma, interleukin 1-alpha and tumor necrosis factor, which cause proliferation of fibroblasts in the orbit and production of glycosaminoglycans (GAGs). As a result of

11

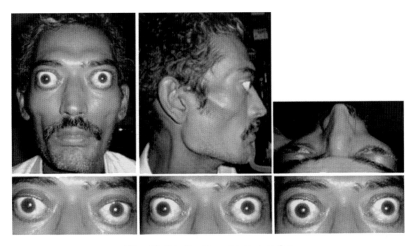

Fig. 11.15: Dysthyroid myopathy.

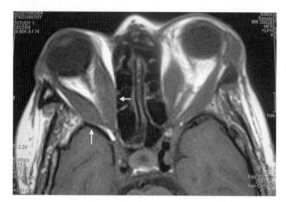

Fig. 11.16: Dysthyroid myopathy on imaging showing fusiform dilatation of EOMs.

abnormal accumulation of these GAGs the orbital pressure rises and the EOM swells up. Cell mediated cytotoxicity has also been implicated. T3 receptors have been seen in high levels in some muscle fibre types demonstrating effects of hyperthyroidism also.

HLA-DR is crucial to recognition of the autoantigen.

Management

Systemic therapy of thyroid imbalance should be evaluated and treated, though it has no bearing on the orbitomyopathy. The deviation in the mean time may be corrected by prisms or occlusion (if large). Severe proptosis with periorbital swelling and chemosis or evidence of compressive optic neuropathy mandate high dose **steroids** which need to be given for a few months and gradually tapered. **Immunosuppressives** and **radiotherapy** have also been tried if steroids fail. **Surgical decompression** by deroofing the orbit is the last resort. If the severity is controlled and the ocular deviation is static for atleast 6 months, **squint surgery** can be done. Maximal recession of inferior rectus, medial rectus or superior rectus (as affected) is required. Adjustable suture surgery has been considered to correct in a more predictable manner. Conjunctival scarring and shortening demand liberal conjunctival recession.

Orbital Myositis

Pseudotumors or nonspecific orbital granulomas, autoimmune myositis and parasitic cysts like cysticercus have been occasionally presented with symptoms of unilateral pain, localised congestion, and ptosis with proptosis, deviation and diplopia. Restriction of eye movements can be confirmed by forced duction test. Ultrasonography and computed tomography can identify solid or cystic lesions and scolex may confirm a cysticercus cyst. The nonspecific inflammations respond to systemic steroids for a few weeks and tapered over a few weeks. In case of cysticercus cysts, albendazole therapy orally 15 mg/kg given for two weeks is beneficial. But in the latter cases, neurocysticercosis should be excluded by computed tomography as also intraocular cysticercus and a cover of systemic steroids should be given.

ORBITAL FRACTURES

Post-traumatic blow-out fractures: Typical or atypical, medial wall fractures are seen after injury with cricket or tennis balls. In the initial phase a black eye, orbital swelling and severe restriction of movements in all directions is seen. Later as generalized tissue edema subsides specific restrictive movements appear. In typical blow-out fractures, the inferior orbital margin is intact but the floor gives way with the inferior orbital contents usually fat and fascia of the inferior oblique, inferior rectus, and sometimes the muscles themselves, prolapse into the maxillary sinus paranasal sinus X-ray and computed tomography are diagnostic.

The clinical features are restricted elevation, restricted depression with hypoesthesia in the infraorbital nerve distribution (Figs 11.17 and 11.18). The medial wall fractures are rarer and present with "pseudo-Duane's" retraction syndrome.

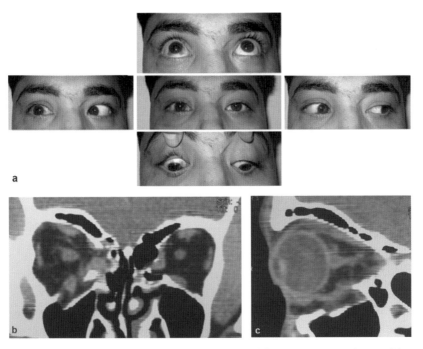

Fig. 11.17: Blow-out fracture—Right medial and inferior wall. (a) Showing clinical picture, (b) anterioposterior view and (c) lateral view showing the fracture orbit floor.

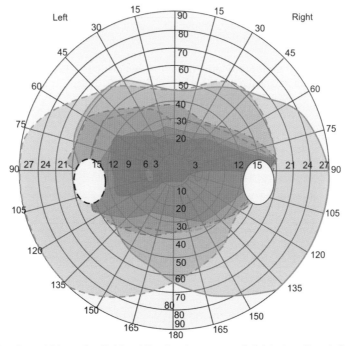

Fig. 11.18: Serial charting of binocular fields of fixation in a case of right elevation deficiency. Elevator and depressor underaction secondary to a blow-out fracture.

Management

No surgery is indicated in the initial two week phase of tissue edema, and even later if the deviation is subsiding unless a large defect in the orbital floor is seen. The latter may present as marked enophthalmos. Follow-up should be meticulous with serial diplopia (Fig. 11.18). Hess charts and binocular fields of fixation. No surgery is indicated as long as sufficient diplopia-free area is available in the primary position and downgaze. In case of severe enophthalmos with fat and orbital tissue prolapse, a subperiosteal approach is made and the defect sealed with 0.3 mm supramid sheath. Ocular deviations are tackled at a later date in stages, first the inferior rectus recessed till the forced duction test is negative and then the superior rectus resected if need be.

Suggested Reading

1. Jampolsky A. Surgical leashes and reverse leashes in strabismus surgical management. In Symposium on Strabismus: Transactions of the New Orleans Academy of Ophthalmology. St. Louis. 1978. Mosby — Year Book Inc.

2. Brown HW. True and simulated superior oblique tendon sheath syndromes. Doc. Ophthalmol. 34: 123, 1973.

3. Burde RM. Graves' ophthalmopathy and the special problem of concomitant ocular myasthenia gravis. Richard G. Scobee Memorial Lecture. Am. Orthopt. J. 40: 37, 1990.

4. Duane A. Congenital deficiency of abduction associated with impairment of adduction, retraction movements, contraction of palpebral fissure and oblique movements of the eye. Arch. Ophthalmol. 34: 133. 1905.

5. Eustis HS, O'Reilly C and Crawford JS. Management of superior oblique palsy after surgery for true Brown's Syndrome. J. Pediatr. Ophthalmol, strabismus. 24: 10, 1987.

6. Huber A. Electrophysiology of the retraction syndrome. Br. J. Ophthalmol. 58: 293, 1974.

7. Noorden GK von and Murray. E: Up-and down-shoot in Duane's retraction syndrome. J. Pediatr. Ophthalmol. Strabismus. 23: 212, 1986.

8. Sharma P Gupta NK, Arora R, and Prakash P. Strabismus fixus convergens secondary to amyloidosis. J. Pediatr. Ophthalmol. Strabismus. 28: 236, 1991.

9. Sprunger DT, Noorden GK. von and Helveston E.M. Surgical results in Brown's syndrome, J. Pediatr. Ophthalmol. Strabismus. 28: 164, 1991.

10. Weinberg DA, Lessner RL and Vollmer T. Ocular myasthenia: a protean disorder. Surv. Ophthalmol. 39: 169, 1994.

11. Wilson ME, Eustis HS and Parks MM/Brown's syndrome. Surv. Ophthalmol. 34: 153, 1989.

12. Wright KW. Superior oblique silicone expander for Brown's syndrome and superior oblique overaction. J. Pediatr. Ophthalmol. Strabismus. 28: 101, 1991.

11

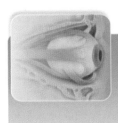

Vertical Strabismus

Vertical strabismus presents a difficult diagnostic problem to the ophthalmologist. Vertical strabismus is a misalignment of visual axes in the vertical direction such that one eye is higher than the other. The higher eye is said to be **hypertropic.** Since whenever one eye is hypertropic, the other eye will always be hypotropic (except in dissociated strabismus), by convention we designate the vertical squint by the hypertropic eye unless otherwise specified (as in incomitant strabismus).

There are four vertical muscles for each eye, the superior and inferior recti primarily acting in abduction and the superior and inferior obliques acting primarily in the adduction, though the recti are primarily elevators and depressors and the obliques primarily intorters and extorters. The vertical rectus muscle of one eye yokes with the oblique muscle of the other eye and vice versa. Ocular motility disturbances of vertical recti and oblique muscles are inseparable and they will be conjointly termed as **cyclovertical muscles.**

Vertical squints are less common than horizontal strabismus, but the vertical fusional vergence being poorer, vertical phorias easily manifest as tropias and are symptomatic.

Pseudovertical squint may give an appearance of vertical deviation but the visual axes are actually in alignment and the eyes have bifoveal vision. This may be due to

- Orbital asymmetry
- Displaced globe by an orbital mass

- Facio-maxillary fractures.
- Vertical angle kappa
- Displaced macula.
- Asymmetric eyelid retraction/ptosis (as in dysthyroid ophthalmopathy or after vertical recti surgery).

Types of Cyclovertical Strabismus

1. Comitant vertical squint (Fig. 12.1)
2. Incomitant vertical squint
   a. Neurogenic palsy
      - Supranuclear (gaze) palsy
      - Nuclear
      - Infranuclear palsy/III and IV, CN palsy
   b. Myogenic dystrophies and myasthenia
   c. Restrictive squints
      - Vertical DRS
      - Brown's syndrome
      - Congenital muscle fibrosis
      - Dysthyroid orbitomyopathy
      - Post-traumatic orbital wall fractures
      - Tumours, pseudotumours, and cysts.
   d. Deviations with primary overaction of inferior oblique
3. Dissociated vertical deviations (strabismus sursoadduction)
4. Cyclovertical motility abnormalities with horizontal deviations: AV group of patterns.

   Most of these conditions have been covered individually in other chapters, we shall deal with certain general aspects.

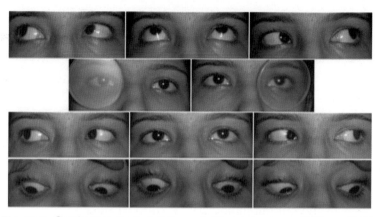

Fig. 12.1: Comitant vertical strabismus left hypertropia, no DVD no IOOA.

Clinical Features

Cyclovertical squints commonly present with:

a. Vertical diplopia which may also have a torsional component.

b. Vertical deviation that is cosmetically unacceptable

c. Head posture that compensates for the squint but is itself cosmetically disfiguring or uncomfortable.

The following points should be specially noted:

1. Find out the gaze-position in which diplopia increases or decreases.

2. The type of head posture should be noted. The duration of head posture should be confirmed with old family photographs, if available.

3. A head posture should be of clinical significance, either allowing binocular single vision and/or getting rid of diplopia. This should be confirmed with the findings on eliminating the head posture.

Interpretation of Head Posture

1. **Face turn**
   a. *To the right side*: Keeps the eyes in levoversion so that the defect of RSR, RIR, LIO or LSO is not manifested.
   b. *To the left side*: Keeps the eyes in dextro-version so that the defect of LSR, LIR, RIO or RSO is not manifested.

2. **Head tilt**
   a. *To the right shoulder*: Compensates for the weakness of extorsion of right eye and/or intorsion of left eye (Table 12.1).

Table 12.1: Inference from Parks three step test

Hypertropic eye in primary position	Hypertropia increases on gaze to	Hypertropia increases on tilt to	Paretic muscle
1. Right	Right	Right	• Left inferior oblique
2. Right	Right	Left	• Right inferior rectus
3. Right	Left	Right	• Right superior oblique
4. Right	Left	Left	• Left superior rectus
5. Left	Right	Right	• Right superior rectus
6. Left	Right	Left	• Left superior oblique
7. Left	Left	Right	• Left inferior rectus
8. Left	Left	Left	• Right inferior oblique

(Courtesy: *Griffin JR Binocular anomalies: procedures for vision therapy. Chicago: Professional Press. Inc. 1982*).

b. *To the left shoulder*: Compensates for the weakness of intorsion of right eye and/or extorsion of left eye (superiors intort, inferiors extort).

3. **Chin-up/down**
   a. *Chin up*: compensates for depressor weakness of either eye.

Ocular Deviation

The alignment of the eyes is tested objectively by Hirschberg's test and cover-uncover test in the nine diagnostic gaze position with each eye fixing alternatively. Subjectively the tests include: diplopia charting with red-green glasses, Hess charting, Maddox rod, double Maddox rod (for cyclotropia), Binocular fields of fixation.

Limitation of Movement

This is checked uniocularly (ductions) as well as binocularly (versions). Habitual or inhibitional palsy improve after patching the paretic eye.

Head Tilt Test

The head tilt test is an important component of the Parks 3 step diagnostic test for diagnosing the abnormal cyclovertical muscle in a case of hypertropia (Fig. 12.2).

- Step 1: Does patient have a right or left hypertropia (RHT/LHT)?
- Step 2: Does the hypertropia increase on dextroversion or levoversion?
- Step 3: Does the hypertropia increase on head tilt to right side or left side?

Points to be kept in mind while interpreting the head tilt test are the possibility of following should be ruled out or **fallacies** will occur.

- Contracture/tethering of a vertical rectus muscle.
- Paresis of more than one extraocular muscle
- Restrictive ophthalmopathy.
- Previous surgery on a vertical rectus muscle
- Myasthenia gravis
- Dissociated vertical deviations.
- Small non-paralytic vertical deviations with horizontal strabismus.

Diplopia Charting

In case of cyclovertical squint, the source of light should be a slit, used horizontally. This maximally separates the images vertically and also allows for observing the tilt. The image which is fainter and farther belongs to the paretic eye.

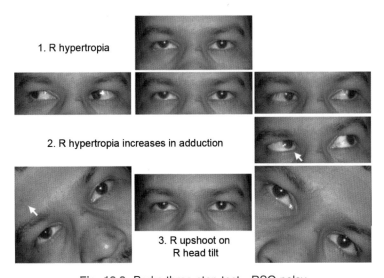

1. R hypertropia

2. R hypertropia increases in adduction

3. R upshoot on R head tilt

Fig. 12.2: Parks three step test—RSO palsy.

In case of dissociated vertical deviations a red filter alone is used, the red image is lower irrespective of the filter being over right eye or left eye. Because the eye behind the filter manifests the DVD, with its image perceived always lower.

Double Maddox Rod

In subjective assessment of cyclotropia, the double Maddox rod test is a simple useful test in cases with binocularity. A DMR utilise a red and white (or both red) Maddox rods. With red before the eye with suspected torsion anomaly and the head tilt corrected, the two rods are aligned at 90° mark, the patient sees two horizontal lines (a vertical prism can be added to separate superimposing lines). If a tilt is present the red line is seen to be tilted. The red Maddox rod is rotated to make the two lines exactly parallel. The misalignment of the red Maddox rod from 90° axis gives the torsion suffered by the affected eye.

Other methods to measure cyclodeviations are synoptophore (using simultaneous macular perception slides with vertical imagery) and by charting blind spot on perimetry. These are all **subjective methods.**

An objective assessment of cyclodeviation can be made by fundus examination on indirect ophthalmoscopy or fundus photography, noting the relationship between the fovea and the disc. Normally the fovea lies 0.3 DD below the horizontal line passing through the geometric centre of the optic disc.

Forced Duction Test (FDT)

FDT is a clinically useful test which distingui-shes between an underaction due to restrictive or paretic cause. In cases with limitation of movement, after anesthetising the eye, the eye is held at the limbus with non-traumatic (Pierce Hoskin's) forceps and passively moved, taking care that the globe is not pushed in the orbit. The latter gives false negative results. Secondly the patient is instructed to look (attempt) in the direction of action of paretic muscle (this is to relax the antagonist or else false positive result will occur). Normally a positive FDT indicates a restrictive element in the opposite muscle or quadrant. In cases of reverse leash due to retro-equatorial fixity, the restriction on the same side can give a similar positive FDT.

Exaggerated FDT

Guyton described exaggerated FDT for obliques. The globe is retracted, abducted, and extorted for superior oblique and intorted for inferior oblique, to make the concerned oblique maximally taut. The eye is then moved from abduction to adduction against the upper lid margin, a tight superior oblique gives a click. For inferior oblique it is moved from abduction to adduction against the lower lid margin and a restrictive inferior oblique is felt (*see* chapter 15).

DISSOCIATED VERTICAL DEVIATION

Dissociated vertical deviation (DVD) is a special form of strabismus characterised by spontaneous upward turning of the dissociated eye. Dissociation may occur by fatigue, day-dreaming or covering of one eye with an opaque or translucent occluder. It may be associated with excycloduction, abduction, and sometimes latent nystagmus. On recovery a slow drifting redressal movement is diagnostic.

It has been attributed with **several names:** alternating sursumduction, alternating hyperphoria or hypertropia, anatopia, double hypertropia, occlusion hypertropia, dissociated vertical divergence. But the most appropriate term is **dissociated vertical deviation** (DVD). However, it has been rightly referred as the **DVD syndrome** which encompasses apart from the vertical deviation, excycloduction, abduction and latent nystagmus. Sometimes excycloduction is the only or main presenta-tion, such cases are termed **dissociated torsional deviation** (DTD). Sometimes dissociated abduction alone is the feature and is called **dissociated horizontal deviation**

(DHD). Rarely a **dissociated esotropia** has been described.

Prevalence

It is rarely seen in infancy, in spite of careful search. It usually presents at 2–5 years age. It is commonly associated with infantile esotropia, and by this time most are operated, however its manifestation has no relation with the surgery. It is usually bilateral but asymmetric. However, in deep amblyopes and sensory heterotropias it is mostly unilateral.

It is commonly associated with infantile esotropia but can also be seen with infantile exotropia, sensory heterotropia and Duane's retraction syndrome. Isolated cases have been seen with normal binocular vision also.

The **inferior oblique overactions** (IOOA) is the condition it needs to be distinguished from, but several times inferior oblique overactions are associated with DVD, but it has different features (Table 12.2). Even superior oblique overactions are associated (Fig. 12.3).

Table 12.2: Differences between IOOA and DVD

Features	IOOA	DVD
1. Hypertropia	Max. in adduction never in abduction	Same in PP abduction/adduction
2. Movement of recovery	Quick refixation on uncovering	Slow drift of eye downwards
3. Superior oblique	usually underacts	May overact
4. V pattern	Present	May be present
5. Pseudo paresis of contra-lateral superior rectus	Present	Absent
6. Incycloduction on reflexation	Absent	Present
7. Latent nystagmus	May be associated	Often present
8. Bielschowsky's phenomenon	Absent	Present
9. Red filter test	Red image higher or lower on alternation	Red image is always lower as eye behind red filter is always higher

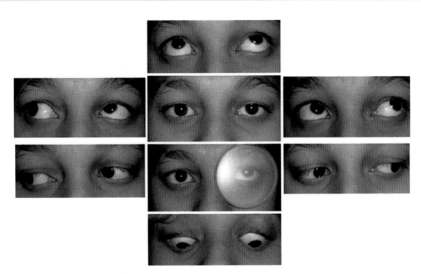

Fig. 12.3: DVD—left eye with IOOA.

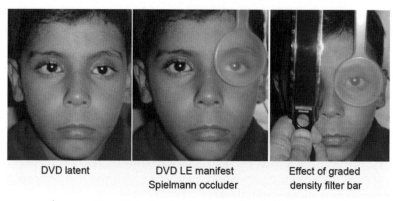

| DVD latent | DVD LE manifest Spielmann occluder | Effect of graded density filter bar |

Fig. 12.4: Depth of suppression in DVD.

Diagnosis

The diagnostic tests are:

- **Spielmann's translucent occluder** demonstrate the updrift and the characteristic slow drifting recovery movement (in hypertropias with inferior oblique overaction there is a refixation movement which is a fast saccade)
- **Bielschowsky's graded density filter bar** demonstrates the pathognomonic light-dependent behaviour of the eye movements. The filter bar consists of increasing density of neutral density filters (Bagolini's graded density red filter bar also suffices). As the density is increased, the eye drifts up and as the density is decreased the eye comes down, even going below the primary position (Fig. 12.4).
- **Red filter test.** This is a simple but characteristic test. The red filter dissociates the eyes. The eye behind the filter drifts up and the subject appreciates diplopia, with the red image lower. When the red filter is put in front of the other eye, this eye deviates up (bilateral DVD) and again the red image is lower.
- Another definitive test is doing **cover test with the fixating eye in sursoadduction,** the eye behind cover still drifts up.

Etiology

The etiology of DVD is an enigma which has yet to be solved. Elastic preponderance of elevators or depressors have been blamed as also the paresis of depressors, imbalances between the amount of innervation from each vestibular organ. Abnormal visual pathway routing similar to albinism or abnormal, intermittent and alternate excitation of subcortical centres could be responsible. The role of the visual stimulation relative to the other eye in the manifestation of the DVD is however, proven beyond doubt. Spielmann has shown that DVD does not occur (or gets neutralised) when both eyes are covered by translucent occluders. Imbalance of binocular stimulation is thus important but it is known to occur in individuals with normal binocular functions, which needs explanation.

Treatment

A plethora of surgical modalities have been tried, sometimes successful, sometimes they fail.

1. **Recession of superior rectus.** More than normal amounts (7–9 mm) are required, and is ideal for bilateral DVD especially when combined with the next modality. In asymmetric cases differential recession is done.
2. **Retroequatorial myopexy (Faden) of superior rectus.** Though it has been temporarily effective even on its own, the best results are seen when 1 and 2 are combined.

12

3. **Resection of inferior rectus.** This approach is the reserve option for some exceptional cases which do not fully respond to first two modalities.

4. **Total anteropositioning of inferior obliques** have been found to be effective and the author's choice in cases of DVD with inferior oblique overaction. The inferior obliques are converted into depressors, because of total anteropositioning.

DISSOCIATED HORIZONTAL DEVIATION (DHD)

This is a recently recognised strabismus with intermittent asymmetric abduction and elevation of the dissociated eye. It may be associated with excyclotropia and latent nystagmus, but may not be accompanied by DVD. Alternate cover test shows less exodeviation than what is seen on "dissociation", also with its characteristic gliding drifts. Cases with DVD in one eye and

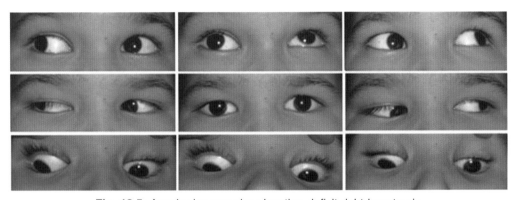

Fig. 12.5: Acquired monocular elevation deficit-right hypotropia.

Table 12.3: Incomitant–supranuclear incomitant vertical squints	
Diagnosis	*Observation*
1. Supranuclear paresis of monocular elevation (Fig. 12.5)	Acquired monocular limitation. No vertical squint in primary position and downgaze. No ptosis. Normal Bells' and Dolls' head movements. Parinaud's syndrome should be excluded.
2. Congenital double elevator palsy	Congenital unilateral limitation of elevation with ptosis (usually) and hypotropia in primary position. 3 types: i. Prominent inferior rectus restriction with FDT positive and normal SR saccades. ii. Elevator weakness with negative FDT and reduced SR saccades. iii. Combination of both
3. Alternating skew deviation (Fig. 12.6)	Episodic alternating skew, with rotary nystagmus. May be associated with brainstem/cerebellar lesions.
4. Dissociated vertical deviation	Most associated with infantile esotropia, characterised by monocular elevation of eye under cover and extorsion. Bielschowsky's phenomenon positive. Improves with recession and Faden of SR

12

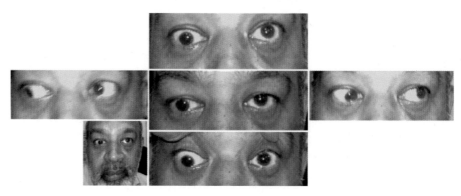

Fig. 12.6: Skew deviation right hypotropia.

DHD in another indicate a common string. Bielschowsky's phenomenon is also present.

The horizontal deviation is **treated** by recession of lateral rectus for the cosmetic aspect. Associated DVD is tackled as above.

Dissociated Esotropia

Spielmann has described a condition in which the eyes are aligned when both eyes are occluded but on covering one eye, the other eye adducts and straightens on uncovering. The **treatment** suggested is retroequatorial myopexy of medial rectus.

DIFFERENTIAL DIAGNOSIS OF CYCLOVERTICAL STRABISMUS

After going through the clinical examination and the special tests enumerated earlier, one would be able to pinpoint the affected muscle or group of muscles. This shall help in formulating the diagnosis and in case of neurological causes help in topically localizing the lesion.

The most common group which shall be observed in practice are the incomitant vertical squints. Tables 12.3 to 12.5 indicate the conditions with their diagnostic findings in a classified form.

Table 12.4: Incomitant infranuclear causes

Diagnosis	Observations
1. Fourth nerve palsy	Head posture present. Diagnosis clinched on Park's 3-step test. Bilateral cases may present with V-phenomenon.
2. Third nerve palsy	
i. Infranuclear	Clinical picture varies with the site of involvement.
	Complete/partial; inorbital lesions the superior or inferior divisions involved.
	Pupillary fibres spared in ischaemic conditions as in diabetic neuropathy
ii. Nuclear lesions	Ptosis and pupillary involvement if present, always bilateral.
	Contralateral or both superior rectus involved.
3. Myasthenia gravis	Variable ptosis with ophthalmoparesis with diurnal variation.
	May involve other muscles.
	Orbicularis "peek" sign and Cogan's lid twitch sign positive.
4. Progressive external	Symmetric slowly progressive ophthalmoplegia especially LPS involvement.
	May have associated tapetoretinal degeneration and deafness.

Table 12.5: Restrictive causes observations

Diagnosis	Observations
1. Dysthyroid ophthalmopathy	Lid lag/retraction with acquired elevation limitation. IR most commonly involved and LR least. Late stages — congestion, chemosis, corneal exposure and optic neuropathy.
2. Orbital floor fracture	Monocular limitation of elevation with enophthalmos, numbness in infraorbital nerve distribution. FDT positive on elevation. X-ray and CT scan helpful.
3. Brown's syndrome	Absence of elevation in adduction. Frequent depression of the eye in adduction for mechanical reasons. V. pattern present. FDT positive.
4. Myositis	EOM movement limitation with periorbital pain, localised congestion, chemosis, may have proptosis. FDT positive and response to steroid is dramatic.
5. Congenital muscle fibrosis	Rare, familial, autosomal dominant. Bilateral ptosis, fixed hypotropia with severe upgaze limitation.
6. Heavy eye syndrome	Association of anisometropia, usually high myopia. The more myopic eye is hypotropic. Called so as the more myopic eye looks low as it were too heavy. No association between the amount of anisometropia and the amount of hypotropia.

Suggested Reading

1. Spector RH. Vertical diplopia. Surv. Ophthalmol. 38: 31–62, 1993.

2. Bender MB, Pasik P, Pasik T et al. Vertical gaze: clinical and experimental considerations with particular reference to oblique movements. Neuro-ophthalmology. 1:79–94. 1981.

3. Bielschowsky A. Lectures on Motor Anomalies. Hanover N.H. Dartmouth College Publication, 1940.

4. Jampel RS and Fells P. Monocular elevation paresis caused by a central nervous system lesion Arch. Ophthalmol. 80: 45, 1968.

5. Jampolsky A. Management of vertical strabismus Trans New Orleans Acad. Ophthalmol. 34: 141, 1986.

6. Keane JR. Alternating Skew deviation. 47. patients. Neurology, 35: 725, 1985.

7. Spielmann A. A translucent occluder for studying eye position under unilateral or bilateral cover test Am. Orthopt. J. 36: 65, 1986.

8. Sprague JB. Moore S. Eggers H and Knapp. P. Dissociated vertical deviation : treatment with the fadenoperation of cuppers. Arch. Ophthalmol. 98: 465, 1980.

9. Wilson ME and McClatchey SK. Dissociated horizontal deviation. J. Pediatr. Ophthalmol strabismus 28 : 90, 1991.

10. Zubcov A, Reinecke RD, Calhoun J.H. Asymmetric horizontal tropias, DVD and manifest latent nystagmus : An explanation of dissociated horizontal deviation. J. Pediatr. Ophthalmol Strabismus. 27: 59, 1990.

12

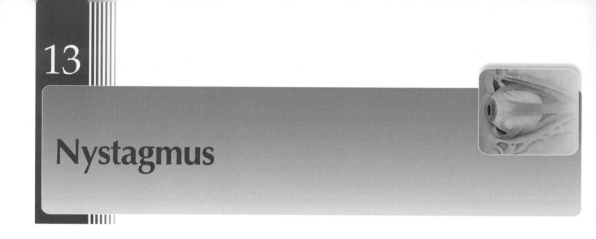

13

Nystagmus

Nystagmus is a regular, rhythmic, repetitive to and fro movement of the eyes. Movements which are not regular and rhythmic are called **nystagmoid movements.** It may be:

- Horizontal
- Vertical
- Rotatory
- Mixed

Description

Nystagmus is usually described on the basis of its **type, direction** (of fast component), **amplitude, frequency** or rate, **conjugacy, unilateral or bilateral** and presence or absence of **null zone.**

The two common types are **pendular** and **jerk** nystagmus (Fig. 13.1). Pendular nystagmus is a smooth sinusoidal oscillation, equal on both sides. Jerk nystagmus has a slow component and a fast component. It may be noted that the primary underlying abnormality causes the slow drift which is corrected by the fast component. However, a jerk nystagmus is characterised by the fast component.

The amplitude is the excursion of the nystagmus and is described as small or **fine** (less than 5°), **moderate** (5°–15°) and **large** (greater than 15°).

The **rate or frequency** is the number of to and fro movements in one second. It is described in cycles per second or Hertz (Hz).

It is **slow** (1–2 Hz), **medium** (3–4 Hz) or **fast** (5 Hz or more).

The **intensity of a nystagmus** is amplitude multiplied by frequency.

It is documented in the nine gazes graphically as shown in Fig. 13.1: *One sided arrow: Jerk Nystagmus; the direction indicating the direction of the fast component; bidirectional arrow: pendular nystagmus; Number of arrow heads: frequency; number of bars in arrow: amplitude; curved arrow: Torsional nystagmus.* Note the nystagmus changes in different gazes and it is documented as such in the different gaze positions in the diagram.

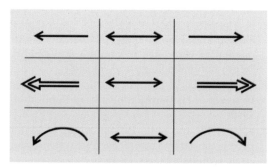

Fig. 13.1: Documenting nystagmus.

Alexander's law states that the amplitude of jerk nystagmus is largest in the gaze of the direction of fast component. Based on this principle **three degrees** of nystagmus are described.

First degree: Nystagmus only in the gaze in the direction of the fast component.

Second degree: Nystagmus also in primary position gaze.

Third degree: Nystagmus in addition to the above two gazes is also present in the direction of slow component.

The jerk nystagmus may have a position when it cannot be elicited. This is the **null zone.** The **neutral zone** is the point where the direction (of fast component) of nystagmus changes from one side to the other. It may be different than the null zone or may be the same. Patients with null zone assume a **head posture** such that eyes are in the null zone. This may be changing periodically over a period of 3–7 minutes and this should be observed constantly to identify a **Periodic Alternating Nystagmus(PAN)** (Fig. 13.2). The head posture can measured by using a scale and protractor as shown in Fig. 13.3.

The nystagmus is mostly **binocular,** rarely it is **uniocular** as in internuclear ophthalmoplegia. Sometimes it is **asymmetric** as in spasmus nutans.

A nystagmus which is symmetric in direction, amplitude, and rate is called **conjugate** when it differs in any one or more parameter, it is called **dissociated.**

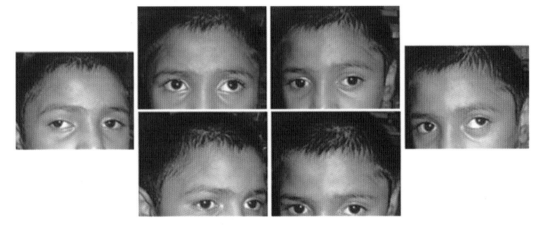

Fig. 13.2: Changing head posture—Periodic alternating nystagmus.

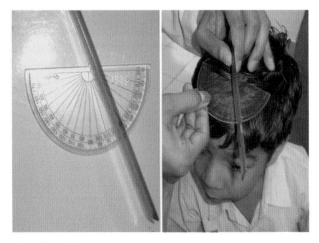

Fig. 13.3: Measuring face turn using scale and protractor.

13

The jerk nystagmus is illustrated by an arrow with dashed lines for the slow component and an unbroken arrow for the fast component. The thickness of the arrow indicates its amplitude and the number of oblique lines on the arrow indicates the frequency. A pendular nystagmus is shown by a bidirectional arrow.

Vertical jerk nystagmus may be **upbeat** (fast component upwards) or **downbeat** (fast component downwards). They are illustrated by arrows upwards or downwards, respectively.

Rotatory nystagmus is shown by curved arrows clockwise or anti-clockwise.

The terms **sensory nystagmus** and **motor nystagmus** were suggested by Cogan. Though most sensory nystagmus (due to poor visual potential) are pendular and most motor nystagmus are jerk nystagmus, this is not always true.

Classification of Nystagmus

- Physiologic nystagmus
  1. End-point nystagmus
  2. Vestibular (caloric or rotational) nystagmus
  3. Optokinetic nystagmus
  4. Voluntary nystagmus

- Pathologic nystagmus.

  A. Nystagmus associated with poor vision (sensory) due to
   a. Retinal diseases (retinoblastoma, retinopathy of prematurity, persistent hyperplastic primary vitreous, retinal dysplasia, Leber's congenital amaurosis, tapetoretinal degeneration, coloboma, retinoschisis, congenital stationary night blindness, achromatopsia, albinism, intrauterine infections like rubella, toxoplasma, etc.)
   b. Optic nerve hypoplasia (Demorsier's syndrome and ONH)

   c. Anterior segment pathology (cataract, mesodermal dysgenesis, aniridia).
  B. Nystagmus associated with neurologic diseases (motor)
  1. Endgaze paretic nystagmus (horizontal gaze center).
  2. Convergence retractorious (vertical gaze, Parinaud's)
  3. Vestibular
   a. Nystagmus central (brainstem nuclei)
   b. Peripheral (labyrinths, VIII CN)
  4. Downbeat (cervicomedullary junction)
  5. Upbeat (cerebellum (vermis), medulla)
  6. Seesaw nystagmus (parasellar lesions)
  7. Periodic alternating nystagmus (acquired).
  C. Nystagmus associated with strabismus
  1. Latent/Manifest-latent nystagmus
  2. Manifest nystagmus
  3. Nystagmus blockage syndrome
  D. Miscellaneous
  1. Spasmus nutans
  2. Manifest nystagmus (congenital motor nystagmus)
  3. Periodic alternating nystagmus.
  E. Nystagmoid conditions
  1. Oculopalatal myoclonus
  2. Opsoclonus
  3. Ocular bobbing
  4. Heimann-Bielschowsky's unilateral vertical bobbing.

Role of Family History

The most common heritable transmission of nystagmus is X-linked. Autosomal dominant is also likely but autosomal recessive is rare. Family history of nystagmus with good vision or poor vision could differentiate hereditary motor nystagmus from conditions with poor vision. Certain conditions like Tay-Sach's occur in ethnic communities like Ashkenazi Jews.

Role of Perinatal History

History of intrauterine infection (rubella, toxoplasma), maternal alcohol abuse or anticonvulsant drugs (optic nerve hypoplasia), neonatal asphyxia or neonatal seizures (cerebral damage) are very helpful.

Systemic Features

Certain systemic features are helpful in diagnosis. Irritability, vomiting, bulging fontanelles may suggest raised intracranial pressure especially in infants after 6 months. Ataxia, seizures or strabismus may indicate posterior fossa disease. Short stature with delayed growth is associated with optic nerve hypoplasia in De Morsier's syndrome. Fair skin with light colored irides suggest albinism. Marked photophobia should indicate achromatopsia. Facial asymmetry, malposition of ears, dental anomalies, skin tags, digital abnormalities (supernumerary, missing or fused fingers) and developmental delay are all associated findings.

Ocular Findings

Visual assessment should be made whenever possible. Pendular nystagmus may have 6/60 or better vision whereas nystagmoid movements have still poorer vision. Brisk pupils are good prognostic signs. A paradoxic pupillary response on "light-off" is seen in cases of congenital stationary night blindness, achromatopsia, optic nerve hypoplasia, and some other conditions with visual potential. After switching off the light, the "paradoxic" pupil constricts in the first 20 seconds and starts dilating after 60 seconds. The ocular features listed in the table in the anterior segment and posterior segment should be looked for.

NYSTAGMUS ASSOCIATED WITH NEUROLOGIC DISORDERS

A brief note is given here.

1. **Gaze paretic nystagmus** is due to parieto-occipital, cerebellar or brainstem lesions affecting conjugate gaze mechanism. It is more coarse than the physiologic end point nystagmus and starts before the extreme gazes compared to them.

2. **Convergence retraction nystagmus** is due to congenital aqueductal stenosis with pinealoma or hydrocephalus in infants. In adults it is due to pretectal, tectal infracts or other lesions.

   An association of paralysis of upgaze, sometimes paralysis of downgaze also, defective convergence, light-near dissociation (pupillary reflexes to accommodation present but lost to light) lid retraction and accommodation spasm, along with repetitive convergence and retraction on attempted upgaze is described as **Parinaud's syndrome.** Such cases require neurosurgery.

3. **Vestibular nystagmus** may be central vestibular or peripheral vestibular. Both are horizontal jerk and rotatory nystagmus on lateral gaze, usually to the side opposite to the lesion. The central vestibular nystagmus have no vertigo, tinnitus or deafness and are usually due to demyelinating diseases, vascular accidents, encephalitis or tumour. The peripheral vestibular nystagmus are due to lesions of labyrinths or VIII cranial nerve. These are intermittent and last for minutes, days or weeks. Fixation tends to decrease the intensity. Vertigo, tinnitus or deafness may be associated. **Oscillopsia** (or perception of spinning around the world) is present.

4. **Periodic alternating nystagmus** (acquired) has a cyclic change of fast component direction. It lasts for about 90 seconds in one direction and then changes after 10–20 seconds pause. It is seen in chronic otitis, albinism, cerebellar compression. Baclofen is helpful in symptomatic patients.

5. **Downbeat nystagmus** is characterised by a jerk nystagmus with fast component downwards. It is due to structural lesions in cervicomedullary junction. Alcohol and

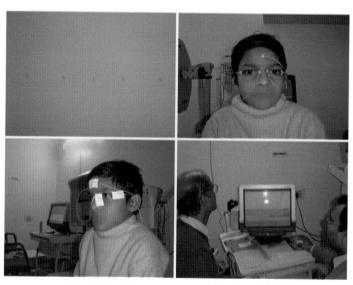

Fig. 13.4: Electronystagmography (ENG)

anticonvulsant consumption can also elicit this.

6. **Upbeat nystagmus** on convergence may convert to downbeat nystagmus. It is due to congenital lesions of cerebellar vermis, medullar or post-meningitis.

7. **See-saw nystagmus** is a special pendular and torsional nystagmus, the eye rises and intorts as the fellow eye falls and extorts resembling a see-saw. It may be congenital or secondary to parasellar tumours expanding within the third ventricle. Usually bitemporal hemianopia is present. Magnetic resonance imaging (MRI) should be done in postneurosurgical symptomatic cases. Baclofen and clonazepam has been tried with some success.

NYSTAGMUS ASSOCIATED WITH STRABISMUS

Three types of non-neurologic nystagmus are associated with strabismus. The most common type is **manifest nystagmus** but amongst the cases of strabismus the most common type is **manifest-latent nystagmus.** A third type **nystagmus blockage syndrome** is a very distinctive type of nystagmus. Another nystagmus presenting to strabismologists is Spasmus nutans with features of Torticollis,

Head nodding and dysconjugate or different eyemovements in the two eyes. These present in infancy and should be subjected to imaging to exclude gliomas of optic nerve or chiasma. If imaging is normal they may have a benign course and resolve by the second or third year.

Electronystagmography

The nystagmus is documented by electronystagmography (ENG), a type of electrooculography using electrodes placed at the medial and lateral canthi (Fig. 13.4) or using infrared camera in **videonystagmography (VNG)** (Fig. 13.5).

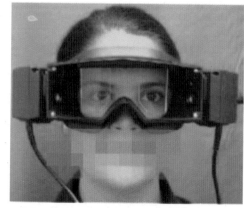

Fig. 13.5: Videonystagmography (VNG).

The ENG tracings depict the movements of the eyes: upward deflection indicates a right sided movement and downward deflection, a left sided movement; the slow component is further studied for its being constant velocity, accelerating velocity or decelerating velocity, (Fig. 13.6). The changes in different gazes are documented as increasing or decreasing in dextroversion or levoversion (Fig. 13.7).

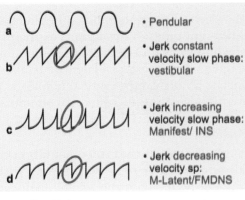

Fig. 13.6: ENG and underlying defects.

Underlying Defects

Three underlying defects have been identified in the slow-eye movement (SEM) subsystem to produce nystagmus.

a. **High-gain instability** in the SEM subsystem results in **accelerating** (increasing velocity) slow phase of the jerk nystagmus or in a pendular nystagmus. Seen in manifest nystagmus (Fig. 13.6c).

b. **Vestibular tone imbalance.** Asymmetric vestibular input on an inherently normal horizontal gaze generator results in a **linear** (constant velocity) slow phase, reflecting a persistent tone to drive the eyes towards the side of "affected" vestibular apparatus. The slow-phase amplitude is reduced by fixation and enhanced by darkness, night, plus lenses or closing eyes. Seen in vestibular nystagmus (13.6b).

c. **Integrator leak.** A leaky integrator causes the eyes to drift away to an eccentric gaze with a **decelerating** (decreasing velocity) slow phase. It is seen in gaze-evoked or gazeparetic nystagmus and in manifest latent nystagmus (13.6d).

Manifest Nystagmus

Manifest nystagmus is called "manifest" as it is present without cover and does not increase on covering either eye. It is usually called "congenital" nystagmus; but is rarely seen at birth, usually in first few months only, so actually it is "infantile" nystagmus (Fig. 13.7). The **characteristics** are:

1. Almost always bilateral and conjugate in direction and frequency.
2. Uniplanar: usually horizontal, even on up and downgazes. Rarely vertical or torsional.
3. Similar amplitude on both sides. The slow phase has increasing velocity = accelerating slow phase.

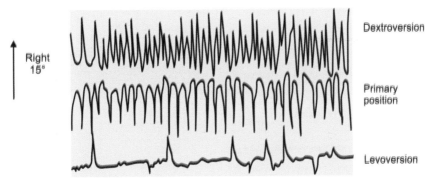

Fig. 13.7: Electronystagmography, ENG in manifest or infantile nystagmus.

4. Distinctive wave forms: Jerk/pendular/mixed. These may vary in different gaze positions, and can vary at different times as they evolve.
5. Dampened by convergence, so near vision is better.
6. Accentuated by fixation effort and improves on eye closure.
7. No oscillopsia.
8. A null-zone is often present and the head posture is assumed to bring the eyes in null zone.
9. Associated head nodding is seen in some cases but unlike true spasmus nutans, it does not offer significant visual gain. It is more like an associated tremor of cephalomotor system.
10. Disappears during sleep or general anesthesia.
11. Inversion of OKN, i.e. on eliciting OKN response the direction of fast component same as that of drum and amplitude accentuated.

Nystagmus blockage syndrome (NBS) and periodic alternating nystagmus are variants of manifest nystagmus.

Latent or Manifest Latent Nystagmus

Latent nystagmus is elicited only on covering the dominant eye. Sometimes a nystagmus is manifest but accentuates on covering the dominant eyes, it is termed manifest-latent nystagmus (Fig. 13.8). Electronystagmographically both are similar differing only in degree.

It presents as a conjugate, symmetrical, horizontal nystagmus with a **decelerating** slow phase. The slow phase of the viewing eye is directed towards the nose (temporal to nasal) causing the fast component to be in the direction of the viewing eye (temporally).

The electronystagmography differentiates the different types of nystagmus explicitly. According to Dell'Osso, 80% of congenital nystagmus is manifest, 15% latent or manifest latent and 5% of mixed variety. While 40–50% of manifest nystagmus have strabismus, 95% of manifest latent nystagmus have strabismus.

It may be noted that documentation of small angle squint may be difficult with nystagmus while charting visual acuity in manifest-latent/latent type it should be noted that eyes are not covered alternately, but a + 6.0 or to + 8.0 D dioptre lens applied before the other eye. Polaroid dissociation can also be used to chart visual acuity of each eye under binocular conditions. The differences between MN and MLN as distinguished by von Noorden are given in Table 13.1.

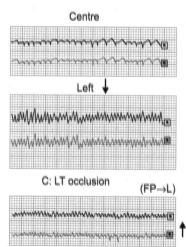

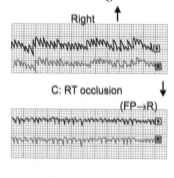

Fig. 13.8: Manifest latent nystagmus (fusional maldevelopment nystagmus).

Table 13.1: Differences between MN and MLN (von Noorden)

Manifest (MN)	Manifest latent (MLN)
1. Biphasic, mostly pendular	1. Jerk mostly, or mixed
2. No change on abduction	2. Increased on abduction
3. Accelerating slowphase	3. Decelerating slow phase
4. No change on covering one eye	4. Increase on covering one-eye
5. Direction independent of fixing eye but may change on either side of null zone	5. Fast phase always towards fixing eye
6. Less commonly associated with infantile esotropia (10–50%)	6. Nearly always associated with infantile esotropia (95%)
7. Binocular visual acuity same as uniocular	7. Binocular visual acuity better than monocular VA.

Nystagmus Blockage Syndrome (NBS)

This is a special form of nystagmus which has an **inverse relationship** with esotropia. Esotropia is a mechanism of "blocking" the nystagmus. As the eye abducts the nystagmus amplitude becomes marked and on adduction as the eye gets locked into an esotropia, the nystagmus gets eliminated. The fixing eye is preferred to be in adduction so that the face turn is in the direction of fixing eye.

It is important to distinguish manifest latent nystagmus with infantile esotropia from NBS. The following differences are to be noted for NBS:

1. Amplitude of nystagmus and degree of esotropia are inversely related to each other.
2. If one eye is patched there is a face turn to the opposite side, to keep the fixing eye in adduction. This reverses on patching the eye.
3. Thirdly, if a base out prism is placed in front of the fixing (adducted) eye, in NBS the eye remains in adduction and esotropia increases, while in infantile esotropia, the eye moves out as the esotropia gets neutralised.

Congenital Periodic Alternating Nystagmus

The nystagmus manifests with the fast phase beating in one direction for 90–120 seconds and then after a pause of 10–20 seconds, it switches its direction to the opposite side which again lasts for 90–120 seconds, which

again reverses. With each alternation the face turn also keeps alternating, (cf NBS in which the alternation occurs only on alternate covering of fixing eye not spontaneously). This condition whenever seen should always exclude the possibility of Arnold Chiari malformation which also presents with PAN.

Treatment of Nystagmus Associated with Strabismus

The exclusion of neurologic conditions in any nystagmus in which the history indicates an acquired nature should always be remembered. In the non-neurologic causes the treatment may be:

a. *Nonsurgical*
   1. Optical devices
      - Glasses
      - Contact lenses
      - Prisms
   2. Occlusion and pleoptics
   3. Medical treatment
   4. Acupuncture
   5. Auditory biofeedback
   6. Botulinum toxin
b. *Surgical*
   1. To shift the null position to primary position
      - Modified Kestenbaum surgery
   2. To induce adduction/convergence
      - Bimedial rectus recession/faden.

13

3. To reduce the amplitude of nystagmus
   - Supramaximal recession or faden on all horizontal recti

Non-surgical Treatment

The use of optical devices has a rational basis. **Overminus lenses** stimulate accommodative convergence and thus dampen the nystagmus. **Contact lenses** are helpful in high refractive errors by giving good visual stimulus for fusional control. In albinism **tinted glasses** or tinted contact lenses, as also in aniridia and aphakia, help by increasing optical blur. A combination of spectacles with contact lenses help in stabilization of retinal image.

The role of soft contact lenses may be by acting by offering a sensory feedback by stimulating the ophthalmic division of oculomotor nerve. Similarly, **acupuncture** applied to the sternocleidomastoid muscles may work to reduce nystagmus. This was observed by the author in a study with the dampening of nystagmus on inserting and twirling the acupuncture needles, but the recordable effect is short-lived (Figs 13.9 and 13.10).

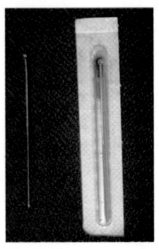

Fig. 13.10: Acupuncture needle.

Prisms can be used for **two** purposes, one to induce fusional convergence by using 7-prism dioptre base out prism in front of each eye.

The other purpose of prisms may be in the preoperative evaluation in a patient with face turn. The prisms are inserted with the **apex in the preferred direction of gaze (base towards face turn).** Thus for a face turn to left, with null in dextroversion, a prism base-in in

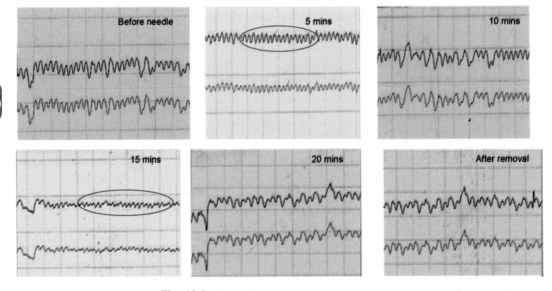

Fig. 13.9: Effect of acupuncture in nystagmus.

front of right eye and base-out prisms in front of left eye, should be used. While prisms are useful for a diagnostic trial in this manner, as a therapeutic alternative they are not helpful. This is because the face turn is usually more than 30–45 pd, and use of such large prisms, even with Fresnel prisms, induces optical aberrations.

Pleoptics by both Bangerter's and Cupper's methods have reported to be beneficial, though this has not been universally accepted. In cases of strabismic amblyopia, any method to improve amblyopia has been found to be effective in decreasing nystagmus. In the past, latent nystagmus was considered as a contraindication to **conventional occlusion** and inverse occlusion was suggested. However, trials with conventional occlusion have been found to be effective in spite of initially increasing the nystagmus. As the amblyopia gets corrected and vision improves, the nystagmus finally decreases.

Penalization with neutral density filters or atropinization may also be used in cases marked by increased amplitude on covering the dominant eye. This may be combined with occlusion.

Auditory biofeedback an attempt to reinforce the ocular motor system by extraocular (auditory) stimulus, have been found to be effective by some workers. The role of Auditory biofeedback was studied by the author with the nystagmus patient made to hear his own audio-conversion of the electronystagmography. This dampened the nystagmus during the period of hearing only with no long term effect. Continuing effects a constant auditory biofeedback with special glasses fitted with an infrared device to detect nystagmus and provide auditory biofeedback may be required (Fig. 13.11).

Medical treatment has eluded a cure. Baclofen is effective in acquired PAN and barbiturates and 5-hydroxytryptophan have been tried by some workers in manifest nystagmus.

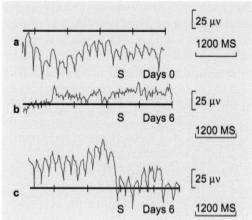

Fig. 13.11: Role of auditory biofeedback—Effect only during the therapy. *(Sharma et al J AAPOS 2000;4: 287–90).*

Botulinum injection in the retrobulbar space has shown to have some subjective relief but requires evaluation. The effect is however short lived and repeated injections would be costly and undesirable.

Surgical Management

As outlined earlier, the surgery for nystagmus is based on **three principles:**

1. To shift the null position, if any, to the primary position.
2. To induce extraconvergence innervation by weakening medial recti, to dampen nystagmus.
3. To reduce the amplitude of the nystagmus by weakening the muscle force of all recti.

Modified Kestenbaum Surgery

Cases of nystagmus that have a null point (other than the primary position) assume a head posture. Surgery of horizontal recti shifts this null point to the primary position. It is indicated in cases that have atleast 20% face turn.

Kestenbaum devised the first surgical approach using recession-resection of all four horizontal recti. He advocated an equal amount of 5 mm for all recti. For a left face turn (null in dextroversion) lateral rectus recession and medial rectus resection of right eye combined with medial rectus recession and lateral rectus resection of left eye is done. Anderson advocated only recessions (Fig. 13.12), thus recessions of right lateral rectus and left medial rectus is done for left face turn. Goto for a similar case advocated resecting the yoke muscles, that is resections of right medial rectus and left lateral rectus.

Later several **modifications** of the Kestenbaum regime have been tried. Parks recommended lesser amount for recessions and for medial rectus surgery compared to lateral rectus surgery. Thus he advocated a 5,

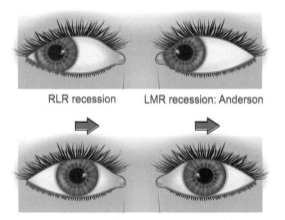

RLR recession   LMR recession: Anderson

Fig. 13.12: Planning for Anderson—Kestenbaum.

6, 7, 8 plan, where recession of medial rectus is 5 mm, resection of medial rectus 6 mm, recession of lateral rectus 7 mm and resection of lateral rectus is 8 mm. von Noorden endorses the same view.

Calhoun and Harley augment the Parks recommendation by additional 2 mm for a 45 degree face turn (i.e. 7, 8, 9, 10 mm). We have got succesful shift of eccentric null position of about 30 degrees by Augmented Anderson's procedure of the yoke muscles (9 mm MR and 12 mm LR recession). For larger 45 degrees eccentric null positions we add the resections (6 mm of MR and 9 mm of LR) of the opposite recti to the above mentioned Augmented Anderson's procedure (Fig. 13.13). In cases of PAN there may be reversal of head posture after this procedure requiring the opposite yoke muscles to be similarly recessed making it a four muscle supramaximal recession (Fig. 13.14).

Some authors perform retroequatorial myopexy (faden) on the recessed muscles for more effect. Any associated squint has to be corrected by making suitable adjustments in the plan.

Vertical Kestenbaum

On the same principle, vertical muscles have been recessed and resected for chin elevation

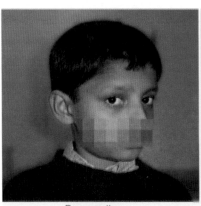
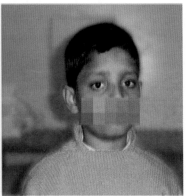

Preoperative   Postoperative 3 months

Fig. 13.13: Augmented Anderson procedure.

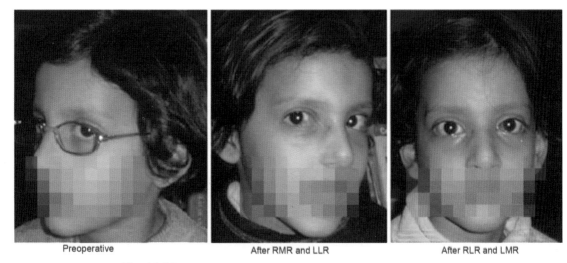

| Preoperative | After RMR and LLR | After RLR and LMR |

Fig. 13.14: PAN—Four Horizontal recti supramaximal recessions.

or depression of 25° or more. For a chin elevation 4 mm resection of both superior recti and 4 mm recession of both inferior recti is suggested. For lesser chin elevations only recession part may be done. For chin depression the surgical plan is reversed with superior rectus recessions and inferior rectus resections (Figs 13.15 and 13.16).

Torsional Kestenbaum

Cases which have a significant **head tilt** have a torsional null position, and shifting the null

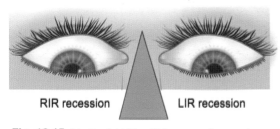

RIR recession   LIR recession

Fig. 13.15: Vertical AHP—Chin up and eyes down.

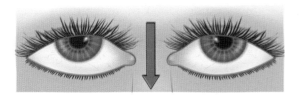

Fig. 13.16: Vertical AHP chin down eyes rolled up.

position by torsional Kestenbaum, is suggested. Three modalities are advocated:

i. The simplest but less effective regime is to **vertically shift the horizontal recti.** For head tilt to right shoulder, the right lateral rectus is shifted up, right medial rectus down. Left medial rectus up and left lateral rectus down.

ii. von Noorden has advocated **shifting the vertical recti horizontally.** It is an effective procedure but runs an inherent risk of anterior segment ischemia in the event of horizontal recti surgery also required, then itself or later. For right sided tilt the right superior rectus is shifted nasally, right inferior rectus temporally, left superior rectus temporally and left inferior rectus nasally.

iii. The third modality is **selective advancement and recession of the anterior fibres of the four obliques.** This approach is technically more difficult but advocated by us, in view of effectivity and no risk of anterior segment ischemia (Fig. 13.17). For a head tilt to right side; advancement of right inferior oblique, recession of right superior oblique, advancement of left inferior oblique and recession of left superior oblique, all by 8 mm, is done. It

13

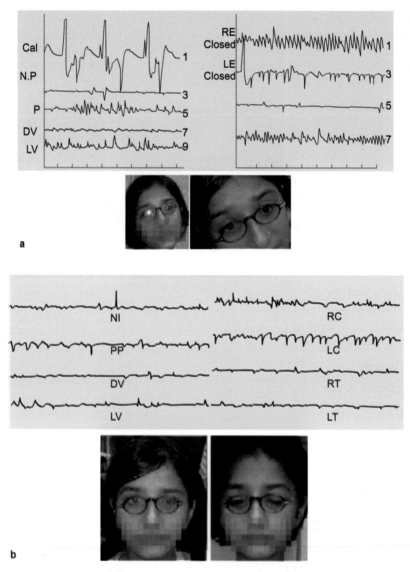

Fig. 13.17: A composite electronystagmogram (ENG) in a case of congenital nystagmus with head tilt to left side. (a) Preoperatively a null was recorded in right head tilt position. (b) Postoperative after the respective oblique muscle surgery.

has been shown to be effective by the shifting of the torsional null to primary position on electronystagmography. **Posterior fixation** and **recession** of medial recti in cases of nystagmus blockage syndrome is an effective surgery. We do not recommmend faden operation on all four horizontal recti to dampen nystagmus. A deliberate plan for more exodeviation postoperatively may be tried in cases with good fusional potential. **Supramaximal recession** of all four horizontal recti has been reported to be effective in lessening the amplitude of nystagmus, without decreasing the extreme ductions or versions. This surgery is useful and really indicated only in cases which have no definite null position. Cases with pendular nystagmus with relatively good visual potential may be a good indication.

Other Surgical Approaches

The retroequatorial myopexy of all four recti, disinsertions of all recti or criss-crossing the adjacent recti to produce impediments to motility or fixating of recti to the orbital periosteum are not desirable approaches, and not recommended. Recently we compared the results of the supramaximal recessions of all four horizontal recti and the Hertle Dell'Osso procedure (disinserting and reinserting the four horizontal recti without any recession or resection) in cases with no eccentric null. We found the two procedures to be equally effective for short durations of about a few months but with no long term results.

Suggested Reading

1. Bagolini B, Penne A and Zanai MR. Ocular nystagmus: some interpretational aspects and methods of treatment. Int. Ophthalmol. 6: 37, 1983.
2. Ciancia. AO; On infantile esotropia with nystagmus in abduction. J.Pediatr. Ophthalmol. Strabismus. 32, 280, 1995.
3. Conrad HG and de Decker W. Torsional Kestenbaum procedure: evolution of a surgical concept. In Reinecke, R.D. editor. Strabismus II orlando, Fla. 1982. Grune and Stratton. p. 301.
4. Dell'Osso LF, Schmidt D, and Daroff R. Latent, manifest-latent and congenital nystagmus. Clin. Vis. Sci. 3: 229, 1988.
5. Dell'Osso LF. Congenital, latent or manifest latent nystagmus. Similarities, differences and relation to strabismus. Jpn. J. Ophthalmol. 29: 351, 1985.
6. Jayalakshmi P, Scott, TFM Tucker SH and Schaffer DB. Infantile nystagmus: a prospective study of spasmus nutans, congenital nystagmus, and unclassified nystagmus of infancy, J. Pediatr. 77: 177, 1970.
7. Noorden GK von Munoz M and Wong SY. Compensatory mechanisms in congenital nystagmus Am. J. Ophthalmol. 95: 387, 1987.
8. Noorden GK von and Wong SY Surgical results in nystagmus blockage syndrome. Ophthalmology. 93:1028, 1986.
9. Noorden GK von, and Sprunger DT. Large rectus muscle recession for the treatment of congenital nystagmus. Arch Ophthalmol. 109: 221, 1991.
10. Yee RD, Wong EK, Baloh RW and Honrubia VA study of congenital nystagmus wave forms. Neurology. 26: 326, 1976.
11. Zubcov AA, Reinecke RD, Gottlob I, Manley DR and Calhoun JH. Treatment of manifest latent nystagmus. Am. J. Ophthalmol. 110: 160, 1990.
12. Zubcov AA, Stark N, Weber A, Wizov SS and Reinecke RD. Improvement of visual acuity after surgery for nystagmus. Ophthalmology. 100: 1488, 1993.

13

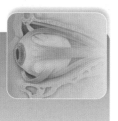

Non-Surgical Management

Management in a case of strabismus may be **surgical or non-surgical.** While many cases require surgical management, almost all will require some non-surgical modality either before surgery, after surgery or both. The quality of non-surgical management reflects the outcome of surgical management also, as the effect of surgery may be mended or spoilt by it. The non-surgical management comprises of:

a. **Optical correction**
   - Refraction and proper prescription including use of bifocals
   - Use of prisms

b. **Orthoptic treatment**
   1. Combating suppression
   2. Managing anomalous retinal correspondence (ARC)
   3. Treatment of amblyopia including pleoptics
   4. Improving fusional vergences and stereopsis

c. **Medical treatment**
   - Topical drugs like miotics, cycloplegics
   - Systemic drugs like levodopa, baclofen
   - Chemodenervation with botulinum toxin.

A. OPTICAL CORRECTION

The first step in the treatment of strabismus is the optical treatment:
   i. It helps to provide a sharp well focussed retinal image which helps fusional control

and proper development of binocular vision.
   ii. Secondly, it corrects and maintains the relationship between accommodation and convergence mechanisms.

A case of amblyopia therapy cannot begin without the proper optical rehabilitation, both for distance and near. A proper prescription even helps a hyperope with intermittent exotropia to facilitate fusional control. While an accommodative esotrope with hyperopia is helped because of relaxation of his excess accommodative convergence.

Proper Cycloplegia

The accommodative convergence mechanisms are so intricately linked that in any case of motility defect or eye strain, the correct refractive status needs to be assessed. This should be done after fully relaxing the accommodation. In children under 8–9 years this is very strong and it is best to use atropine 1% ointment. The use of milder cycloplegics for the sake of exigency or a "shortcut" is undesirable and an injustice to a child. This is really so in the case of dark iris children like ours, as the accommodational tone is stronger than in the light coloured eyes. Atropine 1% ointment is used thrice a day, in rice-grain size applications, for three consecutive days preceding the day of refraction. The use of atropine **drops** is associated with systemic toxicity as they are absorbed through the nasal mucosa. A drop (in each eye) of 1% atropine may contain 0.5 mg atropine, which is almost the adult dose! (The dose for resuscitation of the infant or child is 0.01–0.03 mg/kg only). Manoeuvres like blocking the lacrimal puncta are easier said than done, and so its best to use ointment. The risk of allergy to the ointment itself is rare. The systemic toxicity can be limited if the instruction of rice grain size is noted. It will be extremely rare to see a case who develops systemic effects with the above regime.

In older children with accommodative esotropia also it is advisable to use atropine ointment in cases of doubt (residual variable angle esotropia after milder cycloplegics). Otherwise Homatropine 2%, or Cyclopentolate 1% can be used. The relaxation of accommodation can be checked in older children by their inability to read N-5 on near vision chart (unless they are myopes) or by near-distance retinoscopy (Table 14.1).

Proper Prescription

Prescription should be generally based on the retinoscopy without resorting to under or over-corrections. These may however be indicated in managing small angle esotropia or exotropia, especially after surgery, either residual or consecutive. This is however a temporising measure and needs to be monitored. In every young infant with accommodative esotropia with hyperopia, full correction is advocated, in case of doubt a slight induced myopia may do no harm but a residual esotropia is not desirable. In **infants without esotropia** a refractive error of plus 1 or 2 dioptres may not necessarily be prescribed, as argued by some workers, in the interest of emmetropisation.

A **proper prescription** is usually accepted by children, unless the frame is uncomfortable. Proper attention sould be given to the size, the nasal bridge and the ear supports. Harness frames and elastic tubings which comfortably wind around the infants ears are helpful. It should be noted that the child does not "peek" from the sides of the glasses. Even small infants 3 months onwards comfortably wear glasses, the hesitation is mostly from the parents, who need to be explained properly. After prescription and

Table 14.1: Cycloplegic agents					
Cycloplegic	Instillation regime	On set of peak effect	Duration of peak effect	Retinoscopy allowed	Normal recovery
1. Atropine sulphate 1% ointment	Rice grain size thrice a day for 3 days	18 hour after last instillation	24 hours	3–4 days	10–14 days
2. Scopolamine hydrobromide 0.2%, 0.5%	2 drops 30 min. apart	40 min. after 2nd drop	90 min.	3 days	8 days
3. Homatropine hydrobromide 2%	6–8 drops 10–15 min. apart	40 min. after 2nd drop	50 min.	6 hours	36 hours
4. Cyclopentolate hydrochloride 0.5%, 1%	2 drops 5 min. apart	25 min. after 2nd drop	15 min.	3 hours	18 hours
5. Tropicamide 0.5%, 1%	2 drops 5 min. apart	20 minutes after 2nd drop	45 min.	45 min.	4 hours
6. Combination of • Proparacine 0.4% • Tropicamide 1% • Cyclopentolate 2%	1 drop of each 30 seconds apart	20 min. after last drop	20 min.	4 hours	24–48 hours

14

fitting, regular six-monthly check-ups for vision and at least an annual check of retinoscopy is desirable to adjust for the refractive changes.

Use of cycloplegic drugs is made to relax the accommodation so that the hyperopic glasses are accepted readily. It is best to prescribe a preschool child while he is still under atropine cycloplegia without waiting for post-cycloplegic acceptance.

Bifocals

While refractive accommodative esotropia responds dramatically to their distance hyperopic correction, cases with high AC/A ratio require bifocals, with additional near adds.

The minimum add required is tested in steps of 0.5 D till the convergence excess for near is controlled. A maximum of plus 3.5 dioptre may be required. The type of bifocal should be specified. An executive type, half segment near add is desired, with the lower segment at least covering half of the pupil. This is to ensure the use of near add for all near tasks.

Use of Overminus Glasses

After the suggestion of Jampolsky, overminus glasses have been used by some in cases of intermittent exotropia in under 5 years children. This is helpful in cases with high AC/A ratio, and utilises the accommodative convergence for controlling the exodeviation. This is at best a short-term modality and has found support because of unpredictable results of surgery in intermittent exotropias in very young children with the fear of consecutive esotropia and its consequences of suppression-amblyopia.

Unusually an **inverse bifocal** with a **minus add for near** is required for a convergence insufficiency type of exotropia.

Use of Prisms

The diagnostic use of prism is well understood. Prisms have also been used in

therapy, though not very popular. The reasons for this are:
- Undesirable optical aberrations induced.
- Deterioration of quality of vision.
- Glasses become heavier and unacceptable cosmetically:
  - Plastic and Fresnel membrane prisms are not easily available and expensive as they are susceptible to scratches.

However, small angle deviations, especially residual or consecutive deviations after surgery can be managed during follow-up. Small vertical deviations are also well managed by them. The deviations should be constant and having little incomitance. Usually up to 7–8 prism dioptres (pd) prisms over each eye can be tolerated with glass prisms. With Fresnel prisms up to 25–30 pd may be accepted.

The prisms can be used for combined horizontal and vertical deviations by using prisms rotated obliquely (with horizontal and vertical vectors) as per nomograms. Prismatic effect can also be induced by decentration of spherical glasses especially if the power of glasses is high.

(Prismatic effect induced (pd) = Power of glasses × decentration in cm)

Prisms for Convergence Insufficiency

Apart from correcting deviations, prisms can also be used for fusional convergence insufficiency. These are likes "crutches" and should be used with undercorrection, so that the effort to converge is not fully given-up but strengthened. Gradually they can be tapered off.

Prisms for ARC

Prisms have also been used in anomalous retinal correspondence to alter sensory adaptations. However, this is a restricted use. Jampolsky suggested the use of Prism Adaptation Test (PAT). Esotropes with ARC have been shown to have the phenomenon of "eating-up" prisms, i.e. they require more and more prismatic power each time as they get used to the earlier neutralization. Cases which have "eating-up" prisms require augmented surgery for alignment, compared to cases which are stable.

B. ORTHOPTIC TREATMENT

The orthoptic treatment is indicated for:
- Combating suppression (antisuppression exercises).
- Managing ARC.
- Treatment of amblyopia including pleoptics.
- Improving fusional vergences and establishing stereopsis

Recently, while office orthoptics may be becoming less popular, **home vision therapy** (HVT) is becoming more popular. The role of active vision exercises is an essential part of the strabismology. Orthoptics does not eliminate the deviations but alters the sensory status to make the subject more capable of overcoming the existing deviation. A trained orthoptist is required to handle special situations, but a strabismologist should be able to comprehend and supervise the orthoptic management or he would become a tool in the hands of the orthoptist.

I. Antisuppression Exercises

While suppression may sometimes be desirable in the interest of an uncorrectable or cosmetically acceptable squint, at other times for a functional binocular vision, antisuppression exercises are required. Without going into the types and extent of suppression, suffice to say, that antisuppression exercises are directed in combating foveal suppression. The basic principle is to bring the fovea out of suppression, by differential stimulation favouring the non-dominant or suppressed fovea. Some methods are:
1. **Red filter** is used over the dominant eye and the subject given a task of threading red beads or drawing with red ink. A properly matched red would be invisible to the dominant eye and the task suitably exercises and reinforces the non-dominant eye.

2. **Cheiroscope** is another simple device in which the child is encouraged to trace figures, a mirror septum ensures that both the eyes are used in the task. The target is seen by dominant eye and the drawing surface by the "Suppressed" eye. The procedures utilized are:
   i. Simple drawings to be filled in by crayons
   ii. Tracings
   iii. Interactive games like tic-tac-toe with the therapist marking on the target and the child reciprocating on the drawing surface.
   iv. Increasing fusional vergences are also possible by shifting the drawing paper.

   In all these procedures it should be checked that the patient does not manage by "fast alternation."

3. **Pigeon-Cantonnet stereoscope** is a device based on the same principle of cheiroscope with three flaps with the middle flap having a mirror on one side. It can be used in two positions. In position 1, the two side flaps rest on the desk while the middle flap is vertical. This can be used to train relative convergence and relaxing accommodation, as the subject is made to fuse the two figures (visual axes parallel). In position 2 the right flap rests on desk while the left flaps makes an obtuse angle with the first and the middle flap bisects the angle. In this position the mirror on left side of mirror is used. A chart or figure seen on left flap is seen by left eye (dominant) eye and the right eye (amblyopic) is used to trace the figure on the right flap. It works like a cheiroscope.

4. **Synoptophores** are equipped to impart antisuppression exercises. Suitable slides can be used and the rheostat controls changed to relatively alter the stimulation

14

of two eyes. In addition flasher can be used either in the simultaneous mode or alternate flashing to make the patient appreciate the two images, which can be later fused. Cases with central scotoma in fovea can be taken care of by special techniques like chasing, macular massage (moving the visual target back and forth across the suppressed fovea).

5. **Physiologic diplopia** cases with less dense suppression, can appreciate physiologic diplopia (doubling of a near object when fixation held for distance and vice versa). This is a very useful prerequisite for fusional convergence home exercises.

6. **Bar-reading:** Binocular vision once regained can be maintained with the help of bar-readers. A simple foot ruler held in between the eyes and the book so that it blocks the view of each eye but the subject can read uninterrupted if both eyes are used simultaneously. Head movement should not be allowed. Other bar readers are zig-zag bar reader and Javal grid.

7. **Pleoptics** and **after image transfer techniques** are also a special form of anti-suppression exercise. Anti-suppression exercises should not be imparted to a person having intractable strabismus, who has fortunately learned to suppress. An intractable diplopia is something an orthoptist or strabismologist, does not get credit for.

II. Managing Anomalous Retinal Correspondence (ARC)

As discussed earlier, ARC is a binocular sensory adaptation. An ARC with a small angle deviation that is cosmetically acceptable, should not be treated. This is usually the case and ARC are sparingly disturbed. Cases which require surgery have to be tackled, first by breaking the ARC by occlusion, followed by surgical alignment and later binocular stimulation. Prismatic treatment has also been used in tackling ARC.

III. Treatment of Amblyopia

Amblyopia is a preventable ocular malady occurring due to deprivation of form vision and/or abnormal binocular interaction, which disrupts binocular vision in the sensitive age group of up to 6–7 years. It responds well if treated properly and timely.

The **modalities** of treatment of amblyopia are:

1. Amelioration of amblyopiogenic factor (proper visual rehabilitation)
2. Occlusion
3. Penalization
4. CAM vision stimulator
5. Pleoptics
6. Red filter treatment
7. Active vision therapy
8. Medical treatment

1. Amelioration of Amblyopiogenic Factor

Removal of the amblyopiogenic factor is an essential pre requisite followed by a proper visual rehabilitation both for distance and near. Needless to say that a uniocular (or bilateral) congenital (or traumatic) cataract has to be given both distance and near correction. While this is required prior to occlusion therapy, this may be the therapy for ametropic amblyopia, which do not require occlusion, unless there is a difference in vision in the two eyes (due to anisometropia or strabismus, associated).

2. Occlusion

Since 1743, when de Buffon first described occlusion, it has remained the sheet anchor therapy for amblyopia.

In this therapy the amblyopic eye is given a preferential chance of development, as the dominant eye is totally withheld from the binocular participation. A properly done occlusion with good compliance ensures an almost 100% success rate, especially if treated up to 7 years age. The success rate recedes with increasing age.

Types of occlusion

Occlusion has been classified into different types. In terms of light transmission it is of two types: total and partial occlusion.

a. **Total occlusion:** Which completely obscures both light and form vision and is the type usually advocated for moderate to severe amblyopia. A totally opaque patch can be used in different forms (Fig. 14.1):

  i. **Direct skin patch:** A cotton eye pad patched to the eye with the help of micropore plaster (two inch width). The micropore tape allows sweating and is better accepted.

    Commercially available "opticlude" or "coverlet" are too expensive so also are the commercially available eye pads. Simple eye pads can be made at home for daily use.

  ii. **Spectacle patch:** One glass is made opaque by applying plaster and opaque paper on front and back. A slight extension of the same is made on the lateral side of the glass to prevent side "peeking."

iii. **Doyne's occluder:** A black rubber occluder which sticks on the back of the spectacle glass by suction can also be used.

iv. **Pirate patch:** A black cloth stitched like a pirate patch is preferably sported by some children.

  v. **Contact lenses:** Which are opaque can be used by children who want to avoid the look of an occlusion patch. The tolerance of contact lens is an additional factor and it needs to be worn for full waking hours for good effect.

Use of ground glass by some ophthalmologists needs to be condemned as they can be harmful rather than being useful as they acts as a "Diffusor" almost like a unilateral cataract.

b. **Partial occlusion:** This degrades the vision of the normal (dominant) eye such that the amblyopic eye has the advantage. This is a form of penalization and is used for milder amblyopia or in recovered cases for maintenance of binocular vision. It also

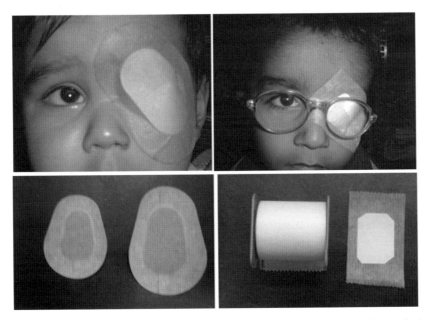

14

Fig. 14.1: Occlusion—eye patches. Direct skin patch, opticlude (left) and home made occlusion patch with spectacles (right).

requires correction of factors like squint anisometropia or aniseikonia suitably. The advantage over total occlusion of this modality is that it offers binocular stimulation. Layers of transparent scotch tape or colorless nail varnish can be applied on the back surface of the glass of dominant eye.

Another way of differentiating occlusion is on the **basis of duration or period of occlusion:**

a. **Full time occlusion:** All waking hours virtually 24 hours.

b. **Part-time occlusion:** This is for graduated duration, different waking hours of the day on the basis of age of the child.

Duration of occlusion: Full time occlusion is advocated by us. It is advised for full day (24 hours) for:

- 2 days up to 2 years old
- 3 days for 3 years old
- 4 days for 4 years old
- 5 days for 5 years old
- 6 days for 6 years old and above.

This is alternated with one day of occluding the amblyopic eye when the dominant eye is opened. At no time are both eyes opened together. Occlusion of dominant eye is called **conventional occlusion** and the occlusion of the amblyopic eye is called **inverse occlusion.**

Follow-up: The course of occlusion is continued till the vision keeps improving or the vision does not improve on two consecutive monthly visits (provided compliance is good). The latter is termed occlusion failure. Usually occlusion yields results in 3 months period. In infants the follow-up is made fortnightly. During follow-ups the vision of the normal eye should be checked to note any deterioration which indicates occlusion amblyopia. This is a form of stimulus deprivation amblyopia and more difficult to treat.

Indications and contraindications

Earlier cases with eccentric fixation, latent nystagmus were considered contraindications. Now, it has been observed that conventional occlusion is effective in unsteady eccentric fixations, in cases under five years and also in latent nystagmus. In cases of intermittent deviations it may cause increase in deviation and also manifestation all the time, which should be pre-warned to the patient. Cases with organic defects should be screened lest they use occlusion in vain. Some cases of organic amblyopia/organic diseases may have an element of functional amblyopia which may improve. Inverse occlusion is rarely used nowadays. Only for steady eccentric fixation therapy with pleoptics above 5 years age.

Maintenance occlusion: All cases after successful amblyopia therapy require maintenance to prevent recurrence of amblyopia. Chances of this are maximal in the first 4 years of life but once a week occlusion should be continued as maintenance till 9 years age.

Occlusion and surgery: Occlusion should always be done prior to surgery, because:

i. A prior surgery with alignment makes the task of assessment of dominant eye by preference of fixation difficult.

ii. Secondly the motivation of parents may be slackened after cosmetic correction.

iii. Finally an occlusion later may induce a squint again.

Occlusion amblyopia is the greatest bug bear of occlusion and should be prevented by proper regime and proper follow-up. Once occurred it is more difficult to treat. Recording of ocular motility has shown pursuit abnormalities developing in the normal (fellow eye of amblyopia) due to amblyopia, even though visual acuity was normal. This could indicate subclinical occlusion amblyopia.

3. Penalization

This is a form of partial occlusion, whereby the amblyopic eye is forced to a greater use,

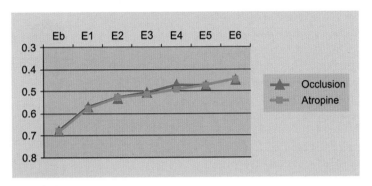

Fig. 14.2: ETDRS visual acuity—Occlusion vs atropine.

while the normal eye is disadvantaged. This may be done by:

i. **Optical penalization:** Overcorrecting with plus glasses (disadvantaged for distance)

ii. **Pharmacological penalization:** Using cycloplegics (disadvantaged for near) (Fig. 14.2).

iii. **Partial occlusion** by sellotape or nail varnish (disadvantaged for both distance and near).

It is also termed **distance penalization or near penalization** depending on for which distance is the dominant eye disadvantaged. A myopic dominant eye is easily given distance penalization by denying proper correction or even fogging with plus glasses. A hyperopic dominant eye is easily disadvantaged by cycloplegic agents.

Penalization is better accepted by patient and parents. It also offers binocular stimulation. But it requires the prior correction of squint with prisms or surgery. The success ratio is also less compared to occlusion.

Penalization has a role for itself especially in non-strabismic milder amblyopias and also for maintenance of the regained binocular vision.

4. CAM Vision Stimulator

Campbell and workers proposed a new modality of amblyopia therapy whereby amblyopic eye is stimulated by slowly rotating, high contrast, square wave gratings of different spatial frequencies for seven minutes. The dominant eye is patched for the period of this treatment. Though it initially received applause due to its promise of a "quick fix" solution, it is no longer popular. At best it is useful as an adjunct to occlusion and impresses the patient by making him feel he is doing some exercise (Fig. 14.3).

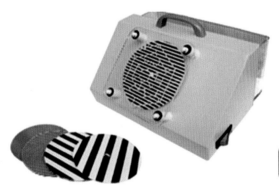

Fig. 14.3: CAM vision stimulator.

5. Pleoptics Therapy

In the aftermath of second world war, amblyopia therapy suffered producing children with dense amblyopia with eccentric fixation. Taking the cue from Comberg (1936), Bangerter (1946) started active stimulation of macula. He coined the term pleoptics from *pleos* = full and *optikos* = sight. In principle,

14

Bangerter dazzled the extramacular retina, including the eccentric point by bright light, protecting the macula by a disc projected onto it. This was followed by intermittent stimulation of macula with flashes of light. He modified Gullstrand's ophthalmoscope and called it the **pleoptophore.** The therapy was continued till the central scotoma weakens and the fixation becomes central.

Cuppers, ingeniously used the **after image** created, centred around the fovea, to give a new sense of direction to the fovea which had lost its straight ahead gaze. He used **euthyscope,** which had discs of varying sizes to create a central after image, apart from dazzling the eccentric point. He also used the alternate flashing of room illumination **(alternascope)** to perpetuate the after images (alternatively forming negative after image in light and positive after image in dark). He also devised **visuscope,** a modified ophthalmo-scope to know the type of eccentric fixation.

The after image is to be projected on the wall or space coordinator where the hand eye coordination is re-learned. This is then followed by exercises with Haidinger brushes on Cupper's coordinator. The latter device uses the property of fovea (due to radial arrangement of outer plexiform Henle's layer or the lutein pigment) to polarise the light. This is not possible by the eccentric point (Figs 14.4 and 14.5).

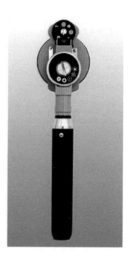

Fig. 14.4: Bangerter's projectoscope.

In a **simple analogy** the two methods may be compared thus: Bangerter's method is like a didactic lecture given to an audience made partially receptive and Cupper's method is like a symposium where the audience is made to interact directly. Rationally, the second approach is better. But unfortunately, pleoptics as such requires a lot of effort from patient and therapist and has become unpopular. Also because occlusion is a simple, technique that is effective.

6. Red Filter Treatment

This therapy was advocated by Brinker and Katz, on the basis of preferentially stimulating

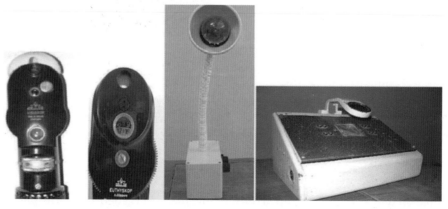

Fig. 14.5: Cuppers' pleoptics instruments—Visuscope, euthyscope, alternascope, coordinator.

the cones of fovea compared to those of the eccentric point, which technically has relatively less cones. The red filter used over the amblyopic eye is Kodak gelatin wratten filter no. 92, which excludes rays of wavelength shorter than 640 nm. The dominant eye (normal eye) is given an opaque patch (occlusion). The eccentric fixation is reported to change, which could be due to the fact that rods and cones mechanism being put on a level a change of fixation occurs. Adler disagreed with the theory of this therapy as the threshold sensitivities of rods and cones for wavelengths longer than 640 nm are almost equal. In practice this therapy is rarely, if ever, used.

7. Active Vision Therapy

Amblyopia therapy and restoring binocular single vision is basically re-educating the perceptual visual cortex and nothing works better than practice. Thus watching television (at optimal distance), reading books (initially larger prints or with pictures) with the amblyopic eye helps.

Eye-hand coordination has to be re-established with respect to the fovea of amblyopic eye and hand.

Near-activity tasks like coloring, cutting, drawing, tracing, joining dots, working through maze, model building games are very useful. Some toys take advantage of the auditory bio-feedback like "talking pens." A simple task can be to draw as many small circles in the large circle of the size of a coin and then subsequently dotting all the small circles. Even letting the child watch TV with his glasses and occlusion patch on, even sitting closer for visibility is acceptable as also letting him play the videogames similarly.

Fast pointing: Aiming tasks are also helpful. Some people advocate strengthening the weak accommodation mechanism by near activities, even utilizing a minus lens spectacle to train it. A combination of plus-minus lenses has also been advocated in a "flipping" exercise.

Another activity described utilizes the after-image transfer technique. An after image is created in the normal eye (with the amblyopic eye occluded), which will be centred at the fovea. Next the amblyopic eye is opened and made to appreciate the same after image (with the normal eye occluded). This too would be centred at the fovea (in NRC). The amblyopic eye is then required to fixate objects to re-learn the space and foveal coordination.

7a. Home Vision Therapy

Most of the activities done in the office of the orthoptist are possible only for short durations, but the learning is fastest if activities can be done at home too. Apart from active vision exercises described above which can be done at home, some card excercises are given for antisupression and relative accommodative-convergence modulation. Double pictures can be used with artificially induced exodeviation (by relaxing the fusion convergence) and stereopsis appreciated, like the popular two double circle (the inner one eccentric) giving the appearance of a bucket in three dimension or incomplete figures which becomes complete on fusion. See comment on watching TV or playing video-games above.

8. Medical Treatment: Levodopa-Carbidopa in Amblyopia

Drugs like levodopa and citicholine are antiparkinsonism drugs that are supposed to facilitate neurotransmission at dopaminergic synapses, which are present in the retina and visual cortex.

Levodopa has been found to increase vision in amblyopic eyes by one or two Snellen lines for short periods of about a month, even in adults, thus increasing the plasticity or effective age group of amblyopia therapy. The systemic side-effects can be reduced by combining carbidopa or probenecid which compete in the peripheral tissues making more levodopa available in the cortex,

14

allowing lower dosages. Trials are being conducted by author in a double blind fashion along with occlusion to see its role of facilitating or shortening the occlusion therapy and not intending to be an alternative to it.

9. Role of Newer Studies of Amblyopia

Several multicentric studies under the Pediatric Eye Disease Investigator Group (PEDIG) have been done in the United States as Amblyopia Treatment Study (ATS). A short summary of these is given below.

ATS-1 (Arch. Ophthal, 2003) – patching for 6 hours v/s full-time - similar magnitude of improvement in VA

But 3.16 vs 2.84 lines and faster in full-time

ATS-2a (Arch Oph, 2003)—2h/d vs 6h/d occlusion in moderate amblyopia and found both had similar visual outcome.

ATS-2b (Ophthal May 2003) - full time v/s 6h patching in severe amblyopia (20/100 to 20/400) and found similar improvement (4.81 and 4.72 respectively) in VA.

ATS-2c (JAAPOS,2004) Recurrence in 21% in 1yr. Less if weaning done 14 vs 42%

ATS-3 (Arch. Ophthal, 2005) compared 2h/d with full time occlusion in older children (13–17 yrs): successful therapy. Atropine not tried in this group

ATS-4 (Ophthalmol, 2004) – Atropine daily vs weekly—similar magnitude of improvement in VA.

Both had 2–3 lines improvemt after 4 mnths

ATS-5 (Ophthalmol, 2006)—Glasses alone had average imp of 2 lines in 5 weeks,

Patching added after 5 wks further improved vision 2.2 vs 1.3 lines

More ATS studies have been published ATS 6–10 which are further refinements about the above findings or in older children. Some more are being conducted like looking into the role of Levodopa (ATS 14 and 17).

IV. Fusional Exercises

Application of orthoptics for treatment of convergence insufficiency and increasing control of intermittent exotropia is so popular that the term "orthoptic excercises" implies this. Even literally *orthos* is straight and *optikos* is eyes. Asthenopia or eye strain is rather common and getting more commonly realized as people work on computer terminals or do a lot of reading work. Early presbyopes, who have been compensating their fusional deficiency by accommodative convergence present with it when given their presbyopic correction.

Convergence insufficiency can be confirmed by noting the near point of convergence (NPC), measuring fusional vergence amplitudes on synoptophore or with prisms. In addition, convergence sustenance should be noted. A sustenance of less than 30 seconds for a 10 cm fixation target is usually symptomatic.

Such cases can be improved by convergence excercises on synoptophore with prism bars. At home the subject is asked to do "pencil-push ups" after becoming aware of physiological diplopia. The pencil push ups are helpful if done properly and regularly. The author's simple home orthoptic trainer (SHOT) is a simple device that can be used.

C. MEDICAL TREATMENT

The use of pharmacological agents, whether in the topical, oral or injectable, have been made in some forms of squint. Miotics have been used in accommodative esotropia, as also cycloplegics. Local injections in the muscles of botulinum toxin achieves chemodenervation an alternative to surgery. And oral drugs like levodopa have been used in amblyopia therapy.

Miotics and Accommodative Esotropia

Initiated by Javal (1896) and popularised by Abraham (1949) miotics act on the ciliary muscle to facilitate accommodation. This

14

reduces the accommodative effort and thus the linked accommodative convergence. The effect on sphincter to cause miosis may also contribute to some extent by reducing accommodative effort by an increase in the depth of focus.

Earlier pilocarpine and eserine were used but were shorter acting and less effective. The longer acting cholinesterase inhibitors now in use are: di-isopropyl-fluorophosphate *(DFP)*, *phospholine iodide (echothiopate), and demecarium bromide (Humorsol)*. Phospholine iodide is available in 0.03%, 0.06% and 0.125% solution, and the minimal dose required to produce desired effects should be used, starting with one morning instillation of 0.03% and increasing if necessary to twice instillation, higher strength. A proper binocular alignment at all times, especially near work with accommodative tasks, is the goal.

The miotics are at best temporary modalities for children who are too small to wear glasses or those who would like to avoid glasses for some special periods like vacations. The bifocals and glasses should generally be preferred as their effect is more constant and predictable. Some ocular side-effects are brow ache, iris cysts, cataract, and retinal detachment. The systemic side-effects are nausea, vomiting, salivation, frequent micturition, diarrhoea and abdominal cramps. The iris cysts are commoner in light colored iris and 2.5% phenylephrine in conjunction avoids them. An important note should be made as the effect of these agents last for a few weeks and can prolong the effect of muscle relaxants like succinylcholine to cause respiratory muscle paralysis during general anesthesia. The drug should be stopped six weeks prior to any surgery under GA and the anesthetist forewarned.

Use of Cycloplegics in Accommodative Esotropia

This may appear ironic but are used therapeutically (apart from diagnostically in refraction) in cases of accommodative esotropia (i) to make them accept the hyperopic correction, (ii) to suppress the accommodative–convergence mechanism and stimulate divergence. The latter is not well accepted and it should be remembered that an accommodational paresis (not total paralysis) may actually increase accommodational effort and aggravate esotropia.

Other Drugs

While in the past some drugs like strychnine, chlordiazepoxide or diphenyl hydantoin have been tried to correct squint but were not well accepted. Recently, however, levodopa is finding acceptability in amblyopia therapy.

Botulinum Toxin A Chemodenervation

The pharmacological correction of strabismus had been a fancy dream for years, which appears to have been realised, at least partially. Alan Scott (1973) published the results of weakening the extraocular muscles in monkeys by injecting botulinum toxin A. This toxin was chosen because 90% of patients of "sausage" poisoning *(botulus* = sausage) contaminated with this toxin had early symptoms of paralysis of bulbar and skeletal muscles. The first results of botulinum toxin in human eye was published in 1980.

Common uses: Botulinum toxin (Botox) a neurotoxic protein synthesised by *Clostridium botulinum* has proved to be effective in Abducens palsy, when early injection of medial rectus prevents its contracture. A few patients have regained paralysis before the effect of Botox passes away. In cases of transposition surgery where vertical recti are being transposed, the botox can be used to weaken the antagonist horizontal muscle by chemodenervation. The horizontal recti are easily accessible in this regard. But cases of dysthyroid orbitomyopathy may be benefitted in early stage when the fibrotic changes have not occurred. Surgical under-corrections and overcorrections and strabismus after retinal

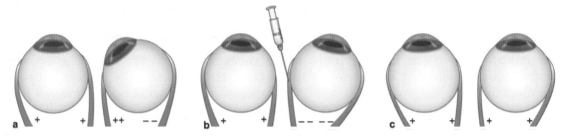

Fig. 14.6: Chemodenervation due to Botulinum injection. (a) Before injection right lateral rectus palsy with esotropia, (b) after injection (2 weeks) of right medial rectus chemodenervation consecutive exotropia created, (c) after few months both eyes aligned with comitance.

detachment also have been tried. Cases of nystagmus have responded favorably to retrobulbar injection. The main disadvantage has been the transient effect which passes off in 3–6 weeks necessitating a repeat injection.

Blepharospasm and hemifacial spasm, cases likewise have been benefitted. The side-effects in the use of extraocular muscles is ptosis.

Recently, their use has been directed in **concomitant strabismus** especially the **infantile esotropes** (Figs 14.6 and 14.7). This is under trial by Scott and McNeer. Some interesting aspects are:

- Infantile esotropes if aligned before six months can have good functional binocularity. If surgery cannot be done, botox may foot the bill.

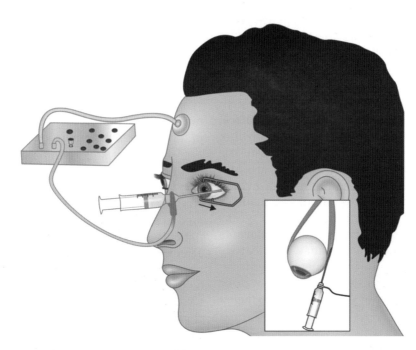

Fig. 14.7: Technique of Botulinum injection in an extraocular muscle under electromyographic auditory control. Ground electrode on forehead. Monopolar (insulated, except bevel) or bipolar needle electrode used. Eye abducted for lateral rectus injection. Avoid global perforation. Injection made at the junction of anterior two-thirds and posterior one-third of muscle.

- While surgical effect of botox in adult eye muscles is transient, effect in early infancy is permanent because of changes in the developmentally immature muscles, specially in the orbital singly innervated muscle fibres.

- Initial overcorrection may restructure the ocular motility balance to yield better result ultimately.

- However, on the negative side, associated changes of oblique overactions or A-V patterns or DVD may still require surgery.

Mechanism of Action

Botulinum toxin A is a 150 kDa molecule. Its carboxyterminus attaches with gangliosides of surface membrane for the **binding step.**

It is **internalised** into intracellular compartment by endocytosis mediated by its amino-terminus. Its light chain inhibits the release of acetylcholine vesicles to produce end point potential (EPP) but miniature end point potentials (MEPP) are allowed. This is the third **intracellular poisoning step.** In this it blocks the acetylcholine release by modifying a substrate that is essential for excitation-release.

The effect starts immediately and peak action takes 5–7 days. The duration of action varies from 2–4 months. The muscle function recovers as new axon terminals sprout to establish new synaptic contacts. Botox does not cause a total inhibition of the non-impulse mediated end point potentials allowing the neurotrophic release of ACh.

Availability of Botulinum toxin: Botulinum toxin is commercially available as oculinum (Allergan Pharmaceuticals, US) and Dysport (Speywood Pharmaceuticals, UK). It is stored in a frozen lyophilized form which is stable. It is reconstituted with normal saline, after which it has to be used within four hours as its shelf-life is short. It is also easily degraded by vigorous shaking, rapid injection, or has changes in pH or temperature. Ing of

Dysport has 40 units and Ing of oculinum has 2.5 units. The lethal dose is 40 units/kg body weight. It is therefore relatively safe. The oculinum vial has 100 units. It is reconstituted with normal saline depending on the strength required for strabismus, usually 2.5 units per muscle has been recommended by McNeer. This is done by using 4 ml of normal saline to reconstitute and using 0.1 ml of the solution.

Methods of injection: The injection in the extraocular muscle must be made under electromyographic control, using monopolar leads (insulated except its tip) (Fig 14.7). The muscle is injected at the junction of anterior two-thirds and posterior one-third. A crackling sound is heard, which quietens the moment the dose is injected. Care must be taken to avoid muscle sheath perforation as spillage to adjacent muscles can cause their paralysis. Perforation of globe should be avoided by keeping the direction of needle away from globe. The subject under local anesthesia is asked to look in the direction of action of muscle. For children ketamine anesthesia is used. McNeer had used nitrous oxide-ethrane insufflation anesthesia and found no difficulty in recording EMG which is not possible under full general anesthesia.

Complications

Ptosis is common occurring in 15–20% cases.

Paralysis of adjacent muscles causing vertical diplopia is also very disturbing. **Dry eyes, reduced lacrimation** and **foreign body sensation** subconjunctival and retrobulbar **hemorrhage** are other side-effects. Pupillary dilatation and accommodational paresis can also occur. Accidental injection in the globe has also been reported but without any neurotoxic effect on retina. The effect of Botox on impulse evoked ACh release can be restored by a dinitrophenol 4-aminopyridine and 4-aminoquinoline. Even decreased temperature facilitates synaptic transmission after Botox poisoning.

14

Newer Studies

A note of other drugs being investigated for strengthening the muscle should be made. Dr. Scott has published improvement after injecting **Bupivacain** (0.5%, 0.75% or even 2.5%) in the paretic muscle. This causes initial muscle fibre damage and later regeneration and fibrosis causing the muscle to be stronger.

Suggested Reading

1. Abraham SV. The use of an echothiophate — phenylephrine formulation (echophenyline-B3) in the treatment of convergent strabismus and amblyopia with special emphasis on iris cysts. J. Pediatr. Ophthalmol. 1 : 68, 1964.

2. Albert DG and Hiles, DA Myopia, bifocals and accommodation. Am. Orthopt. J. 19: 59. 1969.

3. Bangerter A. The purpose of pleoptics. Ophthalmologica 158: 334, 1969.

4. Burian HM. Occlusion amblyopia and the development of eccentric fixation in occluded eyes. Am. J. Ophthalmol. 62: 853, 1966.

5. Calcutt C and Crook W. The treatment of amblyopia in patients with latent nystagmus. Br. Orthopt. J. 29: 70, 1972.

6. Campbell FW, Hess RF, Watson PG, Banks R. Preliminary results of a physiologically based treatment of amblyopia. Br. J. Ophthalmol. 62: 748, 1978.

7. Goldstein JH. The role of miotics in strabismus. Surv. Ophthalmol. 13: 31, 1968.

8. Jampolsky A, Flom M, and Thorson JC. Membrane Fresnel prisms: a new therapeutic device. In Fells P. editor. The First Congress of the International Strabismological Association. St. Louis, 1971. Mosby—Year Book Inc.

9. Kushner BJ. Functional amblyopia associated with abnormalities of the optic nerve. Arch. Ophthalmol. 102: 683, 1984.

10. Noorden GK. von, and Attiah F: Alternating penalisation in the prevention of amblyopia recurrence. Am. J. Ophthalmol. 102: 473, 1986.

11. Noorden GK von, Aula C. Sidikaro Y and La Roche, R. Latent nystagmus and strabismic amblyopia Am. J. Ophthalmol. 103 : 87, 1987.

12. Noorden GK von, Springer F, Romano P and Parks MM. Home therapy for amblyopia. Am. Orthopt. J. 20: 46, 1970.

13. Pigassou R. Prisms in strabismus. Int. Ophthalmol. Clin. 6: 519, 1966.

14. Repka MX and Ray JM. The efficacy of optical and pharmacological penalization. Ophthalmology. 100: 769, 1993.

15. Scott AB. Botulinum toxin injection into extraocular muscles as an alternative to strabismus surgery. Ophthalmology. 87: 1044, 1980.

16. Lyle TK and Wybar KC. Lyle and Jackson's Practical Orthoptics in the Treatment of Squint, (and other anomalies of binocular vision.) 15th Edition H.K.'Lewis and Co. London. 1970.

17. McNeer KW, Tucker MG, Spencer RF. Botulinum toxin management of essential infantile esotropia in children. Arch. Ophthalmol. 115: 1411, 1997.

14

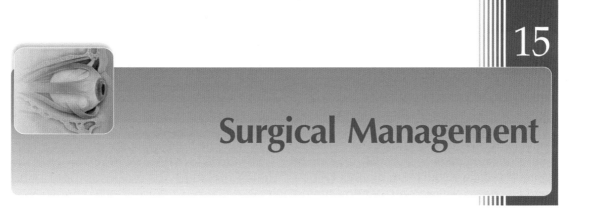

Surgical Management

The instant gratification characteristic of a successful cataract surgery is only paralleled in strabismus surgery, at the sight of two straight properly functional eyes in the immediate postoperative period. But the frustration consequent to a failure to achieve this can also be too soon. This can be minimised only by a thorough understanding of the principles underlying strabismus and proper execution of the procedure. The results of strabismus, surgery depend not only on the intraoperative dexterity but also on the proper preoperative evaluation—and missed or left unattended or the opposite pair of muscles operated can worsen the existing pattern and leave an unsatisfied patient, though the primary position is optimally corrected. Similarly a monocular recession resection where excessive surgery has resulted in optimal correction of deviation, also leaves behind an unsightly narrow palpebral aperture or retraction of the globe. **The goals of strabismus surgery** are two fold:

i. **Cosmetic:** To achieve satisfactory appearance of the parallelism (alignment) of the two eyes and also the adjacent adnexa, in all the gazes of the eyes.

ii. **Functional:** To restore and maintain good and equal visual acuity of each eye as also to restore and maintain a normal single binocular vision, in all the gazes of the eyes.

Strabismus surgery involves two important features; the final goal of surgery is dependent upon the free movement of the tissues after surgery and since there is always a chance of resurgery:

i. The tissue handling should be such as to avoid excessive restriction of the eye, and minimally disturb the strengths and leverage of the muscles.

ii. The tissue planes should be maintained so that a revision is not made difficult.

Preoperative Evaluation

Without going into the details, which should be obtained from the previous chapters on examination, non-surgical management and specific types of squint, only the salient points are being highlighted here.

Assessment of Vision-refraction and Amblyopia Therapy

A scrupulous diagnostic work up includes the assessment of vision by age appropriate tests for recognition of amblyopia and the binocular status full cyloplegic refraction and proper correction is mandatory. A surgery done for the accommodative part cannot be condoned. Any existing amblyopia should be corrected or a case confirmed to be a failure from amblyopia therapy, before deciding surgery. In cases of monocular squint with very poor vision in squinting eye, the refraction of the normal eye is a must. The accommodational innervation is guided by this "normal" eye, and will be relevant for altering the deviation.

Measurement of Deviation

The deviation should be measured with prism bar cover test both for near and distance fixation as also for up- and downgazes (A–V phenomena) and noting for any horizontal or vertical incomitances. Associated inferior or superior oblique overaction or underaction should be noted. The accommodation should be controlled with proper correction, and using a 6/9 size target for fixation, both for near and distance. The surgery is to be done for the **static angle** and not the **dynamic angle.** Similarly in incomitant paralytic squint, both primary and secondary deviations are noted and surgery decided on the basis of the **fixing eye.** If the paralytic eye is dominant the secondary deviation needs to be operated for.

Some Tests Important in Surgery

Forced Duction Test (FDT)

The FDT is a clinical test which needs to be done preoperatively to reveal any restrictive pathology. It also needs to be repeated at various times during the surgery: prior, after conjuctival incision, after dissection of check ligaments and intermuscular septum after looking the muscle (to check the tension of the muscle by hook itself), after disinserting the muscle, after reinserting the muscle and finally after closure of conjunctival flaps.

One should remember, if succinylchlorine is used as a muscle relaxant it may cause contraction of muscle for first 15–20 minutes and make FDT unreliable. Non-depolarizing muscle relaxant like Pancuronium bromide can be used as an alternative to avoid this.

Under typical anesthesia or general anesthesia the conjunctiva is held at the limbus with fixation forceps, or preferably Pierce-Hoskins forceps without retracting the globe by pressure. If the patient is conscious, he is asked to look in the opposite direction of testing to relax the concerned muscle. Any restriction of movement is noted. It is also important to note that both a **direct** and **reverse leash** restriction may be present.

Exaggerated FDT for Obliques

This test described by Guyton tests the tightness of oblique muscles. As against the FDT for recti muscles, the globe is retracted to exaggerate the restriction of obliques.

For **inferior oblique traction test** the limbus is held at inferotemporal and superonasal quadrant positions, the globe is pushed back into the orbit, in full adduction position maintaining intorsion of the globe. It is then brought temporally while continuting to push it backwards. A normal or taut inferior oblique muscle would cause the globe to "pop up" which can be felt and seen. A lax or weakened muscle would not show this response. After a weakening procedure, a positive test indicates insufficient weakening.

For the **superior oblique traction test** (Fig. 15.1) the limbus is held in the superotemporal and inferonasal quadrant positions. The eye is pushed back into the orbit, in full adduction positions, maintaining extorsion of the globe. It is then brought temporally while continuing to push it back in the orbit. A normal or taut superior oblique muscle would cause the globe to "pop up." A click is felt by the examiner. After a weakening procedure a positive test indicates an insufficient weakening done.

Spring-back Balance Test

This test, introduced by Jampolsky, assesses whether surgical adjustment of the muscles has disturbed the balance of passive muscle forces. A marked imbalance would result in comitance under general anesthesia, the eye is passively rotated in the chosen direction with the globe held at limbus by two forceps. After removing the forceps the observer notes whether the globe springs back to the primary position or remains deviated in the eccentric position. The same is then repeated in the opposite direction. It should again spring back with equal force. If it remains in eccentric positions, surgical adjustment is made and the test repeated.

15

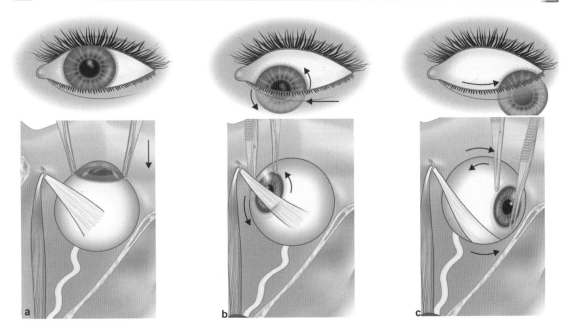

Fig. 15.1: Exaggerated forced duction testing for superior oblique. Right eye shown from top and the anteroposterior section of orbit. Arrows indicate the forced movement. (a) Retropulsion, (b) Excycloduction with adduction and (c) Excycloduction and abduction. In (c) the globe is felt to pass through a feel of resistance with a bump upwards.

Muscle Stretch Test

This is a simple test for checking the elasticity of the recti muscles, intraoperatively. The muscle to be operated upon after disinsertion and passing sutures, is pulled towards the opposite side. A normal muscle, can be advanced up to the centre of cornea with the eye in straight ahead position. If this is not permitted, it indicates a contracture or fibrosis of the muscle.

Ocular Deviation under General Anesthesia

The ocular deviation is altered by the relaxation of convergence tone under general anesthesia. The deviation at the end of the surgery may not reflect the post-surgical outcome correctly. It should therefore be remembered to note the ocular deviation after the anesthesia has been fully achieved (surgical plane), prior to the surgery. The difference between the pre-anesthesia deviation and the deviation after anesthesia should be noted. This difference should be added to the deviation seen after the surgery is completed to estimate the deviation that shall be available postoperatively. This is relevant only for general anesthesia and not for retrobulbar or peribulbar anesthesia.

Communication with the Patient/Parent

The communication between the patient and parent and the strabismus surgeon should be unhindered to answer any queries and also their fears. It should also prevent them from nursing unnecessary or impossible expectations. Some people may have no concept of the extraocular muscles and believe the globe would be exteriosed or exnucleated out of the globe, the muscles operated and then placed back. Another question is whether: it is a minor or major procedure? It is undoubtedly a major surgery, as much as cataract, retina or keratoplasty surgery.

15

In patient admission is not essential, but may be helpful when general anesthesia is required, for proper **pre-anesthetic care.** Some of the children having squint may have associated cardiac, nervous or dental problem, which should be evaluated by the anesthetist. He should be conversant about squint surgery. The occurrence of **oculo-cardiac and oculo-respiratory reflexes** and also **malignant hyperthermia** is more common in strabismus surgery.

The eye to be operated upon should be discussed prior to surgery. At times the patient may feel the "wrong eye" has been operated by mistake. Usually the deviating eye is operated upon, leaving the other normal eye as a reserve for a second surgery if necessary. At times both eyes are operated upon at the same time, and the patient taken into confidence. In constant unilateral squint, the patient may not understand the rationality of operating the other eye and should be explained. Dominant eye surgery has not been known to give significantly better result and usually is avoided. At times surgery is indicated in the other eye, like in double elevator palsy, the elevators of the normal eye may also need to be tackled or a posterior fixation contemplated on the yoke muscle of a paralytic muscle or in Duane's retraction syndrome. These should be explained prior to avoid any litigations.

The operated eye is usually patched overnight for one day only. But if a child is apprehensive, the patch may be opened after six hours. No green shade or dark glasses are required in the postoperative period.

The expectations from surgery should not be undue while dealing with paralytic cases. Similarly cases for cosmetic surgery should be explained about the visual outcome in clear terms. The cosmetic aspect of adjoining adnexa, facial asymmetry, or factors in the anterior segment like corneal opacity, cataract or coloboma with a pear shaped cornea clarified. Strabismus surgery cannot correct these defects. Any associated true ptosis would have to be operated separately.

The possibility and need of **resurgery** should also be conveyed. About 10% cases may be under corrected or over corrected. Some of these may be within the limits of binocular fusion or be cosmetically acceptable, the rest may require resurgery. No strabismus surgery can be 100% predictable and precise, and this should be impressed upon the patient.

Anatomical Considerations in Strabismus Surgery

The knowledge of the anatomy of extraocular muscles is an essential pre-requisite for any strabismus surgeon. Refer to the chapter on anatomy for details. Some **salient points** are highlighted.

The distance of each rectus muscle from the limbus is different for each and is different in infants. While recessions, one should also measure this distance and take into account. The two ends of the recti also differ from the mid point in the muscle-limbal distance. The width of the muscle is about 10 mm (just slightly less than the corneal diameter), this should be restored, for normal physiological actions, after surgery also. While performing vertical transpositions of horizontal recti, care should be taken to keep the muscle shift concentric with the limbus (both ends of muscle equidistant).

A little knowledge of anatomy helps a lot in confirming the **preoperative position of the globe under anesthesia.** A torsion may be induced, which may cause an unaware surgeon to operate on the vertical rectus in place of horizontal rectus. **The points to be noted are:**

• The vertical recti have a slightly oblique insertion (23° obliquity). Their temporal ends are further receded than their nasal ends, whereas the horizontal recti have their upper and lower ends almost equidistant from limbus.

- The relationship of the superior or inferior oblique muscle should be noted. Except the medial rectus, the other three recti have an association of these obliques.
- The lateral triangle of limbus merges more indistinctly with sclera.

The **blood supply of the anterior segment** is contributed by the anterior ciliary arteries which are compromised when the recti are operated. Obliques do not contribute to this circulation. The vertical recti contribute the maximum of the superior and inferior, quadrants. Whereas, the lateral quadrant is mainly contributed by the anterior ciliary artery of lateral rectus, the contribution of lateral long posterior ciliary artery is less significant. The medial long posterior ciliary artery and the two anterior ciliary arteries of medial rectus. **Thus surgery of both vertical recti in combination with lateral rectus can precipitate anterior segment ischemia.** This is particularly in cases of old people with arteriosclerosis syndromes. If essential the surgery on three adjacent recti should be at least spaced by six weeks.

The **sclera** is thinnest (0.3 mm) at the insertion site of recti. So at least 0.5 mm muscle stump should be left for resection resuturing. During recession, during supra-maximal recession surgery or faden surgery special case should be taken to avoid **penetration of the globe.** The **muscle sheath** should also be always preserved. The integrity of Tenon's capsule 8 mm posterior to the muscle insertion should not be violated to prevent **fat prolapsing** and causing fibrofatty adhesions. While working posteriorly the **vortex veins** should be prevented from any damage. The **nerves** to the recti are usually safe as they are about 26 mm from insertion site. But the nerve to inferior oblique is at the crossing of inferior rectus nasal border and the oblique.

Developmental Considerations in Strabismus Surgery

The eye of neonate infant is still growing. The axial length is 70% of the adult eye, the volume is only half and surface area about one-third only. The anterior segment at the birth has developed 80% of its adult size, whereas, the posterior segment develops over the next six months. Any recessions or retroequatorial surgery before six months can be unpredictable.

Choice of Surgery: General Principles

The procedures in strabismus surgery, whether on horizontal recti, vertical recti or obliques, fall into two broad categories: **weakening procedures** or **strengthening procedures.** It may be a combination of the two, where one muscle is weakened and its antagonist strengthened, or one may choose to do a similar weakening procedure on the two eyes. It is not necessary to do **symmetric** procedures on the two eyes but one should try to **establish symmetry** where none exists and **maintain it** where it exists. The aim is to do **symmetrizing surgery.** One has to be guided by the extent of the excursion of various muscles, the versions and ductions.

Another important parameter is the difference in near distance deviation. In esotropia with **convergence excess,** the choice would be bimedial recessions; with **divergence insufficiency,** the choice would be resection of both lateral recti. In case of **basic esotropia** a monocular recession-resection may be done or some surgeons would prefer to still do a bimedial recession. Similarly in exotropia, the **convergence insufficiency type** demands medial rectus resection on both eye; the **divergence excess** mandates recession of lateral recti of both eyes and a basic exotropia a recession resection procedure in one eye. Large deviations require **three** muscle surgery and rarely all four recti need to be operated.

The amount of surgery be preferably split between the two recti being operated, rather than accomplishing a large muscle surgery on one muscle alone. The latter can correct the deviation in primary position but induce incomitance on extreme lateral gaze, as also alter the lid position causing ptosis due to retraction of globe.

The associated oblique overactions need to be tackled, whenever present. In the absence of overactions of oblique but cases having A.V. patterns, vertical shifting of horizontal recti or slanting recession and resections can be done.

The Weakening Procedures

The weakening procedures on the recti muscles (Fig. 15.2) are:

1. Recession
   i. Conventional
   ii. Hang back or hemi hang back
   iii. Adjustable
   iv. Vertical transposition of horizontal recti
   v. Slanting recession
2. Retroequatorial myopexy (Faden)
3. Marginal myotomy
4. Myectomy
5. Free tenotomy or disinsertion

Recession

Recession (Fig. 15.3) is a procedure where the rectus or oblique muscle is disinserted and

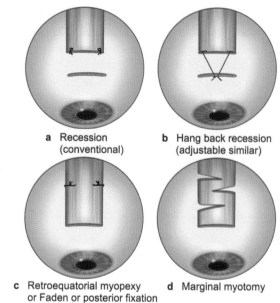

a Recession (conventional)   **b** Hang back recession (adjustable similar)

c Retroequatorial myopexy or Faden or posterior fixation   **d** Marginal myotomy

Fig. 15.2: Weakening procedures.

reinserted to a point closer to its origin. This induces a slack or laxity in the muscle. A lax muscle becomes less effective as its length-tension relationship changes (Beisner's family of curves). As long as the muscle is re-inserted within the length of its **arc of contact**, the

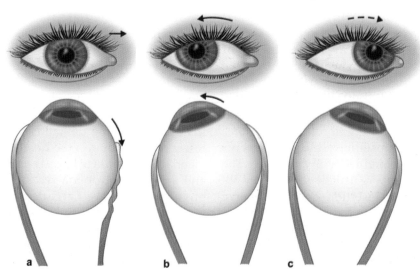

Fig. 15.3: Recession of medial rectus of right eye is shown. (a) Recession causes a slack or laxity of medial rectus, (b) Eye deviates out (exodeviation) to correct the laxity, (c) Adduction becomes weaker only in extreme gaze unless more than maximal limit of recession is done.

15

Table 15.1: Suggested amount of surgical correction

Deviation in Prism Dioptres	Esotropia				Exotropia			
	Recess + MR (One eye)	Resect LR (mm)	Recess MR Both eyes (mm)	Resect LR (mm) Both eyes	Recess + LR (One eye)	Resect MR (mm)	Recess LR Both eyes (mm)	Resect MR Both eyes
15	3.0	4.0	3.0	3.5	4.0	3.0	4.5	3.0
20	3.5	4.5	3.5	4.5	5.0	3.5	5.0	3.5
25	4.0	5.0	4.0	5.5	5.5	4.0	5.5	4.0
30	4.0	6.0	4.5	6.5	6.0	4.0	6.0	4.5
35	4.5	6.0	5.0	7.0	6.5	4.5	6.5	5.0
40	4.5	7.0	5.5	7.5	7.0	5.0	7.0	5.5
50	5.0	7.5	6.0	8.0	7.5	5.5	8.0	6.0

Note: "Statutory Warning"

These values are arbitrary, highly generalised for an "averaged" patient, and have been suggested to initiate a mental formula which has to be individualised, considering the various factors mentioned in the text. **Resections alone are not suggested as a primary procedure.**

torque is not unduly affected, but in case of a recession beyond the arc of contact, a muscle will cease to perform its action. This puts a maximum limit, up to which a recession can be done, which is limited by the **functional equator** (depends on the arc of contact). The functional equator is not the same as anatomic equator, it is 2 mm posterior for the lateral rectus and 2 mm anterior to the anatomic equator in case of medial rectus. Thus the **maximal limits of recession** in adults are 6 mm for medial rectus and 8 mm for lateral rectus (Fig. 15.4). In small children they are 5.5 mm and 7 mm respectively (Table 15.1).

The **minimal** limits of recession depend on the dynamics of ocular motility. A recession of less than 3 mm for medial rectus and 4 mm for lateral rectus may be ineffective.

The recessions are graded weakening procedures and more predictable than any other procedures. They can be undone if necessary or revisited to augment the effect. Their effectivity has made the disinsertion or free tenotomies obsolete procedures to be condemned.

Dis-insertions or free tenotomies are of historical interest, but were highly unpredic-

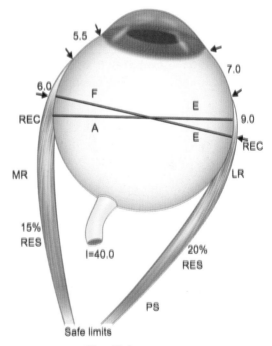

Fig. 15.4: Safe limits.

table as there is no control as to where the muscle will get reattached. They were difficult to be undone or redone to correct the defects. These procedures are now not done, except in dire circumstances of a tight fibrotic rectus,

15

where recessions is not possible as may be in some extreme situations of dysthyroid orbitomyopathy or congenital muscle fibrosis.

SURGICAL STEPS IN RECESSION OF MEDIAL RECTUS

1. After age appropriate anesthesia, the eye and adnexa is cleaned with spirit and betadine and parts draped. An adhesive steridrape is applied. Both eyes should be cleaned and available for visualization. Under GA the other eye is kept suitably hydrated with a wet cotton swab. The surgeon sits on the side facing the medial canthus (Fig. 15.5). The instrument trolley lies over the hand (Fig 15.6).

2. The lids are retracted by a self retaining speculum with blades to prevent lashes coming in.

3. Forced duction testing is done and **shall be repeated at several steps.**

4. Limbal conjunctival incision is made after passing two limbal 6–0 silk or cotton sutures, and incising the conjunctiva after lifting the sutures, to prevent scleral penetration (Figs 15.7 and 15.8).

5. Two radial incisions are made in the conjunctiva with blunt ended spring scissors (90° to each other).

6. The intermuscular septum in the superonasal and inferonasal quadrants, is button holed.

7. The muscle is hooked by Jameson's hook. The hook is passed hugging the sclera to hook the entire muscle (Fig. 15.9).

8. The Green's hook is passed from the other end ensuring the entire muscle being hooked.

9. The check ligaments and intermuscular septum are separated under direct vision, preventing any injury to vessels, or fascia or muscle sheath. Excess of Tenon's capsule in and around the muscle insertion is carefully excised.

10. Two interlocking loops of 6–0 vicryl 5–29 needles are passed and a knot secured, at the two ends of muscle insertion, involving 3–4 mm at either ends.

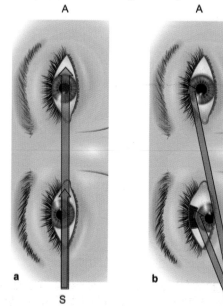
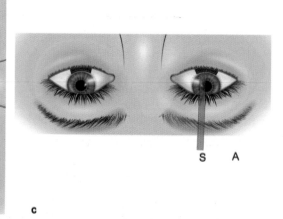

Fig. 15.5: The vantage positions of surgery. (a) On the side facing the medial canthus for same side MR and opposite side LR and IO, (b) On the same side, lower down looking up for same side SR and SO, (c) From the top of the head for inferior rectus. S = Surgeon, A = Assistant.

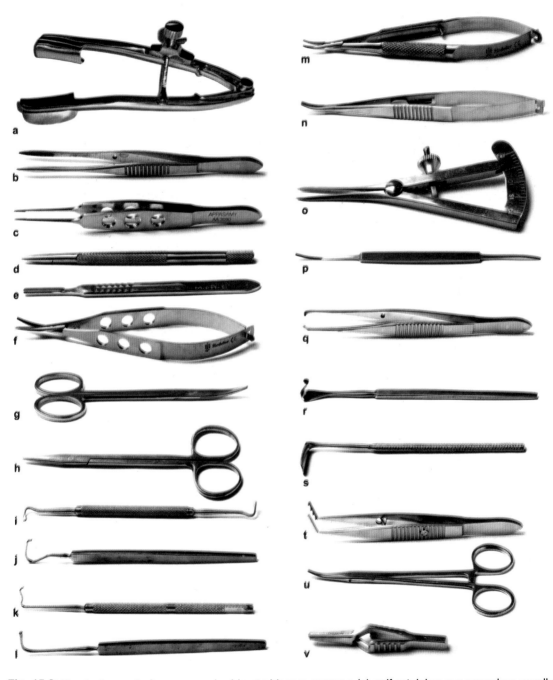

Fig. 15.6: The instruments forceps required in strabismus surgery: (a) self retaining eye speculum usually with blades is preferred, (b) serrated, cupped (Moor field's style), (c) plane forceps, (d) Blade breaker, (e) BP knife handle, (f) Spring scissors, (g) Tenotomy scissors curved, (h) straight tenotomy scissors, (i–l) Muscle hooks, (i) Jameson's, (j and k) Green's, (l) Von Graefe's, (m and n) Needle holders, (o) Castroviejo calipers, (p) Malleable iris repositor, (q) Forceps: fixation toothed, (r) Desmarre's retractor, (s) Deep tissue retractor, (t) Muscle resection clamp, (u) Artery clamps and (v) serrefine.

15

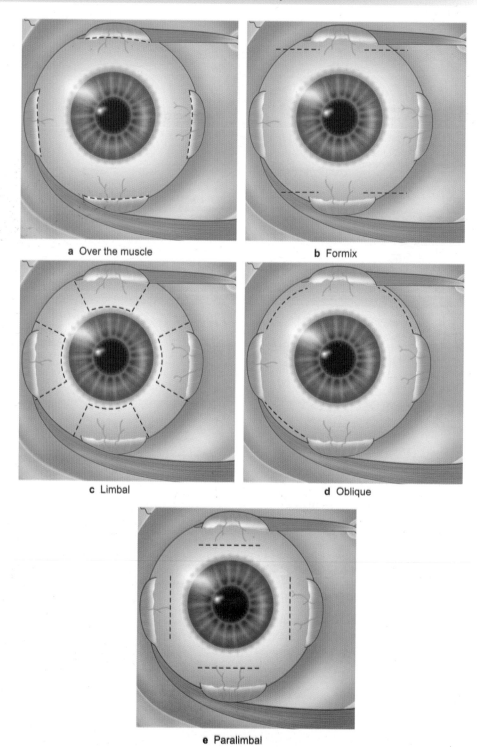

a Over the muscle

b Formix

c Limbal

d Oblique

e Paralimbal

Fig. 15.7: Various types of conjunctival incisions shown for right eye from front.

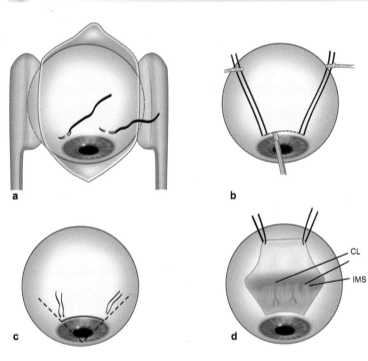

Fig. 15.8: Conjunctival incision: Limbal (von Noorden style) Approaching the right medial rectus. (a) two limbal sutures applied, (b) limbal incision made with blade with the conjunctiva lifted on sutures, (c) two radial incisions perpendicular to each other made with scissors and (d) conjunctival flap retracted showing the medial rectus(M) covered by Tenon's, muscle sheath, check ligaments (CL) and intermuscular septum(IMS) on the sides.

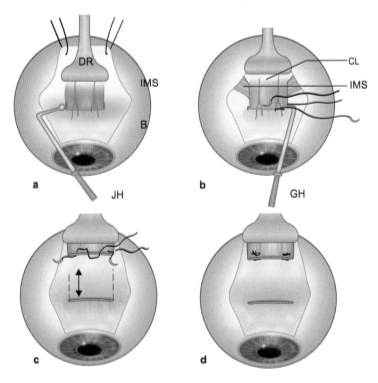

Fig. 15.9: Surgical steps in recession of rectus muscle. (a) After raising the conjunctival flap small button holes B are made in the intermuscular septum (IMS) to hook the muscle with Jameson's hook (JH), (b) The muscle is next hooked by Green's hook from other side and dissection of check ligaments (CL) and IMS accomplished, (c) Two separate interlocking loops on each side of muscle passed. Measurement made from original insertion by calipers and the needles passed parallel to limbus and (d) The muscle is secured with two separate sutures, additional Tenon's excised and muscle freed of any adhesions before closure.

15

11. The muscle is carefully cut with tenotomy scissors leaving a stump of 0.5 mm. Light cautery may be required.

12. The measurement for recession with calipers are made from the upper and lower ends, which are never directly handled with fixation forceps to prevent any induced shift. The fixation forceps hold the insertion at the middle.

13. The two spatulated needles are passed paralimbal away from each other at the marks, ensuring at least 8–10 mm width.

14. The sutures are tied with surgical knots as the assistant holds the knot to prevent any slippage and loosening of the knot.

15. The muscle and its attachments are visualized to rule out any entrapments.

16. The conjunctiva is reapposed with four or more interrupted sutures ensuring no prolapse of Tenon's tissue. The small incision or Fornix incision differs in making the conjunctival incision 7–8 mm from limbus in the lower/upper fornix and then making another small incision in the Tenon's capsule at 90 degrees to the first. The rectus muscle is hooked with the Jameson's hook followed by Green's hook and the muscle is brought in the exposed site by a manoeuver using a lens hook. The upper pole of the muscle insertion needs to be examined to make sure that the entire muscle is in the hook or it is hooked again.

HANG BACK RECESSION

Conventional recession as described above implies re-inserting the rectus muscle with two sutures directly to the scleral points where the insertion is intended.

Hang-back recession is a procedure where recession is done with long ends of the suture between the site of insertion and the muscle (Fig. 15.2b). This is sometimes indicated, when **supramaximal recession** is intended and it is difficult to pass the sutures that posteriorly, as it can risk scleral perforation especially in high myopes. This may also be done in the situations when otherwise a disinsertion or free tenotomy is being considered for reasons given above. The sutures are inserted at the site of original insertion.

Hang back recession incorporates the advantage of recession in that the muscle is not totally free to attach anywhere. But the weakening effect is more than a recession because of a central (midwidth) sag. It also leaves a narrow width of the muscle. A **pseudotendon** may form in the intervening space around the sutures, which may shorten and produce a **late**-under-correction. And at times if the sutures give way or get absorbed it may be as bad as a disinsertion.

Hemi-hang back recession is another modification in which the sutures are passed through a scleral tunnel before being inserted at the original insertion. This may have the advantage of keeping the width of the muscle broader than in hang back and reduce the chance of postoperative creeping forward due to a long hangback.

ADJUSTABLE RECESSION SURGERY

This is a procedure which has the ability to modify the position of a newly operated muscle by the use of adjustable sutures. The adjustment of the amount of recession is allowed when the effect of anesthesia has worn off but before the healing process has commenced.

The classical method is attributed to Jampolsky, whereby the recessed muscle is sutured to the globe in such a manner that the sutures can be loosened and the muscle tendon either drawn forward (less recession) or allowed to retract posteriorly (more recession) at the time of adjustment.

The surgery necessitates a cooperative patient where surgery as well as adjustment can be done under local or topical anesthesia. The indications are:

1. Large angle deviations where the results may be inconsistent.

2. Reoperations in which surgical planning becomes unpredictable due to altered musculofascial factors.
3. Previously injured extraocular muscles where the assessment of muscle function may be inaccurate.
4. Incomitant strabismus with diplopia where a precise postoperative result is desired.
5. Severe mechanical limitations as in dysthyroid orbitomyopathy or musculo-fascial anomalies.
6. Aberrant innervation in III nerve palsy or Duane's retraction syndrome.

Surgical Procedure (Fig. 15.10)

Types of adjustable surgery varies from surgeon to surgeon. A limbal incision is preferred. After hooking the muscle and dissection of intermuscular septum and check ligaments, two separate sutures are passed at the two ends of muscle insertion. The sutures are brought straight or after passing through a scleral tunnel (starting mid distance to allow for forward pull) to the muscle insertion and the two ends tied with each other in a **one and a half knot.** The half knot is opened at the time of adjustment. The ends are cut short (enough for adjustment). The limbal conjuctiva resutured with a 5 mm bare sclera. Some surgeons use a **sliding noose.** This can be adjusted later. Suture material should be strong enough to allow manipulation. 6–0 vicryl can be used or nonabsorbable suture may be used.

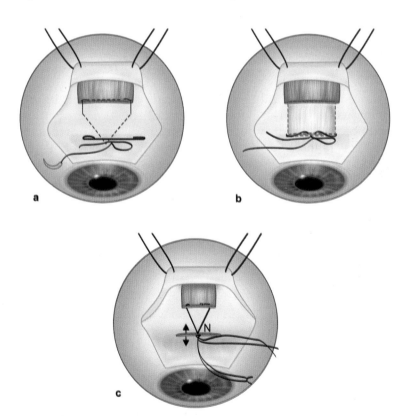

15

Fig. 15.10: Adjustable recession surgery: Three techniques. Techniques (a) and (b) ensure proper width of the recessed muscle, in (c) it is crumpled. (a) Partial distance scleral tunnel made which also limits the forward pulling (reducing recession), (b) Peter Fell's technique of passing suture at insertion, (c) Adjustment by a sliding noose suture (N).

Table 15.2: Adjustments endpoints		
Diagnosis	*Surgery*	*Position of adjustment*
1. Intermittent exotropia	• Recession + resection	• ET 6–8 pd
	• B/E recession	• ET 8–10 pd
2. Sensory exotropia	• Recession + Resection	• ET 4–6 pd
3. Adult esotropia	• Recession + Resection	• Ortho
	• B/E recession	• XT 2–4 pd
4. Sensory esotropia	• Recession + Resection	• Ortho

Readjustment

The readjustment is made within 24 hours of the operation, it may be done on the evening after 5–6 hours of surgery, or the morning after. The eye is topically anesthesized and a lid speculum is inserted. The temporary knot is united and adjustment made. The patient fixates for a distant target and subjectively confirms alignment, as also a cover test is done. The knot is finally secured to lock the suture, and the excess suture trimmed (Fig. 15.11).

It is easier to reduce slack, that is an over-recessed muscle moved forward, rather than to augment an under-recession. (The globe is held with the fixation forceps or a bucket handle loop suture fashioned of 6–0 polyglactin suture as the patient attempts to look in the direction of action of muscle).

The adjustment does not always mean that the same deviation or orthoposition shall remain because the eyes are known to drift postoperatively. In order to counter this postoperative drift, a rough guide for the adjustment is given in Table 15.2.

Some surgeons delay the adjustment to about a week for a more predictable outcome. This is not easy and requires use of visco-elastic substances like Healon or silicon sleeves to allow for such delayed adjustment.

RETROEQUATORIAL MYOPEXY (FADEN)

Retroequatorial myopexy or posterior fixation suture or *faden* (Suture in German) was devised by Cupper (Fig. 15.12). The muscle is sutured posterior to its insertion farther than the limit of its arc of contact (functional equator). This shortens the **lever arm** drastically and severely reduces the action of the muscle in its field of action. However, if no recession is done alongwith, it does not alter the length tension relationship in the primary position and so does not change the deviation in primary position. The posterior

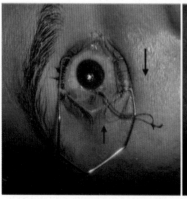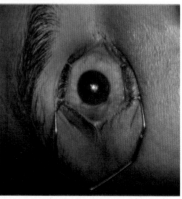

Fig. 15.11: Before and after readjustment.

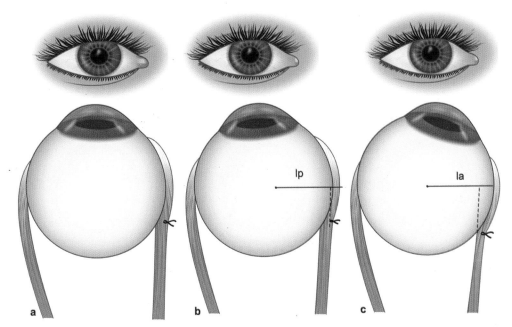

Fig. 15.12: Faden (Retroequatorial myopexy) of medial rectus, right eye. (a) Faden without recession causes no laxity of medial rectus and so no change of ocular deviation in primary position, (b) Lever arm of the muscle force of MR is slightly shorter in primary position (lp), (c) But in adduction the lever arm (la) is significantly shorter causing weaker adduction and progressively more weak in extreme adduction.

fixation has to be really posterior to be really effective. The measurement from the muscle insertions are as follows:

- Medial rectus: 12–14 mm
- Lateral rectus: 16–20 mm
- Superior rectus: 14–16 mm
- Inferior rectus: 14–16 mm

The surgery being most effective on medial rectus and least for the lateral recti. **The indications** for faden operation are:

1. Nonaccommodative convergence excess esotropia (medial recti)
2. Nystagmus blockage syndrome (medial recti)
3. Dissociated vertical deviations (superior recti)
4. Paralytic strabismus (contralateral synergist)
5. Duane's retraction syndrome (contralateral medial rectus)
6. Additional weakening effect over a recessed muscle.

In addition to these indications, some surgeons also performs this surgery for reducing the amplitude of nystagmus (on all the four horizontal recti), for accommodative esotropia with convergence excess (accommodative type).

Surgical Technique

If the faden operation is done without recession, the muscle is passed 5–0 mersilene suture with small half circle needles at the two ends at the marked point on the muscle and the sclera. The knots are carefully applied to prevent any loosening of knot. The bites in the muscle should be 3–4 mm on either side to include at least 80% of fibers in the fixation. A hook is passed to confirm the posterior fixation.

If recession is also done along with retroequatorial myopexy, retroequatorial myopexy, the sutures are passed through the muscle at a point which is faden distance less the recession (*i.e.* for a 14 mm faden and 4 mm recession the muscle is fixed at 10 mm distance). The sutures in sclera are passed at the same (14 mm) distance. The recession of the required amount is then executed (4 mm in above example).

Marginal Myotomy

Another weakening procedure is the myotomy. This may be of two types: **Marginal myotomy** or **Central myotomy.** By making transverse cuts in the muscle of atleast two-thirds widths. Several cuts are made alternately at the two borders of the muscle to effectively leng-then the muscle (like straightening a Z), Central myotomy is not as effective. Artery clamps are applied to crush the muscle before the incision to prevent bleeding from it, Cautery can also be applied.

This procedure is a traumatizing procedure and according to the author, should be considered as the last resort in a maximally recessed muscle still requiring weakening.

Myectomy

The right word is **myectomy** not myomec-tomy (which would mean excising a myoma), is another weakening procedure. It is being done for inferior oblique by some surgeons, otherwise this procedure has become obsolete.

STRENGTHENING PROCEDURES ON RECTI

1. Resection
2. Advancement
3. Double-breasting or Tucking
4. Cinching
5. Transpositioning of adjacent muscles (Fig. 15.13).

Resection

The most common procedure for strengthening is resection. It shortens the muscle

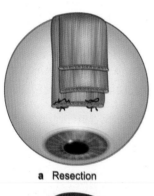

a   Resection

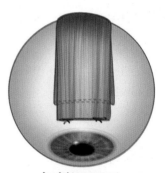

b   Advancement

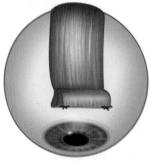

c   Double breasting and cinching

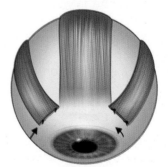

d   Transposition of adjacent recti

Fig. 15.13: Strengthening procedures (a to d).

length effectively making it more taut improving its efficiency by raising it to a higher length tension curve. Resection implies excision of the tendinous part of the muscle only. In fact if the limit is exceeded and muscle mass is excised it will weaken the muscle instead of strengthening it (myectomy). The maximum limit depends on the length of fibrotendinous part of each muscle (inferior oblique which has virtually no tendon cannot be resected to-strengthen). For medial rectus the maximum limit is 6 mm and for lateral rectus it is 9 mm. The minimum limits for medial rectus is 3 mm and for lateral rectus it is 4.5 mm.

Surgical Steps In Resection

The steps 1–9 are the same as for a recession (Fig. 15.14).

10. Measurement of resection is marked with calipers, ensuring that the muscle is not stretched during the marking.
11. Two-double armed 6–0 vicryl sutures (four needles) are passed in an interlocking fashion to hold the muscle. The loose ends held by serrefines or bull-dog clamps.
12. A muscle clamp is applied 2 mm distal to the sutures and the Green's hook removed.
13. The muscle is carefully cut, leaving 0.5 mm stump.

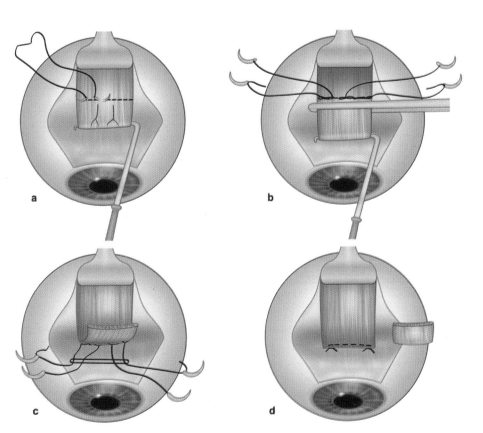

Fig. 15.14: Surgical steps in resection of rectus muscle. (a) After hooking the muscle and dissection as for recession muscle the part to be resected is marked and two sets of double armed needles passed through the muscle, (b) The muscle is clamped and disinserted with tenotomy scissors at the dotted line, (c) The middle two needles are passed-through the muscle tissue and all four needles passed through the insertion, and (d) After tying the knots the excess muscle is resected.

14. The four needles are passed through the stump so that the upper and lower pairs have a 5 mm separation at least. This is to ensure at least 8 mm wide muscle insertion when the knots are tied, preventing any loosing of knots.
15. The muscle is visualized to rule out any entrapments.
16. The conjunctiva is reapposed as for recession. Alternatively after passing the four interlocking bites the muscle is clamped just in front and cauterized and subsequently cut with scissors. The part of the muscle to be resected is excised leaving a stump of 0.5 mm. The muscle is resutured here.

Few changes in surgical steps for small incision fornix procedure for recession and resection are shown in Figs 15.15 and 15.16.

Advancement

This is an alternative strengthening procedure whereby the muscle is re-inserted closer to the limbus, thus stretching the muscle and making it more taut and effective. It is the reverse of recession, but normally has a limitation because of the short limbus-muscle distance and the risk of unsightly congestion in the paralimbal area. However, it is the ideal choice in a consecutive squint, where a recession has been done earlier. In some paralytic squint advancement may be done in addition to the resection.

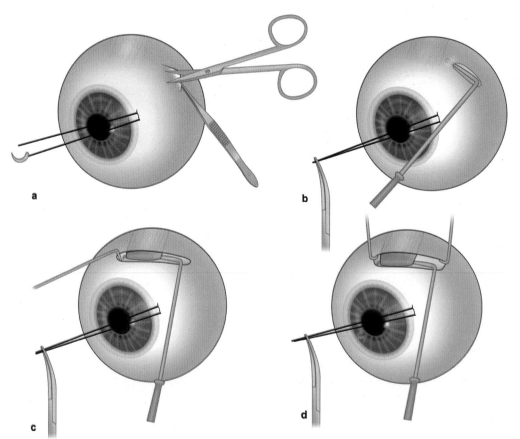

Fig. 15.15: Fornix incision steps: (a) Limbal anchoring suture passed and conjunctival incision in the fornix just temporal/nasal to inferior rectus, (b) muscle hooked, (c) conjunctiva covering the muscle lifted to expose muscle, (d) full muscle hook confirmed by 'pole' test.

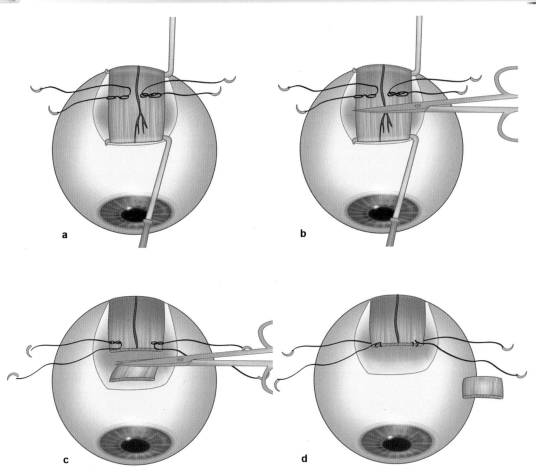

Fig. 15.16: New steps for resection (a to d).

Double breasting or tenoplication is a procedure where the muscle is shortened without excising the muscle mass but this is achieved by double breasting the tendinous/ muscular part (Fig. 15.13c). It is indicated in paralytic squints where thin fragile muscle is present. As a tucking procedure, tenoplication of the superior oblique is a common strengthening procedure for superior oblique.

Cinching is a modified double breasting where the passage of sutures is such as to cause a double breasting of the muscle. The advantage of these two procedures is that the muscle is not disinserted and anterior ciliary vessels not compromised thus not risking anterior segment ischemia.

Anesthesia for Strabismus Surgery

Various types of anesthesia are depending on the age of the patient, type of surgery and the choice of the surgeon.

Topical anesthesia: This is carried out with 1% propracaine or 4% lignocaine drops used topically. It can be used effectively in some highly cooperative patients, for short procedures which do not have posterior manipulations. It is very useful for adjustment on the adjustment day or for adjustment removal in case silk sutures have been used for conjunctiva.

Sub-Tenon's anesthesia: Recently a continuous sub conjunctival irrigation in sub-Tenon's space has been evaluated by

15

Fujishima *et al.* 2 ml of 2% Lignocaine is injected 15 mm away from limbus in the inferotemporal quadrant through a blunt cannula. They found good co-operation of the patients and did not have much chemosis. The advantage is of retaining the motility of eyeball so that correction of the squint can be evaluated on the table itself. The author has no experience to recommend this procedure.

Retrobulbar anesthesia: This is the most commonly used anesthesia in all adults and cooperative adolescents. A dose of 3–4 ml of 2% Lignocaine is injected in the retrobulbar, intraconal space. For prolonged procedures it is mixed with 0.5% Bupivacaine in 1: 1 ratio. Facial akinesia is usually not required.

Some surgeons have used **Peribulbar anesthesia** just as for anterior segment surgery, mainly to decrease the risk of retrobulbar hemorrhage of scleral perforation. But more local anesthetic (8–10 ml) is required and chemosis sometimes can be very difficult to work with. For both retrobulbar and peribulbar anesthesia, care must be taken to avoid injury to the inferior rectus, which has been reported in several cases of anterior segment surgery.

General anesthesia: General anesthesia with intratracheal intubation or with a laryngeal mask, with halothane or nitrous oxide is used in most strabismus surgery in children as also for uncooperative adults. Cases with complications or requiring extensive surgery like slipped muscle or post-traumatic restrictive squints, or post-detachment surgery squints, are better operated under general anesthesia.

Cases of partially accommodative esotropia receiving miotics (cholinesterase inhibitors) should be stopped six weeks prior.

Dissociative Anesthesia

Dissociative anesthesia with agents like ketamine can be used for smaller procedures like adjustment in children as also for botulinum toxin injection in children.

However, they cause undesirable visual hallucinations and forced duction test can be unreliable because the muscle tone is increased by ketamine (intraocular pressure is also increased).

Conjunctival Incisions

The different conjunctival approaches are (Fig. 15.7):
1. Limbal incision of von Noorden
2. Over the muscle incision of Swan.
3. Paralimbal incision of Prem Prakash
4. Fornix incision of Parks.
5. MISS

1. Limbal Incision of von Noorden

This is a segmental peritomy incision with two radial incisions parallel to the palpebral aperture resulting in an unrecognisable scar. It gives good exposure of the recti and makes it easy to work in the correct tissue plane. At the limbus the conjunctiva and Tenons are fused and can be lifted together. It is also advantageous while doing conjunctival recession or while doing adjustable squint surgery. Even for the vertical recti and the inferior obliques, they give good exposure, making the anatomy visible without distortion.

Our technique is to pass two 6–0 silk or cotton sutures at the ends of the proposed peritomy. The limbal incision is made by a blade taking care not to go too deep to cut the sclera tangentially. The radial incisions are made with the blunt spring scissors.

2. Over the Muscle Incision of Swan

This conjunctival incision is concentric with the limbus, for the medial rectus, it is made 1–2 mm anterior to the plica semilunaris, and for the lateral rectus, midway between the limbus and lateral formix. After incision of the conjunctiva, the sclera is exposed superior and inferior to the muscle by cutting through the Tenon's capsule and intermuscular membranes. It leaves a bad scar and can form adhesions between conjunctiva and the muscle if the muscle sheath is ruptured.

3. Para Limbal Incision of Prem Prakash

This is a compromise of the above two techniques, having the advantage of less risk of direct injury to the recti muscles, with good exposure and also allowing passage of two paralimbal sutures 2 mm and 4 mm from limbus, one of which can be used to retract the globe, the other to retract the conjunctiva. The incision is made between the two sutures with spring scissors. The Tenon's has to be dissected before the muscle can be exposed. It also leaves a scar in the visible palpebral area and is not the incision of choice.

4. Fornix incision of Parks

This conjunctival incision is made either in the superior or inferior fornix, usually more on the bulbar conjunctiva and 8 mm from limbus just adjacent to the vertical recti. Bare sclera is exposed after incising the Tenon's capsule perpendicular to the conjunctival incision. This leaves a hidden scar but yields a poor exposure difficult for beginners. However once learnt it is preferred as it is better accepted by the patient, being less irritative

in recent postoperative phase has less visible hyperemia and no visible scarring.

5. MISS

Recently Minimal incision strabismus surgery, MISS has been described by Mojo. It uses two small incisions just at the upper amd lower poles of the insertions of the horizontal recti and the muscle sutured under the conjunctiva. It does not lead to much advantage and is only possible for small recessions and plications in place of resections.

Conjunctival Recession or Resection

In cases of long-standing deviations or those having scars causing a tight conjunctiva, the conjunctival recession is done. FDT done prior to conjunctival incision gets relieved after the incision. A 5 mm conjunctival recession is usually done and is easily incorporated with the limbal incision approach (Fig. 15.17).

Similarly a conjunctival resection of the excess, redundant conjunctiva can also be done.

Choice of Sutures

For recession and resection surgery 6–0 vicryl polyglactin with 5–29 double armed spatulated needles are used.

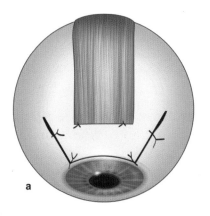 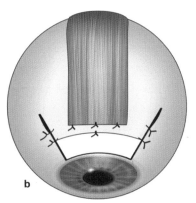

Fig. 15.17: Surgical step showing conjunctival closure. (a) Conventional complete conjunctival apposition in recession and resection, (b) Conjunctival recession of with about 5 mm bare sclera can be done if conjunctival shortening is present. A central suture with the underlying sclera is optional.

15

For inferior oblique the same may be used or 6–0 polyglactin (vicryl) with 5–28 double armed needles (half circle needle) are better.

For posterior fixation (Faden) superior oblique expander non-absorbable 5–0 mersilene suture is used.

For conjunctival closure 8–0 vicryl, same as for recession-resection may be used or 7–0 collagen suture may be used. The latter dissolves earlier and causes less congestion.

Vertical Transpositioning of Horizontal Recti

The horizontal recti can be recessed or resected with vertical transpositioning (shifting). This is done to correct associated A–V patterns or to correct associated vertical deviations along with the horizontal deviations.

The shifting is done such that the muscle insertion remains concentric to the limbus. The following guide is helpful (Fig. 15.18):

i. **A pattern:**
   a. Medial recti shifted up (both eyes) or
   b. Lateral recti shifted down (both eyes) or
   c. Medial rectus up, lateral rectus down in a monocular recession-resection.

ii. **V pattern:**
   a. Medial recti shifted down (both eyes)
   b. Lateral recti shifted up (both eyes)
   c. Medial rectus down and lateral rectus up in a monocular recession resection.

iii. Associated hypertropia: Both medial and lateral rectus shifted down in the hypertropic eye.

iv. Associated hypotropia: both medial and lateral rectus shifted up in the hypotropic eye.

Slanting Recession-resections

The A–V patterns can also be treated by differential recession of the upper and lower ends of the horizontal recti.

i. For A esotropia: Both medial recti are recessed with the upper end recessed more (3–5 mm difference) than the lower ends.

ii. For A exotropia: Both lateral recti are recessed with the lower ends recessed more than the upper ends.

iii. For V esotropia: Both medial recti recessed, lower ends recessed more.

iv. For V exotropia: Both lateral recti recessed with the upper ends recessed more.

A similar slanting resection is made such that the sutures are placed in the muscle in an oblique fashion. For example, for a V

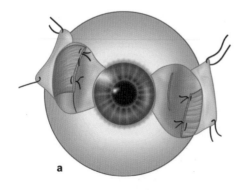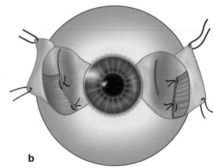

a   b

Fig. 15.18: Surgical scheme of vertical transposition (shifting) of horizontal recti. (a) In A or V pattern both medial or lateral recti may be symmetrically shifted or a monocular recession–resection may be combined with shifting, (b) For hypertropia correction along with horizontal surgery both the recti are shifted in the same direction (down) Reverse for hypotropia.

exotropia: medial rectus is resected such that the resection is more at the upper end, and lateral rectus is recessed more at the upper end (Fig. 15.19).

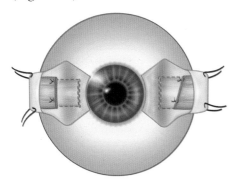

Fig. 15.19: Slanting (differential) recession and differential resection shown for horizontal recti, done for A–V patterns.

Transpositioning of Muscles

Cases in which the function of a muscle cannot be improved by any strengthening procedure, the other adjacent muscles can be transpositioned to aid/improve the action of the paralytic muscle (Fig. 15.20).

Thus in an elevator underaction, the medial and lateral recti are reinserted close to the superior rectus (Knapp's procedure). Indications of muscle transposition are:

1. Paralytic strabismus
2. Slipped or lost muscle
3. Duane's retraction syndrome (rarely).

The essential prerequisite before a transposition is attempted is the absence of any restriction of the antagonist as seen by FDT. If the antagonist is tight, a recession of the same and dissection to free adhesions around it is first done. Care must be taken, however, to not risk having anterior segment ischemia by operating on two vertical recti and lateral rectus simultaneously. A Knapp's procedure (on both horizontal recti with inferior rectus recession) is safe in young adults and children but should be avoided in old people with compromised circulation. The procedure described are many

1. **Hummelsheim's procedure** for lateral rectus palsy: lateral halves of superior and inferior recti are dissected up to 14 mm from their insertion and reinserted adjacent to the lateral rectus insertion. Can also be used for a lost, medial rectus muscle.

2. **Jensen's procedure** for lateral rectus palsy: lateral halves of both superior and inferior recti and the upper and lower halves of lateral rectus dissected free for about 14 mm from their insertion. The lateral half of SR and upper half of LR are tied with 5–0 mersilene sutures at around the equator. Similarly the lateral half of IR and lower half of LR are also tied. This procedure is supposed to have less chance of anterior segment ischemia, but it has still been reported probably due to strangulation by the sutures. To prevent this a modification is suggested where the corresponding edges of the adjacent recti are sutured after splitting as above.

3. **Callahan's procedure:** A modification of the same used for Elevator palsy is called Callahan's procedure where the upper halves of medial and lateral recti are tied with the two halves of superior rectus.

4. **Peter's procedure** for medial rectus in a III C.N. palsy, using the superior oblique. This has been done without removing it from trochlea and shortening the tendon by 16–20 mm.

Other procedures are **listed here:**

- **O' Connor's** lateral rectus cinch with transposition of vertical recti to lateral rectus.

- **Knapp's** procedure for elevator palsy: transpositioning horizontal recti to superior rectus.

- **Helveston's** procedure using preserved sclera to transpose half of vertical recti to the medial rectus. Scott-Foster augmented the effect of the transposed muscle by using posterior fixation sutures on the transposed half 8 mm posterior, to vectorize the forces in line with the paralytic muscle.

15

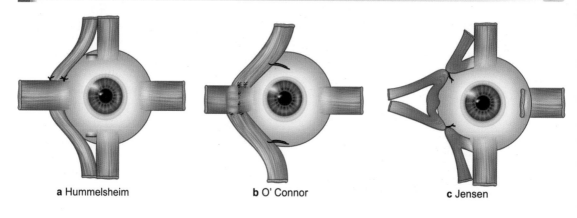

a Hummelsheim   **b** O' Connor   **c** Jensen

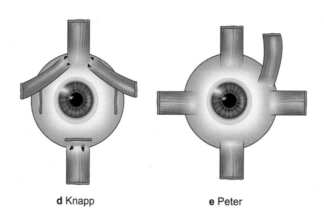

d Knapp   **e** Peter

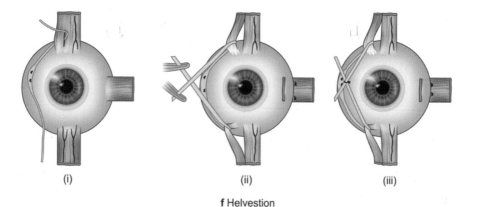

(i)   (ii)   (iii)

f Helvestion

Fig. 15.20: Transposition procedures. (a) Hummelsheim's for lateral rectus palsy, (b) O'Connor's for LR palsy with a cinching of LR, (c) Jensen's for LR palsy with MR recession, (d) Knapp's for Elevator palsy with IR recession, (e) Peter's for adduction in Third nerve palsy and (f) Helveston's: 1.5 mm × 100 mm glycerine preserved sclera used in a case of absent MR (left eye) with recession of LR.

15

Surgery on Vertical Recti

While the weakening and strengthening procedures on the vertical recti are the same as for the horizontal recti, some important differences should be noted.

1. Changes in Lid Position

- The vertical recti are intricately connected to the upper and lower lids. Any surgery more than 5–6 mm without dissecting these attachments can cause changes in the palpebral aperture, also causing:
- Inferior rectus recession: lower lid retraction. Ptosis of the lowerlid.
- Inferior rectus resection: elevation of the lower lid.
- Superior rectus recession: upper lid retraction.
- Superior rectus resection: ptosis of the upper lid.
- This is due to the fact that the check ligaments for the vertical recti are linked to the **Whitnall's ligament** (for superior rectus) and **Lockwood's ligament** (for inferior rectus).

The Lockwood's ligament is a fibrous condensation with the fascia of inferior rectus and inferior oblique.

2. Effectivity of Vertical Recti Surgery

The recession and resection on superior and inferior recti are very effective usually more than 5 mm is not required, the minimal amount required being 2 mm. In cases of congenital muscle fibrosis, large 8–9 mm of recession of inferior recti are called for and if a proper dissection of the attaching fibres is done, no significant lid changes are seen. Slight depression of lower lid may still be seen but are tolerated as bilateral surgery is done. Another condition of large recessions is dysthyroid orbitomyopathy.

As a **general golden rule** the inferior rectus recession should be done conservatively, because the downgaze is more critical to be compromised.

Adjustable recession can be done to ensure better alignment.

Surgery on Oblique Muscles

Surgery on oblique muscles is commonly done either in combination with horizontal muscle surgery as in A and V patterns or for correction of cyclovertical muscle problems like superior oblique palsy, double elevator palsy (contralateral eye inferior oblique), etc. An important fact to remember is that as the oblique muscles do not contribute to the anterior segment circulation they can be combined with horizontal or vertical recti surgery with no added risk of anterior segment ischemia. Thus it is much safer to do a torsional Kestenbaum (for a nystagmus with null in head-tilt position) on all four obliques rather than all four vertical recti with horizontal shifting.

The surgical procedures can be classified as follows:

I. *Weakening Procedures*

a. Inferior oblique (Fig. 15.21)
   i. Generalised weakening
   - Recession
   - Myectomy
   - Disinsertion
   - Denervation
   - Extirpation
   ii. Selective weakening
   - Anteropositioning with recession
   - Pure anteropositioning (without recession)
   - Total anteropositioning
   - Recession of anterior fibres
b. Superior oblique
   i. Generalised weakening
   - Tenotomy (temporal/nasal approach)
   - Tenectomy
   - Recession
   - Translational recession
   - L-lengthening

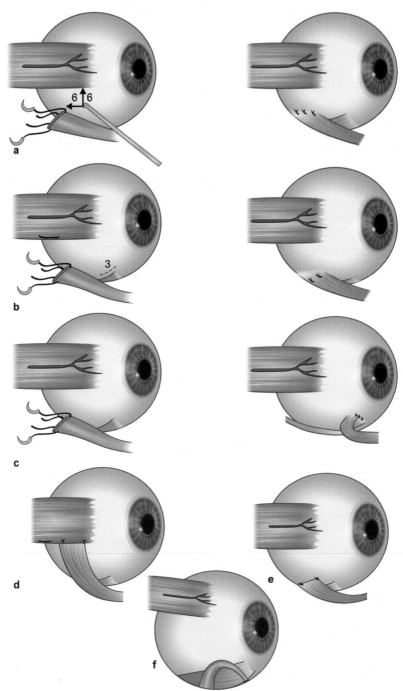

Fig. 15.21: Controlled inferior oblique weakening procedures: (a) Recession Fink's method 6 mm inferior 6 mm posterior to LR, (b) Recession Park's method 2 mm lateral 3 mm posterior to IR, (c) Elliot and Nankin's anteropositioning (total anteropositioning), (d) Pure anteropositioning at inferior border of LR and (e) Modified E and N's anteropositioning (recession-cum-anteropositioning) at lateral border of IR, (f) Stager's anterior and nasal transpositioning.

- Silicon expander lengthening—Loop tenotomy at the insertion

ii. Selective weakening
- Posterior tenotomy
- Posterior tenectomy
- Recession of anterior fibres.
- Anteropositioning.

II. Strengthening Procedures

a. Inferior oblique
  i. Generalised strengthening
  - Advancement
  - Resection and/or double breasting
  ii. Selective strengthening
  - Advancement of anterior fibres.
b. Superior oblique
  i. Generalised strengthening
  - Tucking (tenoplication)
  ii. Selective strengthening
  - Tenting of nasal fibres (Harada-Ito or its modifications)

In the above classification, **generalised** refers to an effect on all the functions of the oblique, whereas selective implies a differential effect on the vertical and abducting function vis-a-vis the torsional effect. It should be remembered that the obliques have a fan-shaped insertion. The anterior fibres of superior oblique cause intorsion, and of inferior oblique cause extorsion. The posterior fibres of superior oblique cause depression and abduction in downgaze. The posterior fibres of the inferior oblique cause elevation and abduction in upgaze. Surgery on one group, sparing others weakens that function selectively without much effect on the other function. Thus a Harada-Ito procedure on superior oblique strengthens the intorsion selectively.

Weakening Procedures on Inferior Oblique

The weakening procedures on inferior oblique are commonly required to be undertaken in the following indications:

1. Superior oblique palsy (ipsilateral inferior oblique).
2. V-pattern deviations with overacting inferior obliques (inferior obliques of both eyes)
3. Double-elevator palsy (contralateral inferior oblique).
4. Upshoots in Duane's retraction syndrome with inferior oblique overaction (ipsilateral inferior oblique).
5. Dissociated vertical deviations (with inferior oblique overaction).
6. Other paralytic/restrictive conditions.
7. Torsional Kestenbaum (in combination with other obliques).

Approach

While the earliest surgery on inferior oblique was done through the skin approach by Bonnet (1841), now the conjunctival approach is chosen. The choice of limbal incision, paralimbal incision or fornix based incision depends on the surgeons's preference. Author's preference is for the fornix incision, as it allows good visualisation of the muscle without disturbing the tissues, and it also allows surgery on lateral rectus surgery if required.

Technique

After the lateral limbal or temporal fornix incision, the lateral rectus is hooked (see recession surgery steps) and the intermuscular septum dissected in the inferotemporal quadrant. The globe is retracted in the superonasal quadrant. The anterior edge of the inferior oblique muscle can be seen as it runs towards the underside of lateral rectus. A blunt hook is passed to lift the inferior oblique gradually till the posterior edge can be seen from the under side as the muscle is lifted. After the entire muscle belly of the inferior oblique is hooked, the intermuscular septum posterior to the muscle is perforated. The fascia between the lateral rectus and the muscle is dissected. The muscle is disinserted

15

with tenotomy scissors under direct vision. The cut ends of the inferior oblique is held with forceps as two vicryl 6-0 sutures are passed one at each end. If available 6-0 vicryl with half circle needles is preferred. The adjacent fasicia is dissected free from the muscle.

The muscle is reinserted using one of the following methods. Each gives a different form of weakening effect; **recession alone, recession with anteropositioning** or **anteropositioning alone** (Fig. 15.21).

i. **Fink's method of recession:** A point 6 mm inferior and 6 mm posterior from the inferior end of the lateral rectus insertion provides the anterior point of insertion for 8 mm recession of inferior oblique. The posterior point is 5-6 mm posterior to the anterior point in the same meridian. For 10 mm recession, the anterior point is 2 mm down from the 8 mm point along the course of the muscle (towards inferior rectus). A 2 mm upward point gives 6 mm recession.

This method reattaches the muscle along the original course of the muscle, only slackening it without inducing anteropositioning.

ii. **Park's method of recession:** A point 2 mm lateral and 3 mm posterior to the lateral end of the insertion of inferior rectus, gives a point of recession of about 10 mm. The posterior point is 5 mm posterior.

This method has slight anteropositioning effect also in addition to the recession.

iii. **Elliot and Nankin's method of recession-cum-anteropositioning:** The anterior end of muscle is positioned at the lateral end of the inferior rectus insertion, with the posterior end being further down (A 5 mm posterior along the lateral border of inferior rectus as modified by the author).

This method in addition to recession, anteropositions the muscle, severely

weakening the elevator and abduction in downgaze. For more effect the anterior end can be inserted about 1 mm or even 2 mm anterior to the lateral end of the inferior rectus. Retaining the posterior end of the muscle 5 mm posterior does not eliminate the elevator function totally. Another variation is Anterior and Nasal transposition described by Stager whereby the IO is reinserted 2 mm nasal to the insertion of inferior rectus.

iv. **Pure anteropositioning:** In this method described from our centre (Prakash, Gupta, Sharma, 1994), the inferior oblique muscle is reinserted just adjacent to the inferior edge of the lateral rectus, with the anterior end of the oblique being at the inferior end of the lateral rectus insertion.

This procedure anteropositions the inferior oblique without producing any recession (a 2 mm or 1.5 mm recession is to counter the resection effect of surgery). The weakening effect is primarily from the anteropositioning affecting the elevator and abduction in upgaze, and is comparable to 8 mm of Fink's recession. It does not change the torsional status (all recessions weaken extorsion).

v. **Total anteropositioning:** The entire width of the inferior oblique is re-inserted anterior to the inferior rectus. This weakens the elevator function almost totally. In fact some depressor action may be produced, with the Lock wood's ligament acting as the new functional origin of the inferior oblique, the muscle running parallel to the inferior rectus. Thus surgery is advocated for dissociated vertical deviation with inferior oblique overaction.

vi. **Myectomy of inferior oblique:** The muscle after being hooked as above is clamped between two artery clamps for 1-2 minutes, then the muscle is cut with tenotomy scissors in between. It may cause bleeding and some surgeons cauterize the cut ends. The author feels this is a very "traumatic' procedure, it cannot be undone, and can give unpredictable results. Moreover, the effect cannot be graduated as in case of recession. In the modern age of controlled procedures, this appears obsolete.

vii. **Denervation and extirpation:** The nerve to the inferior oblique is a fusiform structure on the posterior border of the inferior oblique muscle. This can be hooked and stocked to identify a tight band which is cauterized. This results in the laxity of the muscle. The muscle is disinserted and the entire mess is extirpated. This procedure is to be done only if overaction persists inspite of maximal recession/myectomy.

viii. **Recession of anterior fibres:** The anterior half fibres are separately hooked and split from the rest of the fibres for a length of 12–14 mm and recessed. This will selectively weaken extorsion without affecting the elevator and abductor function. This procedure is done in combination with advancement of the anterior fibres of superior oblique of the same eye plus a similar strengthening (of inferior oblique) and weakening (of superior oblique) anterior fibres of the other eye in torsional Kestenbaum surgery.

Strengthening procedures of inferior oblique

The strengthening procedures on inferior oblique are limited. As it lacks a tendinous portion, resection cannot be done (it will be a myectomy and so weaken it). However, double breasting has been tried and found to be successful.

For **selective strengthening** the anterior half (or entire width) is disinserted and advanced 8 mm upwards from its actual insertion.

Weakening Procedures on Superior Oblique Muscle (Fig 15.22)

The indications for the weakening procedures on the superior oblique are:

1. A pattern deviations with overacting superior obliques (bilateral superior obliques).
2. Brown's syndrome with overacting superior oblique: "Brown's plus" (unilateral superior oblique).
3. Torsional Kestenbaum surgery (as a part of recession-advancement of four obliques).

Special Features

The superior oblique has a long tendon and has its functional origin from the trochlea (running from anterior posterior-wards). It has a fan shaped insertion under the superior rectus. Nasal to the superior rectus the fascia around the superior oblique is not having a distinct sheath and dissection in this area should be tampered with as little surgical manipulation as possible, to prevent any postoperative adhesions. It is much safer to operate from the temporal side.

Surgical Approach

The superior oblique has to be operated with the surgeon sitting on the side of the patient looking towards the upper fornix. The conjunctival incisions is superior limbal (author's choice). Other approaches are fornix incision or paralimbal incision.

The Temporal Approach

After lifting the superior limbal flap and hooking the superior rectus from the temporal side, the superotemporal quadrant is dissected, cutting the intermuscular septum temporal to the superior rectus. The glistening fibres of the superior oblique can be visualized after retracting the superior rectus nasally. There is no need to disinsert the superior rectus as advocated by some surgeons. The subsequent steps are different in the following procedures.

15

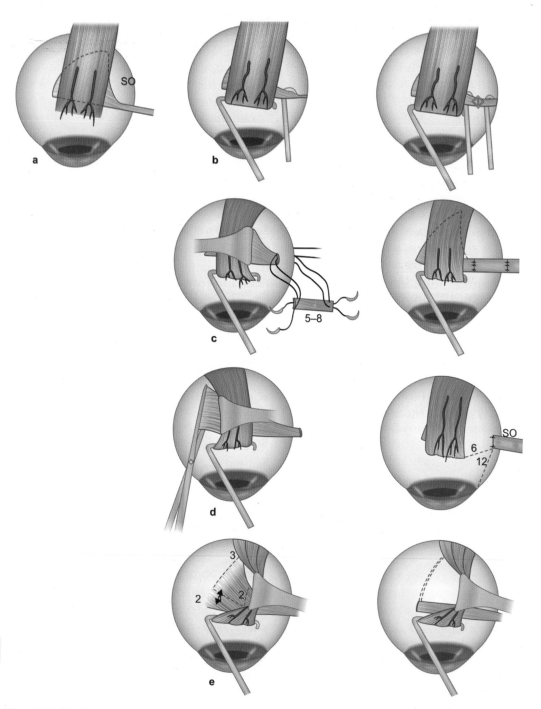

Fig. 15.22: Weakening procedures on superior oblique of right eye: (a) Normal relation of superior oblique and superior rectus, (b) Tenotomy: nasal approach, (c) Silicon expander lengthening 5–8 mm, (d) Translational recession of superior oblique, SO reinserted 6 mm medial to SR and 12 mm from limbus, and (e) Posterior Tenectomy of superior oblique sparing only anterior 1–2 mm fibres, posterior fibres cut in three steps 1, 2, 3.

i. For **tenotomy** the tendon is disinserted at the insertion full width and left to retract. The results are very unpredictable as the free end gets re-attached at any point. In tenecomy a part of the superior oblique is cut between two hemostats.

After identification and hooking the superior oblique the tenectomy may be done nasal to the superior rectus.

This procedure causes a generalised weakening of all functions (including intorsion).

ii. **Tenectomy of posterior fibres (Posterior tenectomy of superior oblique: PTSO).** In this procedure after hooking the superior oblique, the anterior (1 or 2 mm width) fibres are spared and a wedge of the posterior fibres is excised.

This selectively weakens the depressor and abduction in downgaze, correcting the pattern deviations, without significantly affecting intorsion.

iii. **Recession of the full width**

After disinserting the tendon, it is re-inserted 4 mm nasal to the superior rectus. It may be inserted close to the nasal border of superior rectus for less weakening effect.

Prieto-Diaz has suggested inserting the tendon 12 mm from limbus and 6 mm from the nasal end of superior rectus for translational recession. This procedure is supposed to prevent limitation of depression in abduction usually seen with anterior placement of superior oblique.

iv. **Recession of anterior fibres**

A selective recession of the anterior half width can be done for weakening the intorsion alone without affecting depression and abduction in downgaze. This is a part of the torsional Kestenbaum surgery.

The Nasal Approach

After a superior limbal incision or a para-limbal incision (former preferred), the superior rectus is hooked with minimal dissection of nasal intermuscular septum, just button holing close to the nasal end of insertion. A small blunt Steven's hook is passed to hook the glistening band of superior oblique.

For tenotomy or tenectomy the superior oblique is transected after bringing it out of its fascial sheath.

For **silicon band expander lengthening** procedure, prior to transection, two double armed 5–0 mersilene sutures are passed 2 mm apart from each other, the temporal one being 3–4 mm nasal to the nasal border of superior rectus. After transection, the piece of silicon band (2 mm or 2.5 mm wide and 5, 6, 7, 8 mm long) is interposed between the cut ends of the tendon with the help of the sutures. Care being taken to minimally disturb the adjoining fascia, to prevent postoperative adhesions. **The silicon band lengthening is preferably done through the temporal approach.**

The advantage of the lengthening procedure is that it maintains the fan shaped insertion of the superior oblique. The disadvantage is the risk of adhesions.

Another lengthening procedure uses the **split tendon,** split longitudinally for 10 mm length and joining the cut half widths. This procedure was described by Ciancia, but is not very popular.

Strengthening procedures of the superior oblique (Fig. 15.23).

For generalised strengthening the favourite procedure is **tucking,** or **tenoplication. It may be done from temporal or nasal approach but the former is preferred.** A restraint should be exercised with frugal tissue handling to prevent an iatrogenic Brown's syndrome (tight superior oblique). It can be done with the help of a tendon tucker or else a combination of a hook and a resection clamp can serve the same purpose. The tendon is hooked and lifted to double fold over itself and a resection clamp applied. Non-absorbable sutures are passed to secure the double folded tendon. A

15

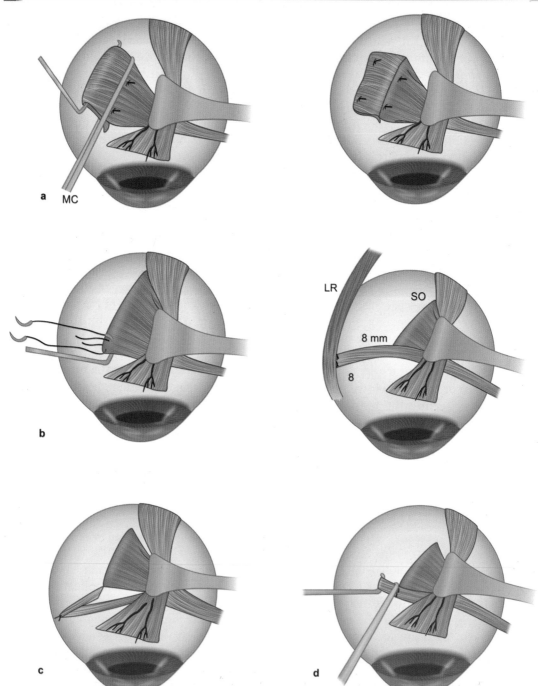

Fig. 15.23: Strengthening procedures of superior oblique. (a) Tucking (full width) with a hook (H) and muscle clamp (MC) instead of a tucker, (b) Classic Harada-Ito procedure, selective advancement of anterior 4 mm fibres close to LR, (c) Modified Harada-Ito procedure, tenting of anterior fibres by a suture close to LR and (d) Tucking of anterior fibres only.

4 + 4 mm double folding produces an 8 mm tuck which is enough for a 3 + superior oblique underaction.

After double folding the loop should be tucked and sutured temporally towards its insertion to prevent any mechanical obstruction. After tucking, an Exaggerated FDT for tightness of superior oblique should be done to confirm the absence of tight superior oblique and the inferior limbus should be able to go up, past the horizontal line joining the two canthi.

For **selective strengthening the Harada-Ito** or its modification procedures are used to selectively strengthen the intorsion. An anterior tenting of the anterior fibres with the help of a non-absorbable suture secures this. The suture is passed close to the temporal end of the superior rectus. The anterior fibres can also be advanced towards the lateral rectus (6–8 mm temporal to superior rectus). This may be done as an adjustable procedure (Metz).

A selective tucking of the anterior fibres can also be done. Such procedures are indicated in superior oblique paresis with intorsion defect as the main complaint. It is also a part of the torsional Kestenbaum procedure.

To conclude, the modern approach is to perform controlled and regulated procedures which can be performed to selectively weaken or strengthen the torsional effect or the elevator and depressor effect along with abduction in upgaze or downgaze to correct V or A pattern.

Newer Procedures

Periosteal fixation of the globe to the medial periosteum in cases of Third neve palsy: The medial periosteum is exposed either through the DCR incision or the retrocaruncular approach and a 5–0 Mersilene suture passed through it, which is brought to the inserion of medial rectus after a medial limbal incision and the globe adducted to produce 5–8pd of esotropia and tightened.

Lateral rectus periosteal fixation: After a lateral limbal incision the 5–0 mersilene suture is passed through the lateral retus and it is disinserted. The lateral periosteum is exposed and the LR secured to it.

Suggested Reading

1. Apt L. and Isenberg S. Eye position of strabismus patients under general anesthesia. Am. J. Ophthalmol 84: 574, 1997.

2. Beisner DH. Reduction of ocular torque by medial rectus recession. Arch. Ophthalmol 13: 85,1971.

3. Buckley EG and Flynn JT. Superior oblique recession versus tenotomy: A comparison of surgical results. J Pediatr. Ophthalmol. Strabismus, 20: 112, 1983.

4. Caldeira JA. Graduated recession of superior oblique muscle. Br. J. Ophthalmol 59, 553, 1975.

5. Cuppers C. The so-called "Faden operation" (Surgical correction by well defined changes in the arc of contact). In Fells P. editor. Second Congress of the International Strabismological Association, Marseilles. 1976. Diffusion Generale de Librairie. p. 395.

6. Dunlap EA. Plastic implants in muscle surgery: A study of the possible use of plastic material in the management of extraocular motility restrictions. Trans. Am. Ophthalmol Soc 65: 393, 1967.

7. Fink WH. Surgery of the oblique muscles of the eye St. Louis, 1951. Mosby—Year Book, Inc.

8. Harada M and Ito Y. Surgical correction of cyclotropia. Jpn. J. Ophthalmol. 8: 88. 1964.

9. Helveston EM. Muscle transposition procedures. Surv. Ophthalmol. 16: 92, 1971.

10. Helveston EM. Surgical Management of Strabismus. An Atlas of Strabismus Surgery ed. 4. St. Louis. 1993. Mosby—Year Book Inc.

11. Jampolsky A. Spring-back balance test in strabismus surgery. In Symposium on strabismus: transactions of the New Orleans Acad. of Ophthalmol. St. Louis, 1978 Mosby—Year Book Inc.

12. Jampolsky A. Adjustable strabismus surgical procedures. (as above).

13. Kushner BJ, Lucchese NJ, Morton GV. Variation in axial length and anatomical landmarks in strabismus patients. Ophthalmology 98: 410, 1991.

15

14. Metz HS. Muscle transposition surgery (20th Annual Frank Costenbader Lecture). J. Pediatr. Ophthalmol. Strabismus 30: 346, 1993.

15. Metz HS. and Lerner H. The adjustable Harada-Ito procedure Arch. Ophthalmol 99: 624, 1981.

16. Metz HS. The use of vertical offsets with horizontal strabismus surgery. Ophthalmology. 95: 1094, 1988.

17. Noorden GK. von. The limbal approach to surgery of the rectus muscles. Arch. Ophthalmol 80: 94, 1968.

18. Noorden GK. von. Indications of the posterior fixation operation in strabismus. Ophthalmology, 85: 572, 1978.

19. Noorden GK. von, Jenkins R.H. and Rosenbaum AL. Horizontal transposition of the vertical rectus muscles for treatment of ocular torticollis J Pediatr. Ophthalmol. Strabismus. 30: 8, 1993.

20. Oliver JM. and Lee JP. Recovery of anterior segment circulation after strabismus surgery in adult patients. Ophthalmology 99: 305, 1992.

21. Park MM. The weakening surgical procedures for eliminating overaction of the inferior oblique muscle Am. J. Ophthalmol 73: 107, 1972.

22. Romans P. and Gabriel L. Intraoperative adjustment of eye muscle surgery. Correction based on eye position during general anesthesia. Arch. Ophthalmol 103: 351, 1985.

23. Prakash P, Gupta A and Sharma P. Pure antero-positioning of inferior oblique. Acta Ophthalmologica 73, 373, 1994.

24. Stager DR. Weakley D.R. and Stager D. Anterior transposition of the inferior oblique-anatomic assessment of the neurovascular bundle. Arch. Ophthalmol 110: 360, 1992.

25. Wright KW. Color Atlas of Strabismus Surgery Philadelphia. 1991, J.B. Lippincott Co.

26. Elliott RL and Nankin SJ. Anterior transposition of the inferior oblique. J. Pediatr Ophthalmol Strabismus 18: 35, 1991.

27. Prieto-Diaz J. Management of Superior oblique overaction in A — pattern deviations. Gracefe's Arch. Clin. Exp. Ophthalmol 226: 126, 1988.

28. Sharma P, Khokhar SK, Thanikachallam: Evaluation of superior oblique weakening procedures. J Pediatr. Ophthalmol Strabismus 1998 (under publication).

15

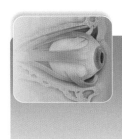

Complications of Strabismus Surgery

Like in any surgery, complications do occur, but can be minimized or at least better managed with proper understanding of technique and experience. They can be considered as in the order of their likely occurrence:

I. INTRAOPERATIVE

a. Surgical

1. *Operation on Wrong Eye*

In horizontal concomitant squints, this may technically make no difference (may even be beneficial allowing the amblyoic eye to be preferred in the postoperative period). But a patient not explained can feel cheated and go for litigation in case of horizontal paralytic squint and in vertical squints it can worsen the problem.

This can be avoided by marking the eye to be operated and checking the surgical plan before surgery.

2. *Operation on Wrong Muscle*

Sometimes due to a torsion of the globe during anesthesia, an unwitting surgeon may operate on the medial rectus instead of inferior rectus or likewise.

This can be prevented by the step described earlier in this chapter. It should be rectified, the moment it is realised.

3. *Wrong Operation Performed*

Recession instead of resection or vice versa can be done by mistake and have disastrous results. One should always check the deviation and surgical plan to prevent this. A recession can be easily converted to resection, as soon as it is realised. While doing this 1 mm less resection should be done. It is therefore always a better idea to do recession prior to resection in a combined procedure. A resection when converted to recession will have to take into account the resection plus extra 1 mm for correction.

Sometimes the vertical shifting of horizontal recti may be done in the opposite direction. This will aggravate the A or V pattern.

4. *Hemorrhages*

If the surgical technique is proper and all dissection done only in tissue planes, bleeding should occur only at two steps:

    i. Conjunctival incision (especially if limbal) and
    ii. At the time of muscle disinsertion.

Both these steps may require light wet field cautery. Slight bleeding may be stopped by pressing a bleeding point for a few seconds.

Regular ooze at every step may also occur due to positive venous pressure which some anesthetists may maintain. This should be communicated to him. Spotting with a swabstick soaked in 1:1000 adrenaline or vasoconstrictor eyedrops can also be used with the knowledge of the anesthetists.

Any major bleeding point should not be left unattended when conjunctival closure is made. One has to be extra cautious while operating posteriorly for retroequatorial myopexy (Faden), superior oblique surgery and inferior oblique recession.

5. Scleral Perforation

It can occur while

  i. Conjunctival limbal incision is made with blade,
  ii. Disinserting a tight rectus muscle with tenting of the thin sclera and
  iii. Passing sutures for muscle fixation.

A proper surgical technique prevents the first. For the tight muscle disinsertion, tenting of sclera should be avoided, if in doubt, instead of scissors use blade to cut the insertion with a hook as the template behind, cutting slowly with direct visualization. The occurrence of needles causing perforation in globe can be minimized with the use of spatulated needles. While working in the deep posterior space, use of small half circle needles help manoeuvring in small space. And for resection a stump of 0.5 mm is left for passage of sutures (sclera is thinnest, 0.3 mm, at the insertion site). Full thickness perforations are rare, most are usually self sealed and nothing needed to be done. But a posterior segment examination should be done immediately and a close follow-up maintained. Usually the risk of retinal detachment or endophthalmitis is extremely rare. And moreover experimental studies have shown that such complications are more likely if cryopexy was done prophylactically. A frank retinal tear however should be cryoed and a buckle applied.

6. Splitting of Muscle Fibres

A faulty technique of hooking may cause splitting of muscle fibres causing laceration of the muscle and subsequent fibrosis. Proper technique and doing under visualization helps. If undetected, half the muscle may only be recessed causing under correction. A proper dissection to ensure that full width is hooked is important.

7. Loose Suture and Partial Thickness Suture in the Muscle

This may fixate the muscle leaving the posterior fibres. A loose suture may cause more weakening than desired. Precision is the keyword in strabismus surgery.

8. Central Sag

It is usual in hang back recession or adjustable surgery as the muscle width is not enough. Two separate bites taken 8–10 mm should ensure a proper width.

However, if a central sag has occurred, a central suture is passed to properly suture this part.

9. Lost Muscle or Slipped Muscle

Rarely a muscle slips while disinsertion, without the sutures having passed, or when the sutures have given way. It is usually not difficult to locate a muscle if the surgeon does not lose his cool. Proper exposure, lighting, retraction of the globe and careful search helps. The adjacent oblique muscle attachments or intermuscular septum can be used as guides. Sutures are passed immediately in the muscle end that is sighted and held firmly. The appearance of muscle fibres (linear pattern) should be helpful. Some suggest use of electrical stimulation or EMG to confirm, but are usually not practically possible or available. If the muscle could not be found in spite of all efforts, a stay suture passed through the sclera on the opposite side or the insertion of the antagonist muscle is passed to keep the globe retracted, to allow muscle to be attached without causing gross squint. The stay suture should remain for two weeks. It the latter does not work a secondary surgery with transposition procedure may have to be contemplated.

Apart from intraoperative lost muscles, and loss during readjustments in adjustable surgery, a strabismus surgeon may have to deal with a previously lost muscle in a referred case. A proper technique has usually been successful in the author's centre. Cases of medial rectus

16

slipped after pterygium surgery has also been observed and successfully managed.

10. *Muscle Sheath, Tenon's Rupture and Fat Prolapse*

Improper technique may cause rupture of muscle sheath, Posterior Tenon's capsule may cause rupture of fat. This may cause extensive fibrosis if too much manipulation is done and can result in a "frozen orbit".

B. Anesthesia Related Complications

1. *Cardiac Arrest*

A serious and fatal consequence, but extremely rare, can occur. It may be due to underlying undetected cardiac disease. Strabismus can have associated cardiac anomalies as in myopathies or congenital syndromes.

2. *Bradycardia*

This is a rather common occurrence in strabismus surgery due to oculocardiac reflex, due to vagal inhibitory influence. Handling of recti muscles, particularly medial rectus can cause it, sometimes even pressure on the globe can cause it. Local 2% lignocaine drops can reduce its probability (even with general anesthesia). It may require intravenous atropine injection.

An oculorespiratory reflex is also reported.

3. *Malignant Hyperthermia*

This is a rare but fatal complication of anesthesia in strabismus surgery. It is supposed to have family history and some children have raised Creatinine Phosphokinase (CPK) levels in serum. A proper monitoring of temperature and noting for signs like trismus during induction itself may be helpful. **Intravenous dantrolene** preoperatively and before induction allows an uneventful anesthesia in such predisposed cases.

4. *Allergy*

Allergy or hypersensitivity to anesthetic agents like suxamethonium should be noted.

II. POSTOPERATIVE COMPLICATIONS

1. Vomiting

Emesis or vomiting is relatively more common in children after strabismus surgery. It may be related to muscle handling or the effect of certain drugs. Recently additional local anesthesia, using peribulbar and acupuncture, have been tried. Antiemetic drugs like droperiodol and ondan setrone are being used.

2. Infections

While slight fever may be seen on the first postoperative day, orbital infections are rare. Orbital cellulitis and suture abscess can occur rarely. They respond well to intravenous and topical antibiotics or antifungals (Fig. 16.1).

3. Suture Granuloma and Reactions

Suture reactions have become less frequent with better suture material available. Earlier silk was used which caused suture granulomas. 6–0/polyglactin (vicryl) has a good track record. It does cause hyperemia, which persists for about two weeks as long as they dissolve.

Allergic reactions can occur both as acute or late allergy to silk sutures. Local steroid drops usually help eliminate such reactions or granuloma. Rarely excision may be required (Fig. 16.2).

4. Tenon's Prolapse and Conjunctival Cysts

Improper apposition of conjunctiva allows Tenon's to prolapse which hampers healing. Implantation conjunctival cysts can occur if malap-position of conjunctiva allows epithelial cells to be embedded. These can be evacuated by needle puncture or excised.

5. Dellen

Corneal dellens due to disruption of tear film and local dehydration are known. The author described scleral dellen in a case of conjunctival recession (bare sclera) which caused localised drying and thinning on exposure and

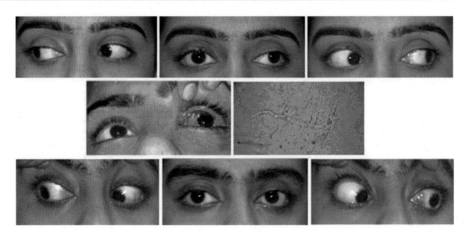

Fig. 16.1: Fungal infection: (top) preoperative view, (middle) fungal infection with fungal hypha, (bottom) after treatment.

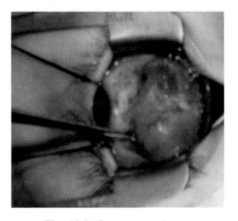

Fig. 16.2: Suture granuloma.

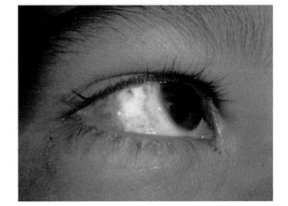

Fig. 16.3: Scleral dellen.

disappeared on rehydration. It required a conjunctival flap. Cauterization should be as light as possible (Fig. 16.3).

6. Anterior Segment Ischemia

This is a rare but serious disorder presenting with corneal edema, corneal thinning, non-pigmented keratic precipitates, segmental iris atrophy with distorted pupil and anterior chamber flare. Late sequelae of cataract and even phthisis bulbi are known. It occurs in cases of three or more adjacent recti surgery being done in one eye, especially in adults with atherosclerosis and hyperviscosity syndromes. Cases with local radiation therapy and cases with previous retinal detachment

surgery are predisposed. As discussed earlier it can be avoided if two vertical recti are not operated along with one horizontal rectus (especially lateral rectus). The obliques do not contribute to the anterior segment circulation and can be used as alternatives.

Treatment is with intensive systemic and local corticosteroids. Most patients show recovery without significant loss of vision, though after a prolonged clinical course.

7. Over Corrections and under Corrections

A cent-percent orthophorisation in strabismus surgery is a surgeon's dream rarely fulfilled. A 10% under correction and about 5% over corrections occur in most expert hands. This

16

may occur in the immediate postoperative period or be delayed due to a post-surgery drift.

Small residual (under corrections) or consecutive (over correction) exotropias are easily managed by orthoptic fusional vergences or by manipulating the spherical correction in young children with high AC/A ratio. Postoperative esodeviations may be similarly managed or may require prism neutralization.

A marked over correction after a recession especially adjustable suture may be due to muscle slippage and should be managed without delay. Otherwise resurgery should be done after 6 weeks or three months. Cooper's dictum of undoing what was done may be required or it may be treated as a fresh case. This is evaluated after observing versions for any incomitance and FDT (Fig. 16.4).

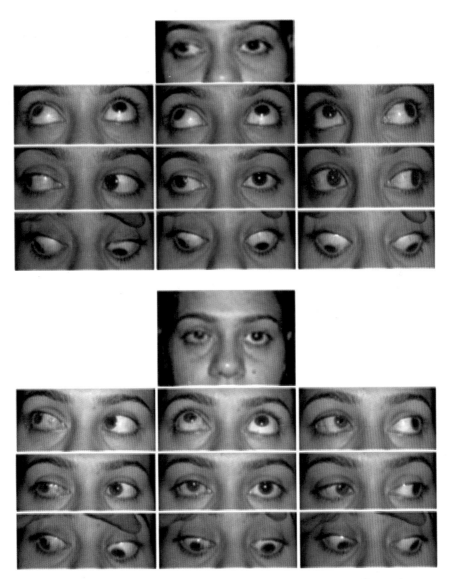

Fig. 16.4: Residual squint (top) and corrected after surgery (bottom)

16

A note of caution may be made as demonstrated by author's experience of an intermittent exotrope who was over corrected. He started having increasing convergent squint. On suspicion, fundus examination showed papilledema and computerized tomography revealed internal hydrocephalus, requiring immediate neurosurgical intervention. This case highlights the need to keep an open mind and evaluate for neurological changes even postoperatively.

Suggested Reading

1. Bergman JA. Idiopathic malignant hyperthermia Arch. Ophthalmol 93: 232, 1975.

2. Brown HW. Complications in surgery of the extraocular muscles. In Fasanella R.M. editor: Management of complications in Eye Surgery. Philadelphia, 1957. W.B. Saunders Co.

3. Brown HW. Complications of the surgical management of strabismus in Haik GM editor. Strabismus Symposium of the New Orleans Academy of Ophthalmology. St. Louis, 1962. Mosby–Year Book Inc.

4. Cooper EL. The surgical management of secondary exotropia Trans. Am. Acad. Ophthalmol. Otolaryagol 65: 595, 1961.

6. Prakash P, Verma D and Menon V. Anterior segment ischemia following extraocular muscle surgery Jpn. J. Ophthalmol 30: 251, 1986.

7. Salamon SM, Friberg TR and Luxenburg M.N. Endophthalmitis after strabismus surgery. Am J. Ophthalmol 93: 39, 1982.

8. Saunders RA, Bluestein EC, Wilson ME, and Berland JE. Anterior segment ischemia after strabismus surgery. Surv. Ophthalmol 38: 456, 1994.

9. Sharma P. Arya AV and Prakash P. Scleral dellen in strabismus surgery. Acta Ophthalmol 68:493, 1990.

10. Simon JW, Lininger LL and Scheraga JL. Recognised scleral perforation during eye muscle surgery: incidence and sequelae. J. Pediatr. Ophthalmol Strabismus. 29: 273. 1992.

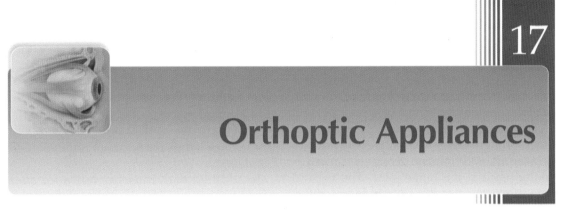

Orthoptic Appliances

INTRODUCTION

The objects seen under conditions of binocular vision are seen by both eyes, and one cannot know which eye is seeing what? Or whether one eye is not functioning at all. This is possible if the two eyes can be **dissociated** so that the single "physical space" (the real three dimensional world) is broken into **two "physical spaces"**, one visible to each eye. This can be done by:

1. **Septum** so that one half of the field is seen by one eye exclusively and the other half by the other eye.
2. **Two tubes** one in front of each eye.
3. **Red-green glasses,** which are totally complementary in the sense that one eye with red filter sees only red light and the other with green filter sees only green light.
4. **Polaroid dissociation,** each eye views through polaroid filters each one at 90° to the other.
5. **Bagolini's striations,** a spot light scattered by striations, the two glasses set at 90° to each other.

The idea is to control the image presented to each eye (in intensity, colour, etc.) as well as in relation to each other (in physical location), so that different parts of the retina of each eye, as desired, can be stimulated.

Uses of Orthoptic Appliances

They can be used for:

i. Diagnosis like-measurement of deviation (subjectively/objectively), range of fusion, accommodation-convergence/ accommodation ratio

- The status of binocular single vision (suppression, amblyopia anomalous retinal correspondence),
- The evaluation of stereoacuity and
- Appreciation of entoptic phenomena.

ii. **Therapeutics** in providing fusional exercises

- Correction of anomalous retinal correspondence,
- Relative accommodation or relative convergence and
- Amblyopia therapy to teach coordination with the Haidinger brushes.

Some of the important orthoptic instruments are described here, their use is also described in the relevant sections.

1. SYNOPTOPHORE

This is a complete orthoptic instrument which is based on the principle of haploscope (two physical locations projected to create one physiological localization). The oldest model was called **Amblyoscope** devised by Worth and later modified by Black, so it is called **Worth-Black amblyoscope.**

Worth-Black amblyoscope consists of two sets of tubes hinged to one another. Each set consists of a short tube joined to a longer tube at an angle of 120° with a mirror placed at the point of union, slide or object is projected at the distal cut of each tubes, viewed through a convex lens having a focal length of 12.5 cm, so that it simulates seeing a distant object and accommodation is not required. The two sets can be brought closer to simulate convergence or taken apart to simulate divergence, rotation taking place at the hinge joint. The vertical deviation can also be adjusted, but inter-pupillary distance cannot be adjusted. This basic model is not used in the orthoptic sections but can be used for Home Vision Therapy for various orthoptic exercises.

Instrument Design

The basic design of the synoptophore is shown in Fig. 17.1. There are different modifications of synoptophore with added features. Thus in addition to measuring deviation and management of binocular vision function, there are provisions for afterimages, automatic flashing and Haidinger's brushes.

Clement-Clarke International Ltd., makes three designs 2051, 52, 53 of which 2051 is the most comprehensive one with all the above mentioned additions. 2052 has autoflashing and after image attachments but not the Haidinger brushes attachment. And 2053 is the basic model without any of these additions.

The instrument has a **base** which houses the transformer (AC-DC) and voltage selector, on-off switch. The switches and controls of other additions are also on the base unit.

Supported by two columns attached to the base unit are two **optical tubes.** These house low voltage lamps for normal illumination of the slides.

In addition high intensity bulbs for after image creation and Haidinger brushes are also available. The slide carrier has a plastic diffusing screen and an iris **diaphragm** (used to control the field of vision along with Haidinger brushes). At the junction/bend of the tube is a reflecting mirror. A convex lens of + 6.50 D spherical power is placed at the eyepieces. The slide lies at the focal point of the eyepiece lens, so that it simulates viewing of a distant object, so that accommodation is not stimulated. In case accommodation needs to be stimulated (as in measuring AC/A ratio) −3.0 Ds lenses can be housed in the slots in front of the eyepieces.

The optical tubes can be brought closer or farther to align with the **interpupillary distance** and this position can be locked. In addition the tubes can be rotated horizontally relative to each other (both can be moved independently or one locked in any position and the other moved to check deviation in different gaze positions). The tubes can be both together or any one can separately be rotated **vertically** also. The slide carriers can be tilted in the longitudinal axis of the tube to simulate an intorsion or extorsion of any or both eyes.

A wide **variety of slides** are available:
1. Series A, Maddox test slides, white binding.
2. Series S, Special purpose slides, blue binding (used with automatic flashing, after images) or with Haidinger brushes.
3. Series D, stereoscopic vision slides, yellow binding.
4. Series F, Fusion slides, Green binding.
5. Series G and H, simultaneous perception slides, Red binding.
6. Mayou series of 8, simultaneous perception slides, orange binding.

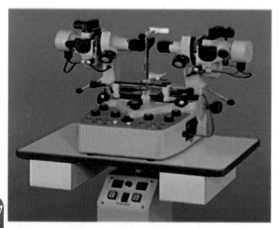

Fig. 17.1: Synoptophore.

17

The slides are available for different visual angles to test foveal, macular or paramacular perceptions while testing the binocular status.

Functions of Synoptophore

a. Diagnostic

1. Measurement of deviation:
   a. With each eye fixing (paralytic squints).
   b. Objective angle and subjective angle (ARC).
   c. In different gaze position (incomitant squints).
   d. Horizontal, vertical and torsional deviations can be measured, (the last only subjectively).
2. Measurement of range of fusion.
3. Assessment of binocular status: Simultaneous perception, fusion and stereopsis, for foveal, macular and paramacular retinal areas.
4. Special functions as adaptability to function in aniseikonia (even monocular aphakia of 33% aniseikonia) with the help of special slides.
5. "After image" testing.
6. Cases with incomplete suppression can also be tested by using differential illumination and by using flashing devices.
7. Appreciation of entoptic phenomena, with Haidinger brushes.

b. Therapeutic

1. Fusional vergence exercises.
2. Management of suppression-antisuppression exercises.
3. Treatment of anomalous retinal correspondence.
4. Amblyopia therapy with the help of Haidinger brushes.

Technique

1. The patient is seated with his chin and forehead adjusted so that his eyes are at the level of the eyepiece.
2. The interpupillary distance is adjusted, with the fixing eye aligned with the line on top of the eyepieces. Each eye is adjusted separately (so no effect of squint).
3. The appropriate slides for the test are put and the test done. For measuring deviations simultaneous macular (or foveal) perception slides are used. For subjective determination of deviation the patient decides the end point and for objective determination the examiner does so by on-off light (like cover test). Adjustments in the position of tubes in horizontal, vertical, directions is made for horizontal and vertical deviations. For torsional deviations the slides are tilted so that they appear straight (subjective assessment).
4. For measuring the fusion ranges, after the above steps and neutralization of the deviation (phoria or tropia), the two tubes are locked. Convergence (adduction) divergence (abduction) is induced till the patient sees binocularly single (subjective) and one of the eyes is seen to deviate out (objective). This is the break point. Reversal of this is done to test the recovery point, when he starts seeing binocularly single.
5. Special functions are described at relevant areas.

2. CHEIROSCOPE

This is used for anti-suppression exercises on the principle that the patient's hand reinforces the stimulus for the "suppressing" eye (Fig. 17.2).

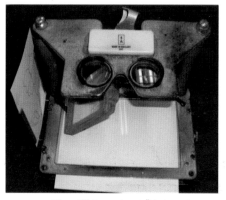

Fig. 17.2: Cheiroscope.

17

Instrument Design

Basically it consists of a working base, a vertical picture carrier on the side, two eye pieces (+ 8.0 DS each) mounted on the stand which is 12.5 cm from the working base, and an oblique septum-cum-mirror which may be designed to be tilted.

Uses

The subject sees the picture through one eye (a reflected image, projected on to the base) which is superimposed by the picture on the base unit seen directly with the other eye.

It may provide simple games like putting a net on the butterfly, or tracing the picture on a blank paper on the base unit.

In case of a manifest squint suitable prisms can be used with the eyepieces, but it may not be suitable for cases with large deviations.

3. PIGEON-CANTONNET STEREOSCOPE

This is a simple inexpensive alternative to synoptophore and cheiroscope for anti-suppression exercises in cases with normal retinal correspondence. It can also be used to measure deviations for near.

Instrument Design

It consists of three stiff cardboard flaps hinged to one another. The outer flaps can be made to lie flat (180° position) (position-1) or at angle of 120° to each other (position-2) by means of a cord, which can be hooked to the middle flap or septum. The septum has a mirror on one side, which can be covered if not in use. The septum is 25 cm long and determines the working distance. The outer two flaps have gradations in centimetres (Figs 17.3a and b).

Uses

Position-1 is used to practice **alternation to overcome suppression** by chasing, superimposing tracing or stereogram exercises. In this position the Pigeon-Cantonnet stereoscope (PCS) acts as a Remy's separator, basically dividing the binocular field into two monocular hemifields. **Position-2** is used for

i. Measurement of deviation, which can be done with each eye fixing separately. With orthophoria the objects placed at identical gradations (distance from the septum) are seen superimposed. If there

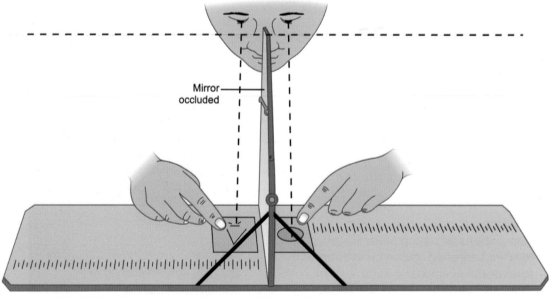

Mirror occluded

Fig. 17.3a: Diagram to show the use of Pigeon-Cantonnet stereoscope in position 1.

17

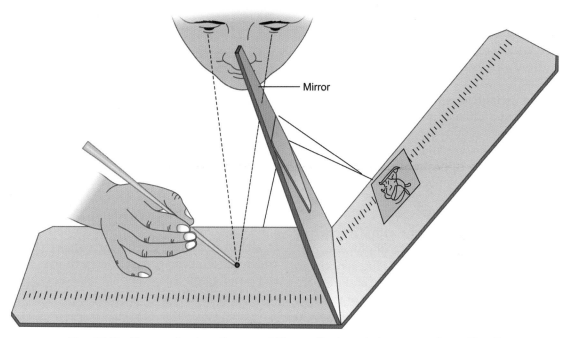

Fig. 17.3b: Diagram to show the use of Pigeon-Cantonnet stereoscope in position 2.

is a difference in the gradations on the two flaps, as the patient superimposes the objects, it indicates a heterophoria. Reading on the fixing side minus reading on the other side gives the deviation. Esodeviation has a positive sign and exodeviation a negative sign. The reading **multiplied by four** (25 × 4 = 100 cm) gives the deviation in prism dioptres.

ii. Antisuppression exercises.

iii. Fusion vergences can be determined as well as vergence exercises be given.

iv. Stereopsis can be tested with the help of stereograms.

4. STEREOSCOPES

Stereoscopes are instruments incorporating lenses or rotating prism, whereby two monocular images can be superimposed and seen as binocularly single or fused. They are used for giving vergence exercises in heterophoria, intermittent divergent squints and for training relative accommodation or relative convergence in treatment of accommodative or relative convergence in treatment of accommodative esotropia.

Instrument Design

The **Holmes, Keystone** and **Asher-Law stereoscopes** basically consist of:

i. A 5 dioptre lens split into two halves with the halves placed such that the central parts are outwards (with decentration they give a **base-out** effect).

ii. A central bar and a septum.

iii. A mobile card-holder.

Uses

When the cardholder is at 20 cm distance, the rays from the object are parallel (as if coming from infinity). As the card is moved closer, more accommodation and convergence is

17

required. Since the cards on the cardholder can be closer to the midline or away, the vergence requirement can be altered with the accommodation being constant. Conversely the accommodation can be altered with the vergence controlled. Thus relative accommodation and relative convergence can be trained.

The **variable prism stereoscope** and **Cruise stereoscope** utilise a rotary prism to change the vergence requirement.

The Pigeon-Cantonnet stereoscope, though not having any optical parts serves like one and so is called a "stereoscope".

5. REMY SEPARATOR

This is a simple instrument with a wooden or metal septum and a fixed cardholder.

It has objects separated by the septum so that one eye sees one object only, and they are superimposed if the visual axes are parallel, i.e. there is no squint. A person with mild exodeviation can be made to accommodate and converge, and later taught to relax his accommodation with convergence being still exercised. This will correct his exodeviation. Similarly esodeviations can be taught to relax convergence.

6. DIPLOSCOPE

This is an orthoptic instrument used for treatment of horizontal heterophoria, accommodative esotropia and intermittent exotropia (Fig. 17.4).

Instrument Design

It consists of a metal shaft 25 cm long with a metal pad to rest on the nose at one end and a fixed card holder at the other end. A metal septum with four apertures is transversely placed 6.5 cm in front of the cardholder. The four circular apertures are 8 mm in size, two are horizontal 15 mm apart on either side of the mid point, the other two apertures are vertical, one below the left hand aperture and the other above the right hand aperture. The

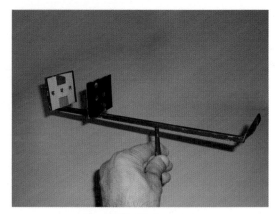

Fig. 17.4: Diploscope.

card has three letters D, O, G inscribed horizontally, with a green square above O and a red square below O. **O** stands for **oeil** (eye), **D** for **droit** (right), and **G** for **gauche** (left), which are French words. The right eye sees D, O, and green colour and left eye sees O, G, and red colour.

Uses

To use the instrument, the patient is made to change fixation, which changes his vergence and his perception. These **points of fixation** and their **perception** are:

1. Central letter O on the card, 25 cm sees D, O, G.
2. Metal septum, midway between horizontal apertures, 18.5 cm sees DO, OG.
3. At a point placed half way between metal septum and eyes. 9.25 cm sees OG, DO.
4. At an object located some distance behind the card, sees, DO, OG.

The positions 1, 2, and 3 require convergence of increasing amount and position 4 requires relative divergence relative to the printed card.

7. STEREOGRAM CARDS

These are pairs of objects printed on a card such that their images can be fused to form a single image and some with disparity create a three-D-effect. They are used in a manner similar to Remy Separator, but without the

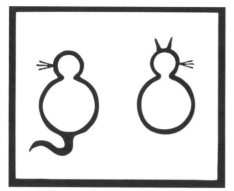

Fig. 17.5: Stereogram card.

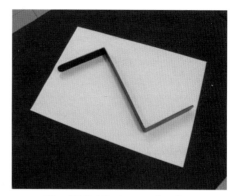

Fig. 17.6: Zigzag reading bar.

septum. The patient is asked to exercise relative divergence (or relative convergence) relative to the printed card, so that physiological diplopia creates four images, and the two adjacent middle image get superimposed and fused. Finally the patient sees three figures, a central fused figure and two monocular figures. This is used to train relative convergence or divergence (Fig. 17.5).

8. READING BARS

These are simple orthoptic tools, which work on the principle of introducing a bar or obstruction in the field. This obstruction is for a small vertical strip of words for one eye and a different vertical strip of words for the other eye. If the patient sees with both eyes, he can read the text uninterrupted without horizontally shifting his head. This is used to ensure usage of both eyes simultaneously and helps in anti-suppression.

Different types of bar-readers are: a thumb bar reader, Priestley-Smith's zigzag bar reader (Fig. 17.6), **adjustable Mayou-Bar reader, Mayou, head band bar reader and the Javal grid.**

9. MADDOX TANGENT SCALE

The Maddox tangent scale is a wooden cross with a central fixation bulb and markings on its horizontal and vertical limbs, used to measure deviations with binocularity. The markings are in degrees, the larger figures correspond for a **5 metre** fixation distance. (Maddox the English strabismologist who contributed so much to orthoptics had his examination room of 5 metres, this set the convention of the tangent scale). The smaller markings are for one metre fixation distance.

It is usually used with the Maddox rod.

The **Maddox rod** (Fig. 17.7) is a red coloured disc with several parallel grooves, (mounted like a trial lens). It converts a point of light viewed through it into a line perpendicular to its axis (of grooves). This is used to dissociate the two eyes. The right eye with the Maddox rod sees a line (vertical for horizontal deviations as the rod is kept horizontal and sees a horizontal line for vertical deviations), while the left eye sees the spotlight and the scale. The marking on the Maddox scale (Fig. 17.8) crossed by the line gives the deviations. Both horizontal and vertical deviations can be measured.

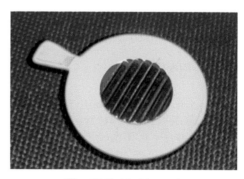

Fig. 17.7: Maddox rod.

17

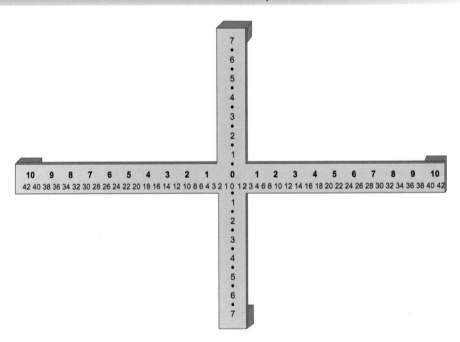

Fig. 17.8: Maddox tangent scale.

The Maddox rod usually used without the tangent scale, in which case a prism bar or rotary prism is placed over the other eye, as the patient fixates fixation light. The prism power required to make the line cross the fixation light measures the deviations. The **Maddox hand frame: uniocular** and **binocular** also has rotary prism which can be used for this purpose, without extra prism bar.

10. MADDOX WING

This is a simple appliance to measure the heterophoria for near fixation in prism dioptres. It can measure horizontal, vertical deviations as well as cyclophoria (Fig. 17.9).

Instrument Design

It consists of a metal screen which has markings in prism dioptres both for horizontal and vertical deviations. At the other end of the metal screen is a face piece with two apertures for the eyes and a slot for the nose. Two metal septa, one vertical and the other oblique are "wing" like giving the name to the

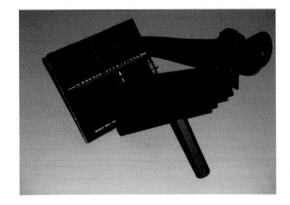

Fig. 17.9: Maddox wing.

instrument. These dissociate the view of the two eyes so that the scales are seen by the left eye and the white vertical and horizontal arrows by the right eye.

Uses

It is used with its direction slightly downwards. If there is orthophoria the arrows point at 0 for both scales. If there is an **heterophoria** the

17

patient reads out the digit, at which the white arrows point towards.

For **cyclophoria** the movable red arrow is adjusted to appear parallel to the horizontal scale. This is measured in degrees.

The face piece has slots to introduce lenses for presbyopes or refractive error.

It should be remembered that the Maddox wing measures heterophoria for near (34 cm, 14 inches), which may be different from the heterophoria for distance.

11. NEAR POINT RULER

There are several ways of measuring the near point of convergence and near point of accommodation. The simplest is a **linear rule** with a sliding or moving target preferably a linear one. Other more accurate methods are **Livingston's binocular gauge** and **RAF** (Royal Air Force) **binocular gauge,** the latter has small print targets for accommodation control (Fig. 17.10).

The linear rule is 36 cm long, the target is kept far and, the subject asked to focus his attention on the line. It is gradually brought closer to the eyes. For **subjective** recording the patient is asked to indicate when he starts seeing double (for near point of convergence) or when he starts seeing **blurred** (for near point of accommodation). The reading is taken as the **break point.** The object is slided back and the reversal is noted as **recovery point.**

For **objective** recording of near point of convergence the point where one of the eyes starts deviating out is noted.

The normal near point of convergence (NPC) is 6–10 cm. The near points of accommodation are recorded monocularly for both eyes and also binocularly. Preferably a reading test type should be used. In adults the Near point of accommodation is less than 10 cm and recedes with age especially after 40 years.

12. BISHOP HARMAN DIAPHRAGM TEST

This is a fine instrument to detect the strength of the fusional response and is used to screen pilots where exophoria and its control is very critical.

Instrument Design

It consists of a cardholder which has a row of letters (ABCDEFG) or number (1234567) viewed through an adjustable diaphragm (Fig. 17.11).

Uses

The IPD is adjusted for the subject prior to the test and he is asked to read the numbers. The examiner gradually closes the aperture of diaphragm and the subject indicates an interruption of binocularity. The **possible** responses are:

   i. A dividing bar separates the numbers into two groups **(exophoric** or **bar response).**

   ii. Crowding or overlapping of central numbers occur **(esophoric response).**

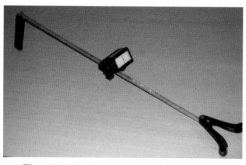

Fig. 17.10: RAF binocular gauge/ruler.

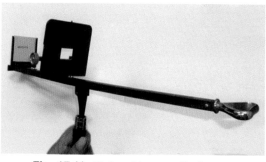

Fig. 17.11: Bishop Harman diaphragm.

17

iii. The numbers separate into two levels, one being higher than the other **(hyperphoric response).**

iv. The numbers at one end disappear **(uniocular response).** If they disappear on left side, it indicates a right suppression.

Apart from this observation the reading on the **ocular poise scale** is recorded. Any reading **above 4** is indicative of abnormal binocular function.

13. PRISM BAR AND LOOSE PRISMS

These are the most important tools in the hands of the strabismologist or orthoptist. A set of glass or plastic prisms available as loose prisms in different denominations is used. The prism bar is a linearly arranged set of prisms of increasing dioptric power. Two bars, one for horizontal deviations and the other for vertical prisms are required. Additional loose prism of 30 and 45 prism dioptres should be available along with the prism bars (Fig. 17.12).

Wafer prisms, clip on prisms, or prisms mounted in trial lens discs are very useful for prism neutralization. Membrane prisms (Fresnel prisms) which can be stuck onto the glass of the subjects are also available.

14. BAGOLINI'S STRIATED GLASSES

These are simple glass or plastic discs with regular linear striations. They are used in pairs (the axis of which are at right angles). These

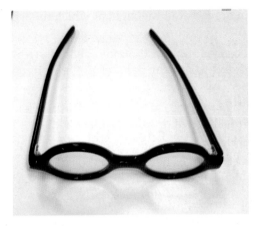

Fig. 17.13: Bagolini's striated glasses.

pairs may be mounted on a binocular frame or may be available as loose pairs. These are least dissociative and most physiological and therefore they are the most valuable for assessment of binocular functions (Fig. 17.13).

15. NEUTRAL DENSITY FILTERS AND GRADED DENSITY BARS

The neutral density filters are special photographic filters and are used for assessing the depth of suppression. They are also used for grading the relative afferent pupillary defects.

A ladder or bar of increasing density filters (neutral or red filters) is used for assessing the depth of suppression and in cases of dissociated vertical deviations, its manifestation and grading.

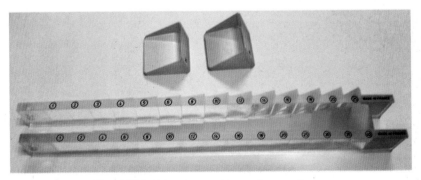

Fig. 17.12: Prism bars with two loose prisms.

16. RED AND GREEN GLASSES

These are also called diplopia goggles and consist of a pair of red and green glasses. The colours being mutually exclusive, that is, a red light is seen by red filter but not the green one and vice versa. A white light appears as a distinctive red with one eye and green with the other. This helps in making the patient aware of his diplopia. By convention red is used for right eye and green for left eye. **Diplopia testing** utilizes these goggles to chart the separation of the double images in the nine different positions at a fixed distance. This helps in documenting incomitance.

Red green goggles are also used with **Worth-four-dot test, Hess screen** testing, **Lancasters chart testing** and with **stereoscopic tests** of **TNO** and **Awaya.**

17. WORTH-FOUR DOT TEST

This is a set of four circles (dots) arranged in a rhombus form. The top dot is red, two horizontal dots are green and the bottom dot is white. This is usually incorporated in most of the self-illuminated Snellen chart boxes. When viewed with red-green goggles, at a distance of 6 metres, the following responses are seen (Fig. 17.14).

i. All four dots seen in a rhombus pattern, the white appears pink or light green to most people with one red dot and two green dots. This is a normal binocular **response** with orthophoria.

ii. Five dots (two red dots and three green dots): seen displaced in two sets depending on horizontal (crossed or uncrossed pattern) or vertical deviations. This is seen in incomitant **or paralytic squints** with **binocular vision.**

iii. Two red dots only seen. This indicates **left suppression.**

iv. Three green dots only seen. This indicates right suppression.

In case of central macular scotoma if the worth four dot test is not possible at 6 metres distance, the same can be done at 1 metre distance (this increases the angle subtended on the retina).

18. HESS SCREEN AND LEES SCREEN

Hess screening (Fig. 17.15) is used to document the **relative incomitance,** underactions and

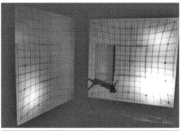
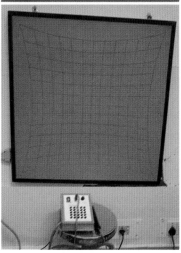

Fig. 17.15: Lees screen (top) and Hess screen (bottom).

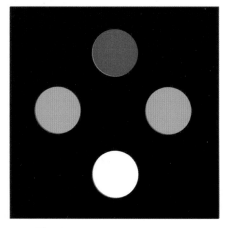

Fig. 17.14: Worth-four dot test.

17

overactions of the yoke muscles of the two eyes. The excursions of the fellow eye are charted as the fixating eye is made to fixate in different gaze positions.

Instrument Design

The original **Hess screen** consists of a black cloth three feet wide and three and a half feet long marked with a series of red lines forming squares of 5° each. From the central zero point three squares (15°) in each direction marks the inner square formed by 8 additional points. An outer square of sixteen dots has excursion of 6 squares (30°) in each direction. The outer square is used for mild incomitances not detected on inner square charting. The pointer is a junction of three short green threads knotted to form a Y. This is freely movable over the screen and is handled by the subject, by means of a black rod 50 cm long.

Uses

The subject wears red and green goggles and sees the points on the inner square with right eye (red on right eye) and aligns the green Y on the red dots one by one. The observer records the points he charts (which differ if there is a relative incomitance between the two eyes). This charts the excursions of the muscles of left eye. Next the test is repeated with red glass over left eye which charts the excursions of the right eye muscles.

The **Electric Hess screen** utilises red dots shown one by one as the subject overlaps these with a green pointer.

Lees Screen

Lees screen test is based on the same principle but does not require red-green goggles as it utilises a septum (mirror) to dissociate the two eyes.

Instrument Design

It consists of two square translucent screens set at 90° to each other. In between the two lies a mirror septum. This has a chinrest such that the patient is seated at 50 cm from either screen (Fig. 17.13).

Uses

One screen is viewed straight and the other through the mirror. The fixating screen is illuminated (it shows the Hess chart) and the examiner points at the 8 points of inner square one by one with a metal wand. The subject superimposes these points by another wand. For a moment the other screen is illuminated to show the Hess screen and the notation made on the chart. First the left eye is charted with right eye fixating. Next the right eye is charted with the left eye fixating, by switching the illumination on the other screen.

Hess charting of common ocular motility problems is shown at the end of this chapter.

19. VISUSCOPE

This is a modified ophthalmoscope devised by Cuppers of Germany. Now this has been incorporated in all modern ophthalmoscopes. It has a central star for fixation around with concentric circles of 3° and 5° are present. These are projected on to the retina as the patient is asked to fixate. The fixation is noted as **central** or **eccentric** which may be steady, unsteady or wandering. Eccentric fixation may be para foveal (outside 2°), paramacular (outside 5°) or peripheral (beyond 10°–12°).

The visuscope can also be used along with the tangent scale to check **correspondence.** The patient fixates at the central light of the tangent scale through an obliquely placed mirror with the normal eye, as the other eye (amblyopic) is seen through the visuscope and the star projected onto the fovea. If the patient has **bifoveal** (normal) **retinal correspondence** he sees the star on the spotlight otherwise the star is projected on one side indicating anomalous **retinal correspondence.**

20. PROJECTOSCOPE

This is a modified Keeler Ophthalmoscope used for pleoptics therapy. It has a Nutt autodisc with three graticules. In position-1 it has a Linksz star with green filter. In position-2 the central 3° (or 5°) is shielded by a black disc as a bright flash dazzles the extra foveal point. In position-3 the foveal area is stimulated by white light. These three positions are automatically shifted by the Nutt autodisc. Instead of the passive stimulation in position 3, the fovea may be centred on a black cross on the wall, by centring the cross with the circular after image created around fovea. The initial method is Bangerter's method of pleoptics therapy. The training of fovea-space coordination is the Cupper's method of pleoptics therapy (see text and Figs 14.4 and 14.5).

21. EUTHYOSCOPE

This is also a modified ophthalmoscope used for the Cupper's method. It is similar to Projectoscope with omitted position 3. This apparatus depends on dazzling the extra foveal point (positionl) and then creating an annular after image centred around the fovea. This is achieved by shielding the foveal area (2° or 5°) and dazzling the eye with bright light for 20–30 seconds. The after image thus created is prolonged by using the **alternascope,** a device which allows switching on and off of room illumination, so that alternately the positive and negative after images are created each perpetuating the other. The patient is given the task of centring his after image (and that's foveal) with a cross in space. This re-educates the space-eye coordination, which is shifted in cases with eccentric fixation.

22. COORDINATOR

This is an instrument to re-educate the coordination between fovea and the straight ahead gaze, which is taken up by the eccentric point in eccentric fixation. It utilises the Haidinger's brushes in which rotating cobalt blue polarised light is used. Since the fovea alone has the property of appreciating polarization (due to its lutein pigment or the orientation of Henle's nerve fibre layer), the fovea perceives a "rotating two-blade-fan," centred at the fovea. To ensure that the patient is seeing it, its speed and direction can be altered and verified.

The coordinator is used to teach the amblyopic eye hand-eye coordination on **Cuppers binocular coordinator,** in which the patient does simple tasks like centring the rotating fan (or fovea) on the aeroplane or other such figures. A diaphragm is used to increase or decrease the field seen by the patient. During the exercises the aperture is gradually reduced to guide him in centring (see Fig. 14.5).

Space coordinator is used to teach coordination on space on a polished white steel screen (magnetic) illuminated by 500 watt light, at about 1–6 metres. Five magnetic optotypes (E) are used in a row as the patient learns to centre the central optotype without "separation difficulty". A crowding or overlapping or a gap may be seen. One of the five Es may be suppressed.

Haidinger brushes attachment is available with the **synoptophore,** and they are used in conjunction with after images for binocular coordination. For this Haidinger brushes are seen by the fovea of the amblyopic eye and the afterimage is created in the normal (fellow) eye centred at the fovea.

TESTS FOR STEREOPSIS

(Compiled with the help of Lt Col Dr Anirudh Singh)

Stereopsis is a hallmark of the human race that has bestowed on it the supremacy in the hierarchy of the animal kingdom. It is the ability to fuse images that have horizontally disparate retinal elements within Panum's fusional area resulting in binocular appreciation of visual object in depth, i.e. in the third dimension.

17

Tests for stereopsis

Stereopsis test for near	Equipment	Stereopsis grade tested
1. TNO test	TNO booklet containing 7 plates and red green spectacles	15–480 seconds of arc
2. Titmus Fly test	3-dimensional polaroid vectograph and polaroid spectacles	Fly-3500 arc seconds Graded circle test-800-40 seconds of arc animal test for children-400, 200 and 100 seconds of arc
3. Stereo Butterfly test	3-dimensional polaroid vectographand polaroid spectacles	Upper wings 2000 sec of arc, lower wings 1150 sec of arc and abdomen 700 sec of arc. Graded circle test and animal test is same as Titmus fly test
4. Random dot stereogram	Polaroid spectacles	400–20 seconds of arc
5. Lang test	Test plates:	Car-550, seconds of arc
	Stereo I	Star-600 seconds of arc and Cat-1200 seconds of arc
	Stereo II	Moon-200 seconds of arc Truck-400 seconds of arc Elephant-600 seconds of arc
6. Lang 2 pencil test	2 pencils only	3000–5000 seconds of arc
7. Stereopsis slides placed in synoptophore carrier	Synoptophore with stereopsis slides	720–90 seconds of arc

Stereopsis test for distance	Equipment	Stereopsis grade tested
1. AO vectographic project-O-chart slide	Phoropter with polarizing lenses	480–30 seconds of arc
2. Mentor B-VAT II SG video acuity tester	Video system with monitor using Random dot E(BVRDE) and Contour circles(BVC)	240–15 seconds of arc
3. Frisby Davis Distance Stereotest(FD2 test)	Box with four translucent objects at varying distances	5–50 seconds of arc at 6 m
4. Distance Randot stereotest	3-dimensional polaroid vectograph and polaroid spectacles	400–60 seconds of arc

PRINCIPLE OF STEREOPSIS

The basic mechanism is dissociation of the two eyes so that each gets a slightly different view of the same object and then fuses to form a single image with third dimension.

- **Haploscopic principle**

  In this principle the dissociation is achieved by placing angled mirrors in front of each eye so that right eye sees the right temporal field while the left eye sees the left temporal field. This principle is used in Synoptophore.

- **Anaglyph**

  A stereogram in which dissociation of image is produced by using colour is known as the anaglyph. The anaglyph consists of stereo paired object formed by using conjugate colours like red and green. These objects when viewed with special glasses, one lens being coloured red and the other coloured green a three-dimensional scene is perceived. The test based on this principle is TNO test.

- **Vectographic principle**

  The vectograph permitted two stereo paired pictures developed in such a way that light passing through one is polarized in one direction while light passing through the other is polarized in the other direction. This permits a viewer to use special glasses consisting of Polaroid filters to see the three-dimensional scene. Vectography has the advantage over anaglyphic photography that avoids the annoyance of seeing the red-blue tint in the scene. This principle is used in tests like Titmus fly test and Randot stereopsis test.

- **Panographic principle**

  This stereogram is real depth stereogram, which incorporates grid of cylinders with random dots in its pattern, that will cause the deviation of the image to give real time depth perception. Lang's test is based on this principle.

TESTS FOR NEAR STEREOACUITY

The Netherlands Organization/TNO TEST

Test material: There are 7 plates to be viewed with red-green spectacles (Fig. 17.16).

Uses: The three initial plates enable the examiner to quickly establish whether gross stereopsis (1980 sec of arc) is present at all. Plate IV is a suppression test. Plates V-VII are used for qualitative estimation. When used for screening purposes, plate V can be used as a pass-fail criterion. It the test plate is presented in a reverse form, test items will be seen in reversed depth.

Method—present the plates serially at 40 cm distance in a well lit room.

Advantage: Can be used in children as young as 3 years old

Can be used as a screening tool for various occupations

Limitation—tests only near stereopsis the images appear in shades of red and green

TITMUS STEREO TEST

Principle: The test consist of vectographic stereograms which has contour patterns that use crossed polarized filters located at axis of 45 and 135 in front of either eye (Fig. 17.17).

Equipment: Stereo fly card and polarized glasses.

Uses: Allows effective screening of gross stereopsis and fine depth perception especially in strabismus

Age: 3 years onwards

Advantage: Offers no monocular clues to discourage guessing

Limitation

i. Some patients may point out to the specific disparate image as they look different from the rest and not due to stereopsis

ii. Only checks near stereopsis

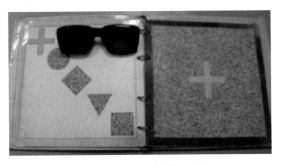

Fig. 17.16: TNO Plate III.

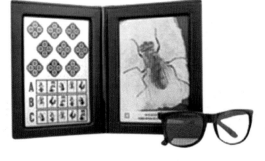

Fig. 17.17: Titmus fly card with polarized glasses.

17

STEREO BUTTERFLY TEST

This test is quite similar to the Titmus fly test but instead of the fly it has hidden configuration ofbutterfly within the random dots (Fig. 17.18).

The range of stereoacuity tested are upper wings 2000 seconds of arc, lower wings 1150 seconds of arc and abdomen 700 seconds of arc.

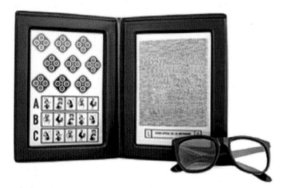

Fig. 17.18: Stereo butterfly card with polarized glasses.

RANDOT STEREOTEST

Principle: This test consists of random dot stereogram rather than contour patterns. This removes the lateral displacement cue found in the Titmus fly test (Fig. 17.19).

Uses: Allows effective screening of gross stereopsis and fine depth perception especially in strabismus

Age: 3 years onwards

Advantage: Offers no monocular clues to discourage guessing.

Limitation

Only checks near stereopsis

LANG TEST

Two versions of the test plates are available, whichdiffer only according to the 3D objects to be recognized. The LANG-STEREOTEST I displays a star, a cat and a car, while the LANG-STEREOTEST II displays a moon, a truck and an elephant,each of them appearing on a different level (Fig. 17.20). In addition, the LANG-STEREOTEST II contains a star that can be seen with only one eye.This test costs about rupees 8000.

Principle

This test is based on panographic presentation of a random dot pattern. Glasses are not needed in this test. A separate image is provided to each eye through cylindrical lenses imprinted on the surface lamination of the test card.

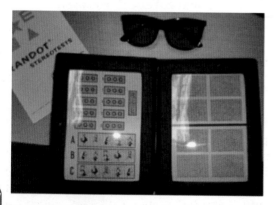

Fig. 17.19: Randot stereotest for near with key for the right page.

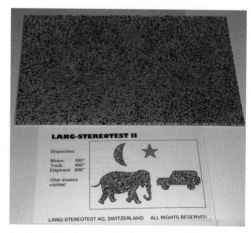

Fig. 17.20: Lang-stereotest card stereoscopic images embedded in the random dots.

Advantage

Can be used in children who refuse to wear Polaroid or red-green spectacles.

This is a relatively cheap test which can be conveniently performed.

LANG TWO PENCIL TEST

The two pencil test was popularized by Lang but was known long back. This test has no false negative responses and a 100% sensitivity and negative predictive value (NPV), this test may be used as a potential screening test for detecting gross stereopsis (*see* Fig. 5.17).

Advantage

   i. Easily performed
  ii. No stereoscopic test material required
 iii. No Polaroid or red-green glasses required

STEREOPSIS TESTING WITH SYNOPTOPHORE

Stereopsis slides are placed in the slide carrier and patient instructed to view with full refractive correction in place (Fig. 17.21). Two

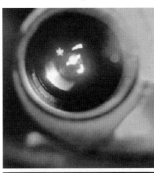
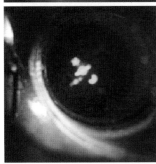

Fig. 17.21: Stereopsis slides as seen through right and left eyepiece in a synoptophore.

slide types are available; one with a paratrooper and the plane where the patient is asked whether the paratrooper is in front of plane or not. Second slide type has four stars each and one of them when seen binocularly appears in front of the other.

CONFIRMATION OF STEREOACUITY RESULT

1. To confirm a result, ask the child to close one eye while looking at the stereoscopic figures. Immediate disappearance of the figures will be noted.
2. When in doubt whether the patient already knows about the test, then use the test card upside down, the figures will appear in depth rather than being raised.

STEREOTESTS FOR DISTANCE

Distance stereotesting is proved to be highly sensitive to smallrefractive error changes, heterophorias and strabismus. Distance stereopsis evaluation aids in assessment of control of deviationand deterioration of fusion in cases of intermittent exotropia.Normal distance stereoacuity indicates good control with little orno suppression while detoriation in same may be an indication of surgery in such cases.

AO Vectographic test and Mentor B-VAT-II video acuity tester are no longer used nowadays.

FRISBY DAVIS DISTANCE (FD2) TEST

Principle: This is a free space test of real depth invented by Mr JP Frisby and H Davis. It is based upon the near Frisby Stereo Test but with various modifications arising from the need for distance presentations (Fig. 17.22)

The test material consist of a box containing four back illuminated and differently shaped plastic objects mounted on rods. These are either four animal or four geometric shapes set in a transparent frame pointing towards the observer. The shapes are translucent but sufficiently dark to obscure the rods, giving the appearance that the shapes are free floating.

17

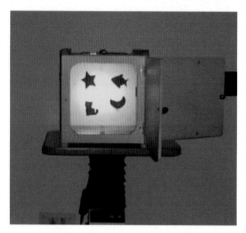

Fig. 17.22: Frisby Davis Distance (FD2) stereotest with four shapes.

Advantage

i. Easy to administer particularly in children from age group of 3 years onwards
ii. Repeated testing possible without learning how to pass for the wrong reasons
iii. Possible to demonstrate the task to ensure task understanding prior to testing
iv. Not using stereograms as these have disadvantages for some patient groups where use of dissociating glasses (Polaroid/red-green) breaks the fusion.

DISTANCE RANDOT TEST

Principle: based on vectographic random dot stereogram.

Advantage

i. Offers no monocular clues to discourage guessing
ii. Deterioration of distance stereoacuity in intermittent exotropia is taken as a sign of poor control and gives an early indication for surgery (Fig. 17.23).

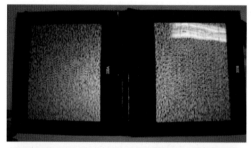

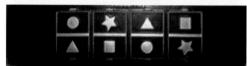

Fig. 17.23: Distance Randot stereotest card with the key on back cover.

HESS CHARTING OF COMMON OCULAR MOTILITY PROBLEMS (Figs 17.24a to k and 17.25)

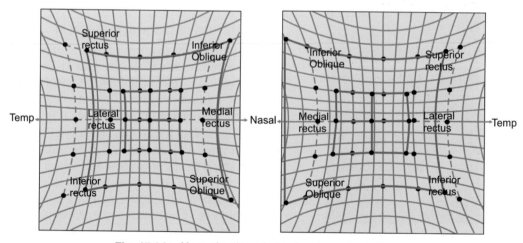

Fig. 17.24a: Hess charting—Lateral rectus palsy left eye.

Note: Hess charting shows green before left eye on left charts and green before right on right charts

17

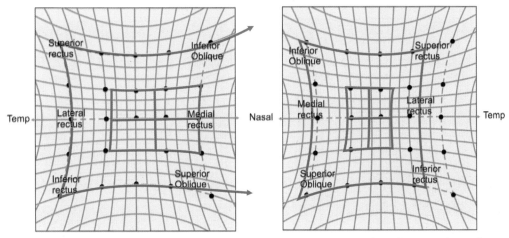

Fig. 17.24b: Hess charting—Right eye lateral rectus palsy LR underaction recent onset.

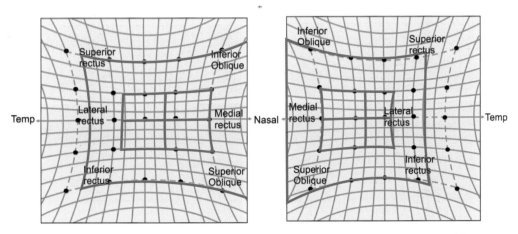

Fig. 17.24c: Hess charting—Right eye lateral rectus palsy RLR underaction old.

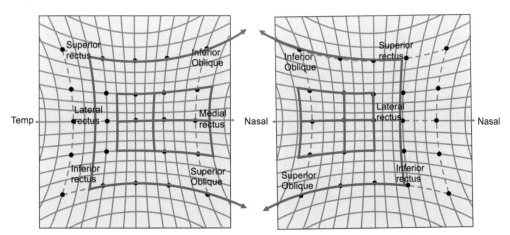

Fig. 17.24d: Hess charting—Bilateral asymmetric lateral rectus palsy.

17

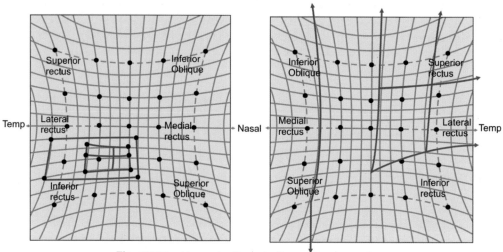

Fig. 17.24e: Hess charting—Left eye III nerve palsy.

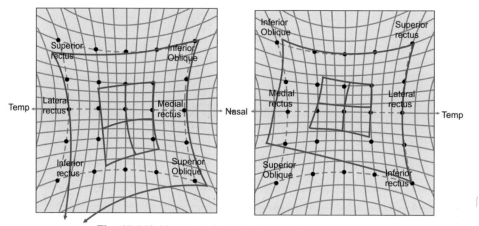

Fig. 17.24f: Hess charting—Right eye IV nerve palsy.

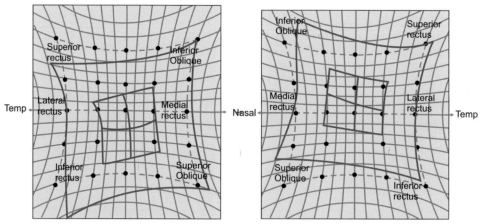

Fig. 17.24g: Hess charting—Right eye IV nerve palsy SO underaction old.

17

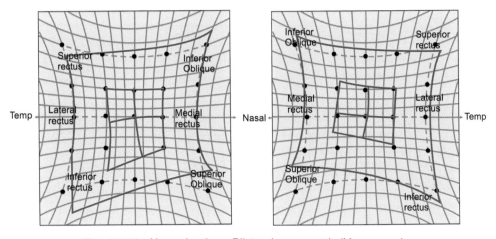

Fig. 17.24h: Hess charting—Bilateral asymmetric IV nerve palsy.

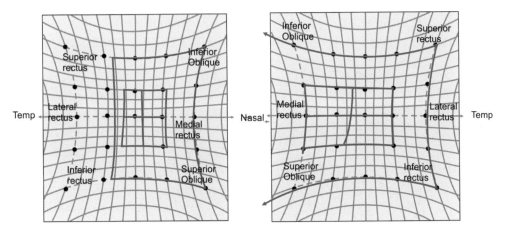

Fig. 17.24i: Hess charting—Left Duane retraction syndrome.

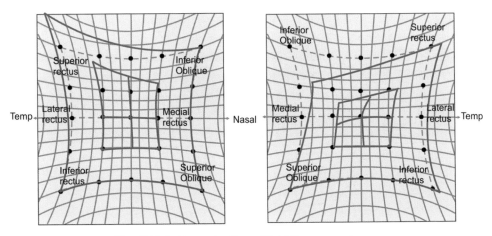

Fig. 17.24j: Hess charting—Right Brown syndrome.

17

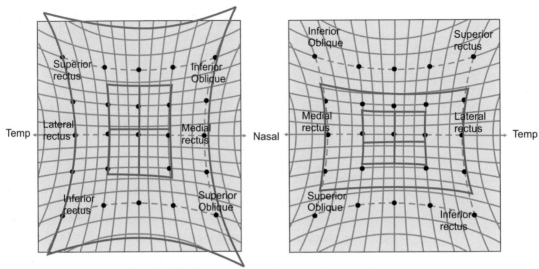

Fig. 17.24k: Hess charting—Blow out fracture right eye.

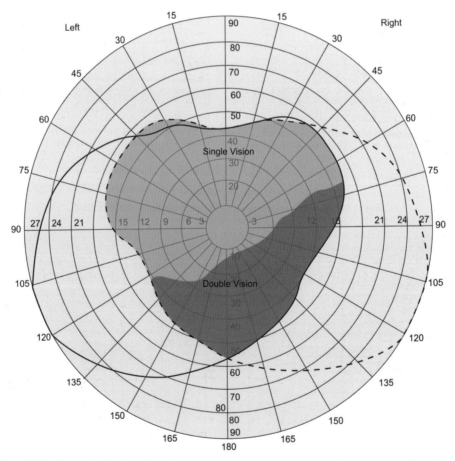

Fig. 17.25: Binocular fields of fixation showing areas of binocular single and double vision.

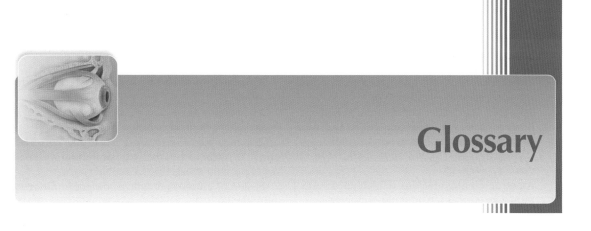

Abduction (Latin, *ab* - away from, *ducese* = move) unilateral movement of the eye horizontally outwards, away from the primary position.

Abnormal Retinal Correspondence
See Anomalous Retinal Correspondence

Accommodation: The ability of eye to focus near objects by increasing the convexity of the crystalline lens by increasing the tone of ciliary muscle.

- **Amplitude of accommodation:**
  The difference between far point and near point, in dioptres.

Anomalies of accommodation:

- **Accommodative (ciliary) spasm:**
  Overaction of ciliary muscle bringing the far point closer to the eye causing **pseudo myopia.**
- **Accommodative insufficiency:**
  Underaction of ciliary muscle receding the near point of the eye (away from the eye).
- **Accommodative fatigue:**
  Tendency of recession of near point due to excess near work.
- **Accommodative inertia:**
  Inability of the eyes to adjust the accommo-dation according to the object distance.
- **Accommodational paralysis:**
  Total inability of the eyes to focus for near objects.

Accommodative Convergent Strabismus, Accommodative Esotropia: Esodeviation of eyes due to use of accommodation over and above the requisite amount for the object distance. May be due to uncorrected or under corrected hyperopia, or high accommodative—convergence to accommodation ratio or weak accommodational mechanism. It may be fully accommodative or partially accommodative (where there is a non-accommodative element also).

The esodeviation increases with accommodational effort.

Adaptation: Adjustments to overcome the consequences of a squint. It may be sensory or motor. The former are suppression and anomalous retinal correspondence. The motor adaptations are: head posture and blind spot mechanism.

Adduction (Latin, *ad* = towards, *ducese* = move): Unilateral movement of the eye horizontally inwards, towards the midline or nose.

Adnexa (Latin, *ad* = to, *nexa* = neighbouring): Refers to adjacent structures. Ocular adnexa refers to eyelids, lacrimal apparatus, paranasal sinuses, etc.

Advancement: A surgical procedure in which the muscle is reinserted at a position further away from its origin. This is a strengthening procedure as it makes the muscle taut. For recti the new insertion becomes closer to the limbus and for obliques it is further backwards and up (inferior oblique) or down (superior oblique).

Alternating squints: A squint which switches freely between the two eyes, as each eye is capable of maintaining fixation. Examples: Alternating esotropia, A. Exotropia, A. sursumduction (*see* Dissociated Vertical Deviation).

Amblyopia (Greek, *Amblyos* = blunt, *ops:* vision): A condition of diminution of best corrected vision of one or both eyes which is not due to any organic cause of the optical media, fundus or visual pathways. It is a developmental anomaly due to obstacles in the visual development in the formative years of neural plasticity (amblyopiogenic age). It may be due to form vision deprivation or abnormal binocular interaction in this critical period and is usually correctable if treated in this period.

Types of amblyopia:

- **Strabismic amblyopia:** Amblyopia due to abnormal interaction due to strabismus.
- **Anisometropic amblyopia:** Amblyopia due to form vision deprivation and abnormal binocular

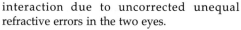

interaction due to uncorrected unequal refractive errors in the two eyes.

- **Stimulus deprivation amblyopia:** Amblyopia due to form vision deprivation and also abnormal binocular interaction (in unilateral/asymmetric cases) secondary to cataract, corneal opacity, ptosis, etc.
- **Ametropic amblyopia** due to high uncorrected refractive error is a type of this amblyopia.
- Terms like **amblyopia of arrest** (due to arrested development of visual acuity) or **amblyopia of extinction** (due to secondary loss of visual acuity) are not used nowadays.
- **Amblyopia exanopsia** (amblyopia due to media opacities like cataract, etc.) is better called stimulus deprivation amblyopia.
- **Meridional amblyopia** is amblyopia of a particular meridian due to astigmatism.
- **Aniseikonic amblyopia** corrected anisometropia having aniseikonia causes amblyopia of this type.

Ametropia (Greek, *a* = not, *metron* = measure, *ops* = vision): Refractive error of the eye.

(**Isometropia:** equal refractive error in the two eyes).

Anisometropia: Unequal refractive error in the two eyes.

Antimetropia: One eye myopic, other hyperopic.

Angles: Alpha, gamma, kappa, lambda:

These are the angles between the optic axis (geometric, anatomical) and the visual axis (line joining the fovea and the object of regard) at various points of subtense, as follows.

A. alpha	:	at the nodal point.
A. gamma	:	at the centre of the eye.
A. kappa	:	at the mid point of pupil.
A. lambda	:	angle kappa measured with

cornea as reference point. (This is usually called **A. kappa,** though A. lambda would be more appropriate.

A **positive** angle kappa (lambda) is when the optical axis is more temporal than the visual axis. Normally a positive 5° angle kappa is seen in emmetropic eyes. In hyperopes it is more positive and in myopes less or even **negative** (optical axis nasal to the visual axis). A positive angle kappa gives a look of exodeviation **(pseudoexotropia)** and a negative angle kappa, a look of esodeviation **(pseudoesotropia).**

Anaphoria, Anatropia: (*see* Dissociated Vertical Deviations).

Anisometropia: Unequal refractive error in the two eyes.

Aniseikonia (Greek, *an* = not, *iso* = equal, *ikon* = image): Unequal images in the two eyes.

This may be due to **optical causes** like corrected unequal refractive error (e.g. unilateral aphakia corrected with spectacles) or **retinal** causes.

Fusion of aniseikonic images differs in different individuals.

Anisophoria: Unequal heterophoria with each eye fixating.

Anisotropia: Unequal deviation of eyes between looking up and looking down positions (*see* A–V phenomenon).

Anomalous (Abnormal) Retinal Correspondence: A binocular condition in which the fovea of one eye develops correspondence (common perceptive visual direction) with the extra-foveal point of the other eye, under binocular conditions of stimulation. This is an adaptation to a constant small angle squint occurring early in childhood and provides binocularity (anomalous or abnormal) in spite of a manifest squint.

The shift of the perceptual visual direction from the fovea to the extra foveal point of the other eye is called **angle of anomaly** (difference between objective and subjective angle).

In **harmonious ARC,** the angle of anomaly is equal to the angle of deviation and the subjective angle of deviation is zero.

In **unharmonious ARC,** the subjective angle is less than the objective angle of deviation. The difference between the two is the angle of anomaly.

Anteropositioning, an operation in which the oblique muscle is reinserted anterior to its original insertion (which is behind equator). This alters its vertical and abducting effect profoundly with less effect on its torsional effect. It may be combined with a recession or done as a "pure" anteropositioning.

A selective anteropositioning of anterior fibres alone may also be done as in Harada-Ito procedures (sagittalization of superior oblique).

"A" phenomenon, "A" pattern, refers to the ocular deviation which have more relative divergence in down gaze and/or more relative convergence in upgaze. This may be associated with superior-oblique over actions.

Apparent strabismus: (*see* pseudo strabismus)

Asthenopia (Greek, *a* = not, *sthenos:* strength *op* = vision, *see*).

A condition in which the eyes get fatigued or strained on near work or use of eyes. This may be due to uniocular causes like accommodational weakness or binocular causes like extraocular muscle (fusional) weakness.

Astigmatism (Greek, *a* = not, *stigma* = point) A kind of refractive error when the point source of light can not be brought to a point focus on the retina. This is due to unequal refractive power of the two meridians of the eye.

It may be **compound astigmatism** (both the meridians myopic or hyperopic) or **mixed astigmatism** (one meridian myopic and other hyperopic) or **simple astigmatism** (one meridian myopic or hyperopic, the other being emmetropic). It may be **regular, oblique** or **irregular.**

Bifocals: A type of spectacle lenses which have two segments of different dioptric power. The upper segment is for distance and the lower segment for near fixation. It is usually prescribed in presbyopia, accommodative esotropia with convergence excess for near, and aphakes. It may also be used for divergence excess or convergence insufficiency exotropia. Trifocals, and multifocals are also used.

Binocular function: The ability of the two eyes to function simultaneously to add the field of vision have fusion and also perceive stereopsis (three-dimensional vision).

In the presence of ocular deviation binocular function causes diplopia.

Binocular Single Vision: Normal Binocular Single Vision (NBSV) is the ability of the two fovea to normally correspond with each other, simultaneously to have a normal range of fusion and stereopsis. This is also called **Bifoveal Single Vision.**

In the presence of squint with anomalous retinal correspondence, **Abnormal (anomalous) Binocular Single Vision** (ABSV) is possible, which is not bifoveal (it is foveal-extra foveal). This also has fusion and stereopsis but of a poorer quality.

Binocularity can be tested by using some form of dissociation of which the least dissociating are Bagolini's striated glasses, polaroid glasses and phase difference haploscope.

Blind spot mechanism (Swan's): This is an adaptive mechanism in esotropes of 12°–18° deviation, where the diplopia is avoided, because the point of regard falls on the blind spot in the deviating eye.

Brun's nystagmus: Nystagmus in both directions of gaze; vestibular in one direction and gaze paretic in the opposite direction, due to cerebellopontine angle lesions.

Caloric testing: Introduction of hot (44°C) or cold (30°C) water into the external ear canal to induce vestibular nystagmus.

COWS: Cold opposite warm same (fast component direction)

Centrad prism: A unit of prismatic power (*see* prism dioptre).

Cogwheeling (saccadic pursuit): Interruption of smooth pursuit movements by small saccades giving a jerky, uneven movement.

Concomitance, comitance (Latin, *con* = with, *comes* = companion).

This refers to a type of strabismus in which the deviation (relationship between the two eyes) remains the same in different directions of gaze. The strabismus is called **concomitant or comitant strabismus.**

Confusion is said to occur when the two fovea in a person with normal retinal correspondence have two different objects.

Conjugate movements (Latin, *con* = with, *jug* = yoke).

This refers to the yoked movements of the two eyes in the same direction (version) e.g.: dextro-version, laevo-version, sursum version, deorsum-version, Dextro-elevation, dextro-depression, laevo-elevation, laevo-depression.

Convergence (Latin, *con* = with, *vergere* = bend). This refers to the simultaneous movement of both eyes inwards (nasally). Convergence may be **voluntary** or **involuntary** (reflex). Involuntary convergence may be **tonic** (resting tone), **proximal** (due to the nearness of object), **accommodational** (associated with accommodative effort) and **fusional** (ability to align a tendency of exodeviation).

Convergence anomalies

C. insufficiency (deficiency): Difficulty in maintaining adequate convergence. This results in eyestrain on near work. This refers to week **fusional convergence** and can occur in exophoria orthophoria or even in esophoria. This is different from the convergence insufficiency type of exodeviation of Duane.

Convergence Sustenance: Inability of convergence to be maintained for an adequate length of time. Usually less than 30–40 seconds at near point of convergence (8–10 cm).

Convergence spasm: Overaction of the medial recti on both sides causing convergence excess deviation.

Contrast sensitivity: This refers to the reciprocal value of the least (lightest) distinguishable contrast (difference between light-dark band or letter and back ground).

The contrast (**Weber fraction**) for letters is defined as $(L_t - L_b)/L_b$, where L_t and L_b are the luminance of the target and background, respectively. The contrast for sine-wave gratings is (**Michelson contrast**) = $(L_{max} - L_{min})/(L_{max} + L_{min})$, where L_{max} and L_{min} are luminances of light and dark bands, respectively.

A plot of contrast sensitivity over a range of spatial frequencies gives the contrast sensitivity function. It shows a peak at intermediate spatial frequencies of 2–6 cycles/deg, with a rapid fall-off at higher spatial frequencies and a gradual decline at lower frequencies, under photopic conditions.

Arden's, Regan's and **Cambridge contrast sensitivity charts** use gratings and **Pelli-Robson** charts use letters.

Cover test: It is an objective test to confirm or exclude the possibility of a manifest squint (tropia). The apparently fixing (straight) eye is covered and the apparently deviating eye observed for its behaviour. A change of fixation of this eye confirms tropia.

This assumes that the deviating eye is not blind (can fixate), is not fixed due to paralysis or restriction, and does not have eccentric fixation.

It also helps in detecting latent nystagmus, and binocular diplopia.

Cover-uncover test: This is an objective test in which the behaviour of the eye is observed after removing the cover (which had dissociated the two eyes). This is to detect the presence of an heterophoria (latent strabismus), a tendency of deviation which becomes manifest on dissociation.

The basic presumptions of cover test should be kept in mind.

The cover-uncover test also provides information about the fusional status, depending on the ability of the deviated eye behind cover to have realignment.

- **Alternate cover test** is an extension of cover-uncover test in which the cover is rapidly alternated (switched) between the two eyes. It is helpful in quicker dissociation, but it cannot distinguish between a heterophoria and heterotropia on its own.
- **Prism Bar Cover Test** (PBCT) utilises this test to measure the deviation between the two eyes.
- **Distant Cover test:** This is a variant of cover test used in children who will not permit the occluder close to his face.

Correspondence: It is the relationship between the retinal points of the two eyes which share a common visual direction. Normally the fovea of the two eyes correspond with each other and share the common principal visual direction, this is called **Normal Retinal Correspondence** (NRC), or foveo-foveal retinal correspondence.

As an adaptation to a small angle constant deviation in early childhood, a correspondence develops between the fovea of one eye and an extra-foveal point of other eye (foveo-extra foveal) and is called **Anomalous Retinal correspondence** (ARC).

Apart from the fovea, each point of the retina corresponds with its fellow eye retinal points that share its visual direction. These are **corresponding points**. The **non-corresponding points** are called **disparate points**.

Crowding phenomenon: The phenomenon in which letters or optotypes displayed closely together are read with greater difficulty as compared to single optotypes. This difficulty in discrimination is due to the adjacent optotypes or their surrounds having less separation than the critical separation required. In normals this is 1.9 to 3.8 min of arc and in amblyopic eyes, this is 8.4 to 23.3 min of arc. Because of growing phenomenon, **single letter acuity** is better in amblyopes compared to **line-acuity.** This difference becomes less as amblyopia is treated.

Cycloparesis, Cycloplegia (Greek, *kyklos* = circle). Weakness of the ciliary muscle. Paresis refers to partial and plegia to total weakness.

Cyclodeviation, Cyclophoria, Cyclodeviation. This refers to a torsional deviation of the eyes, phoria (latent) and tropia (manifest). The nasal turning of the 12 o' clock corneal meridian is called **intorsion** or **incycloduction.** The outward turning of the 12 o' clock meridian is called **extorsion** or **excycloduction.**

Cycloversion: A simultaneous conjugate torsional movement of both eyes. Right eye extorsion and left eye intorsion is **dextrocycloversion.** The reverse of this is **laevocycloversion.**

Cyclovergence: A simultaneous disjugate movement of the two eyes, in opposite direction is called **cyclovergence.**
- **In-cyclovergence** (intorsion of both eyes)
- **Ex-cyclovergence** (extorsion of both eyes).

Cyclic squint, circadian or clock-work squint.

This refers to the manifestation of a squint at regular intervals of time. It may follow a 24–48 hour cycle. The esodeviation of a cyclic esotropia is present on squinting days, while on non-squinting days, there is no squint not even esophoria.

(**Note: Cyclic** term has been used in **three** different connotations: **ciliary body, torsion** and **periodic**).

Delta or inverted Y pattern: A type of horizontal squint in which the exodeviation is present in down gaze while upgaze and primary position is normal.

Deorsum refers to downward.

Deorsum version: Straight downgaze.

Deorso-adduction: Down gaze in adduction (the field of action of superior oblique)

Depressor: Refers to a muscle that moves the eyeball downwards, e.g. inferior rectus and superior oblique.

Dextro-version: A version movement in the right direction (right lateral rectus and left medial rectus action).

Dextro-depression: A version movement in the right and down ward direction (right inferior rectus and left superior oblique action).

Dextro-elevation: A version movement in the right side and upward direction (right superior rectus and left inferior oblique overaction).

Dextro-cycloversion: A torsional movement of right eye extorsion and left eye intorsion.

Diamond-pattern: A type of exodeviation present only in the primary position, up- and downgazes being normal.

Dioptre: A unit of measure of the power of a lens. It is equal to the inverse of the focal length in metres. A lens with a focal length of 1 m (100 cm) has a refractive power of 1 dioptre (D).

Dioptric: Refers to refractive changes (compare **catoptric** for reflective and **entoptic:** perception of contents within the eye).

Diplopia (Greek, *diplos* = double, *ops* = sec): Refers to an appreciation of two images of one object.

It may be **monocular** (due to astigmatism, subluxation of lens or optic nerve problems) or **binocular** (due to misalignment of visual axes.

Physiological diplopia occurs with the binocular single vision arid is appreciated as doubling (crossed diplopia) of a near object (bitemporal disparity) when a distant object is fixated; or doubling (uncrossed diplopia) of a distant object (binasal disparity) when a near object is fixated.

Pathological or binocular diplopia occurs when a squint occurs, and the object of regard is fixated by one fovea and stimulates an extra-foveal point **(disparate point)** of the other eye.

- An esodeviation has uncrossed diplopia (homonymous) due to stimulation of the nasal retina of other eye.
- An exodeviation has crossed diplopia **(heteronymous),** due to stimulation of the temporal retina of the other eye.

- In vertical squints the diplopia is vertical due to stimulation of upper or lower area of the retina.

Incongruous diplopia refers to the separation of images assessed subjectively not corresponding to the objective angle of squint (UHARC).

Paradoxic diplopia refers to a diplopia that is reverse of what is expected of a deviation, e.g. crossed diplopia in a convergent squint and uncrossed diplopia in a divergent squint.

A monocular diplopia or **binocular triplopia** is seen in some operated cases of anomalous retinal correspondence.

Disjugate, Disjunctive movements (Vergences): Movements of the two eyes in opposite directions to each other, e.g. convergence, divergence, vertical divergence and conclination (incyclovergence) and disclination (excyclovergence).

Doll's eye movements: Movement of eyes opposite to the direction in which the head is tilted or twined side to side, in the conscious patient when fixation is maintained and also in unconscious patient without fixation due to nonoptic reflexes.

Eccentric fixation: An uniocular condition in which some point of retina other than the fovea (central fixation) assumes fixation. The extra foveal eccentric point usurps the straight ahead gaze property and zero-retinomotor value of the fovea.

Eccentric viewing: An uniocular condition in which some extra-foveal point assumes fixation but does not have the property of straight ahead gaze, which is still with the fovea.

Electromyogram (EMG) recording of electrical activity of a muscle by introducing electrodes in side the muscle tissue.

Electronystagmogram (ENG): Recording of nystagmus in the eyes by recording the resting potential - change in the corneo-retinal potential which changes as the eye moves side to side, recording electrodes placed at medial and lateral canthi.

Electro-oculogram: Recording of eye movements by recording the change in the electrical activity at the lateral and medial canthi due to a moving eye. The eye acting as a **dipole,** corneal potential being positive relative to the retina which is negative.

Elevator: A muscle that moves the eyeball upwards, e.g. superior rectus and inferior oblique.

Emmetropia (Greek, *en* = within, *metron* = measure, *ops* = see): A normal refractive condition of the eyes in which parallel rays of light from infinity are brought to a focus at the retina, with the accommodation relaxed.

Enophthalmos (Greek, *en* = within, *ophthalmos* = eye): Posterior retraction of the eyeball in the orbit.

Esodeviation, esophoria, esotropia (Greek, *eso* = inner, *pherein* = bear, *trepein* = to turn). A nasal ward (convergent) deviation of the eyes. Such a latent tendency is **esophoria,** and a manifest convergent squint is **esotropia.**

Essential alternators: Cases of symmetrical freely alternating strabismus dating from early infancy (before 6 months) in which no neurological or accommodative factors is the cause and the potential for good binocular vision is poor. However, vision of each eye is good and equal.

Exodeviation, exophoria, exotropia (Greek *ex* - out, *pherein* = to bear, *trepein* = to turn). A lateral ward (divergent) deviation of the eyes. Such a latent tendency is exophoria and manifest deviation is exotropia.

Exophthalmos (Greek, *ex* = out, *ophthalmos* = eye): Anterior protrusion of the eyeball also called **proptosis.** Earlier the former term was restricted for active causes like endocrine dysfunction with the belief that it was due to the some active muscular contraction. This is not true and both terms can be used.

Extrinsic ocular muscle, Extra-ocular muscle: The six muscles which move the eyeball, *viz* the superior, inferior, medial and lateral recti and superior and inferior obliques. The levator palpebrae superioris is also sometimes included in extraocular muscles (EOM). (c.f. **Intrinsic ocular muscles).**

Facultative Suppression (see suppression) **Faden, Posterior fixation, Retroequatorial myopexy:** An operation in which fixation sutures are applied posterior to the functional equator to reduce the effective force of the muscle in and only in its field of action.

A recession can be combined with faden for a change of deviation in other positions.

Feedback, ocular: This refers to the outcome of position change that makes accuracy adjustments for short-term and calibrates the motoneuron output for long-term after an eye movement. Three potential ocular feedbacks are available.

- **Vision** — The retinal target discrepancy provides accuracy although with long latency.
- **Efference copy** or the corollary motoneuron discharge (from nucleus prepositus hypoglossi, NPH) which goes to the control centres.

- **Muscle proprioception.** Unlike typical skeletal muscle, the Golgi-type tendon organs, though described are not the primary sensor receptors (resection of muscle would lose them!) The palisade terminals are the main receptors, which are with distal myotendinous junction especially the global multiply innervated muscle fibres (these are not present in levator muscle).

Fixation: This refers to the ability to look at an object and maintain the gaze on it. To prevent retinal adaptation (Troxler's phenomenon) the eye drifts and refixates with microsaccades during a fixation, making fixation an active mechanism maintained by the **position maintenance system.**

Fixation types:
- **Central** or foveal fixation.
- **Eccentric**—parafoveal, paramacular, peripheral.
- **Wandering.**
- **No fixation**
- **Cross-fixation:** Foveal, but right eye for left field and left eye for right field.
- **Quinquipartite fixation** — a five part (compartment) fixation: Extreme right and left by the respective eyes, intermediate zone on each side by the opposite eye (cross fixation) and the central zone by either eye alternately.
- **Tripartite** fixation, a three parts fixation pattern: right side by left eye and left side by right eye and central part by either eye alternately.

Fixation disparity: Under binocular conditions a slight misalignment (disparity) of one fovea in relation to the other is still fused and seen as a single image. This disparity is in minutes of arc. The appreciation of a disparity by special tests (polaroid dissociation of fovea with fusion lock) is called the **associated phoria.** (c.f. dissociated phoria seen on cover-uncover test).

Fusion disparity: This term has been used interchangeably with fixation disparity by Jampolsky.

Forced Duction Test (FDT): A passive duction test conducted under topical anesthesia or general anesthesia to detect any restrictive limitation of movement, by using forceps to hold at the limbus, and moving the eye.

Exaggerated FDT has been described to test the restrictive element of oblique muscles, i.e. tight superior and inferior obliques.

Active Force Generation Test (AFGT) is a test in which the ability of the muscle to contract and generate a tug on the globe held by the forceps is felt. This detects whether the muscle is paretic or normal in the presence of limitation of movement by a restriction, and the power of the muscle.

Fusional convergence can mask an exodeviation into an exophoria and **Fusional divergence** can mask an esodeviation into an esophoria.

The **sensory fusion** refers to the cortical mechanism which blends the two images and **motor fusion** to the motor misalignment which can be withstood artificially.

Weak fusional reserves cause manifestation of a squint.

Fresnel prisms: Thin membrane prisms made of polyvinyl chloride with multiple small prisms etched on it. They are available for up to 30 prism dioptres but visual acuity becomes less above 12–14 pd.

Frenzel's glasses: High plus (+20 D) lenses used in looking for small magnitude nystagmus. Eliminat fixation and provide magnification.

Fusion refers to the ability of the two eyes to blend its images in spite of a motor misalignment.

Hering-Hillebrand deviation *see* Horopter.

Hering's law of motor correspondence, the yoke muscles (synergists) receive equal and synchronic innervarion for any particular eye movement.

Heterophoria (Greek, *heteros* = other, *pherein* = bear) or Latent strabismus: A tendency of the visual axes to deviate from the position of alignment.

Heterotropia: Manifest strabismus.

Hirschberg's test: A semiquantitative estimation of ocular deviation by observing the shift of corneal light reflex (1 mm = 5°–6°).

Horopter: It refers to an imaginary plane formed by joining the projection of all corresponding points of the retina at a fixed distance. It was referred to as the "horizon of vision" (boundary of vision) by Aguilonius.

Longitudinal horopter refers to the locus in space of object points imaged on "subjective longitudes" of the retina. It is the same as the horopter of horizontal correspondence.

Objects located on the horopter are seen as single and outside the horopter are seen as double. (But see Panum's area).

The **theoretical** or **geometric** horopter is a geometric construct of the corresponding points of the retina (Vieth-Muller circle). It is not the same as the longitudinal horopter in actual practice (also called empirical horopter). The latter is flatter. The difference or deviation is called the **Hering-Hille brand deviation.**

Horror fusionis refers to avoidance of bifoveal stimulation. It is a phenomenon described by Bielschowsky. It is seen on synoptophore as increase in deviation, called "chasing" by orthoptists. It has been considered as a etiologic factor of strabismus: "Purposive strabismus" (van der Hoeve).

Hyperacuity: Hyperacuity refers to certain types of visual function like **stereoacuity** and **Vernier acuity** which are finer than the resolution potential of the foveal cones (half minute = 30 seconds of arc), and are therefore called **hyper** (higher) **acuity.**

Hypermetropia, Hyperopia (Greek, *hyper* = over *metron* = measure, *ops* = eye): Refers to a refractive error in which parallel rays of light are brought to a focus behind the retina, with the relaxed accommodational mechanism. It is also called "Long Sightedness."

Hyperphoria, Hypertropia (Greek, *hyper* = over, *pherein* = bear, *trepein* = to turn): Refers to upward vertical deviation, *hyperphoria* is a *latent* upward vertical deviation (tendency) and *hypertropia,* a manifest upward deviation.

Hypophoria, hypotropia (Greek, *hypo* = under): Refers to a downward vertical deviation, phoria is a latent downward deviation and tropia a manifest downward deviation.

Hz, Hertz: Unit of frequency, cycles per second.

Incomitance (Latin, *in* = not, *comes* = companion): This refers to a squint which is not concomitant. The deviation in different gazes are different and there is a limitation of movement in one field of action. It may be **paralytic, restrictive** or **spastic.**

Incongruous diplopia (*see* diplopia).

Intermittent Squint: This refers to a squint which manifests at certain times and is controlled at other times or which manifests only for a particular fixation, distance.

Interpupillary distance (IPD): This is the distance between the two pupillary centres. This is approximately the same as the **interocular distance** (distance between the centres of rotation of the two eyes, when person is looking at far distance). For near fixation the IPD is less than the IOD. IPD determines the **vergence** required for near fixation. Average IPD = 60 mm (55 – 65 mm).

Intrinsic ocular muscles: The muscles inside the eyeball, namely sphincter pupillae, dilator pupillae and the ciliary muscles.

Iso ametropia: Equal refractive error in the two eyes.

Jaeger test types: Refer to reading test type introduced by Jaeger. They are not regularly arranged in definite octave difference. The Times Roman or N-types are commonly used.

Krimsky test: Prism neutralization of the ocular deviation by centering the corneal light reflex in cases which do not have central fixation, light perception or ability to move the eye. It is also called Prism Reflection Test.

Laevo-version: Left sided horizontal movement of eyes.

Laevo-depressor: Left ward and downward movement of eyes.

Laevo-elevation: Left sided and upward movement of eyes.

Length-tension curves: These are plots of the tension in the muscles for each length (stretch, seen in different gazes) for an effort as seen by the movement of the other eye. A muscle is strengthened by raising its length tension curve (advancement or resection) and weakened by lowering its length tension curve (recession, myotomy expander) (see muscle physiology chapter for details).

Macropsia, Micropsia, Metamorphosia: Distortion of retinal images, macro = larger, micro = smaller and metamorphopsia = irregular.

Miosis (Greek, *myein* = to shut) constriction of pupil.

Mydriasis: Dilatation of pupil.

Myectomy (Greek, *myo* = muscle, *ex* = out, *tomy* = to cut): This refers to removal of a part of the muscle. (**Myomectomy** is a misnomer).

The removal of **entire** muscle is called **extirpation.** These are weakening procedures.

Myopia: A refractive error in which the parallel rays of light are focussed in front of the retina, with the relaxed accommodation.

Myotomy: This refers to cutting a muscle (but **not** removing any part of it) like **marginal myotomy.** It is a weakening procedure.

Near test types: These are optotypes used for testing the near vision, e.g. Reduced Snellen, M. units, jaeger types, Times Roman or N types, etc. They are usually tested at 35 cm or 40 cm.

Normal Retinal Correspondence: *See* correspondence.

Nystagmus (Greek, *nustadzein* = to nod): A regular, rhythmic to and fro oscillation of the eyes. It may be **Pendular or Jerk or Mixed.** It may be **latent, manifest-latent** or **manifest.** Acquired nystagmus may have specific pattern and usually an underlying neurological cause.

Occlusion: A specialised way of covering an eye for a particular period of time to prevent or reduce visual stimulation of one eye and relatively stimulate the other. It acts by stimulating **form vision** and preventing **abnormal binocular interaction.** Other diagnostic uses of occlusion are also known.

Occlusion may be **total** or **partial** (depending on transparency of the patch). It may be **constant** or **part-time** (depending on the duration of the patch). It may be **conventional** (dominant eye patched) or **inverse** (amblyopic or eccentric fixation eye patched). Various types of **occluders** are known.

Ocular Movements, Eye Movements: These are described as **Voluntary, Command** or **Reflex** eye movements. There are six types of eye movement systems:

1. Saccadic (Fast eye movement).
2. Pursuit (Smooth eye tracking).
3. Vergence.
4. Vestibular and tonic neck reflexes.
5. Position maintenance or fixation.
6. Optokinetic eye movement.

Ocular movements are also described as **ductions** (uniocular) versions (binocular conjugate) and vergence (binocular disjugate). And also a **horizontal, vertical** or **torsional.**

Orthophoria: An ocular posture which has no latent deviation on cover-uncover test at near or distance fixation. This is the perfect state of ocular motor equilibrium. The ideal goal of strabismus surgery.

Orthoptics: This refers to the diagnostic methods in the detection and quantification of ocular deviation and anomalies of binocular vision and the therapeutic methods in the maintenance and restoration of (normal comfortable binocular single vision (bifoveal). This **excludes** optical, medical and surgical procedures.

Paralysis, paresis, plegia: The **underaction** or weak action of muscle is termed **paresis** when it is partial and **paralysis** when it is complete. Plegia is usually used as a suffix for paralysis.

Past pointing (False projection): This refers to the false **localization** of an object in space beyond its actual **location** due to faulty sense of neuromuscular effort.

Physiological diplopia, Pathological diplopia: *See* diplopia.

Phoria: An abbreviation of heterophoria in common usage.

Presbyopia (Greek, *presbys* = old age, ops = to *see*): Age-related decline in accommodational ability causing difficulty in reading fine print at normal reading distance (35–40 cm). It usually occurs between 40 and 45 years, earlier in tropical and equatorial areas.

Principal Visual Direction: This is the line of fixation from the fovea to the point of regard. It is independent of the position of the eye in the orbit or the fixation object in relation to the body. Each eye thus has its own principal visual direction and under binocular conditions, a **common principal visual direction,** a line in between the two centres at the median point between the eyes, is present. Objects on the two principal visual direction are seen superimposed though located separately in space.

Prism: A wedge shaped lens (piece of glass, plastic or any refractive material), which deflects the light rays towards its base. The amount of deflection depends on the relative difference of the refractive index of the two media and the angle between the two refractive surfaces of the prism.

Prism dioptre (pd) is the unit of measurement of the deflection of light rays caused by a **prism.** One prism dioptre is the power of a prism that deflects the rays of light at a distance of one metre by one centimeter. One pd is equal to half degree (4/7th of a degree). Being measured on a tangent, at longer distances, the units of prism dioptres are not equal, therefore another unit is described: **centrad prism,** in which the units are measured on the circular arc at 1 metre distance.

PBCT, Prism bar cover test: *See* cover test **Prism Reflection Test:** *See* Krimsky test.

Proprioception: *See* Feedback, ocular.

Pseudomyopia: Artificially induced myopia due to accommodational spasm, a result of retinoscopy done without proper cycloplegia.

Pseudostrabismus: Apparent squint. An appearance of squint when no manifest deviation (misalignment of visual axes) exists. This may be due to a large positive angle kappa **(Pseudoexotropia),** a negative angle kappa, epicanthus, telecanthus (all causing pseudo- esotropia. Hypertelorism and euryblepharon (long palpebral aperture) may cause pseudo-exotropia. An ectopic macula (ROP) also can cause pseudostrabismus, usually pseudoexotropia.

Ptosis: Drooping of the upper eyelid, due to weakness of levator or mechanical factors.

Purposive strabismus: A squint that serves a purpose, like increased deviation to avoid diplopia.

Recession, retroplacement: An operation in which the muscle is re-inserted at a point nearer to its origin (posterior for recti muscles). This slackens the muscle, shifting it on a lower length tension curve and so weakens the muscle.

Refractive error, Ametropia: An ocular condition in which the parallel rays of light (from infinity) do not meet at the retina, with the accommodational mechanism relaxed, e.g. hyperopia, myopia and astigmatism.

Resection: An operation in which a part of the muscle (distal fibrotendinous part) is excised decreasing its effective length and thus stretching it, lifting on a higher length tension curve, strengthening the muscle. If more than 20–25% of a muscle is excised it may actually weaken the muscle.

Retinal Rivalry, Foveal rivalry, Cortical rivalry: An active competition at the level of cortex, whereby one of the two dissimilar images on fovea or corresponding points is not appreciated at certain times and is appreciated at other times.

Separation difficulty: *See* crowding phenomenon.

Simultaneous perception: The ability of the corresponding points of the retina to perceive both the images simultaneously. This is the basic requirement for any fusion to be elicited. For testing simultaneous perception, dissimilar images are used. These are of different sizes: for simultaneous **foveal** perception it is up to 1°, for simultaneous **parafoveal** perception it is 1°–3° size, for simultaneous **macular** perception it is 3°–5°, and for simultaneous para macular perception it is more than 5°. (Because of dissimilar images SP may not be elicited while fusion is elicited.)

Synoptophore slides: Slides are used for simultaneous perception (dissimilar images) fusion slides (similar images with monocular controls), stereopsis slides (similar images with some parts dissimilar causing nasal/temporal disparity). Slides may test foveal, parafoveal (1°–3°), macular (3°–5°) para macular areas (more than 5°). Special slides for angle kappa, after images aniseikonia, torsion are also available.

Stereopsis, stereoscopy (Greek, *stereos* = solid, skopein, *ops* = to see): The binocular ability to fuse similar images with some parts slightly disparate, producing appreciation of depth. Monocular clues may give a 3-D effect but not true stereopsis.

It is one of the **hyperacuity** and is measured in seconds of arc. Normal stereoacuity in adults is finer than 40 arc seconds, usually up to 16–20 arc seconds.

It can be tested by real depth instruments **(Frisby)**, two-2 dimensional vectographic images **(Randot, litmus, TNO)** or by panography **(Lang's stereotest)**. It may be tested for near and distance both.

Strabismus, Squint (Greek **strabos** = crooked) refers to an ocular condition in which the visual axes of the two eyes do not meet at the point of regard (misalignment of visual axes).

Strabismus fixus (Convergens or divergens): A musculofascial anomaly in which the eyes are "anchored" in a fixed position, convergent or divergent, rarely vertical.

Strabismus surso-adductorius: A strabismus in which hypertropia of the eye in adduction and upward movement (sursum—adduction) is seen. It is due to primary inferior oblique overaction.

Suppression: A condition in which the image formed upon one of the retina is not perceived. It is partially or completely ignored or neglected from cortical perception. It may be **physiological** as in **binocular single vision** in avoiding physiological diplopia, cortical rivalry or the neglect of peripheral field. Or it may be **pathological** in the presence of a manifest deviation, this is in two forms:

a. **Suppression of fovea of the deviating eye** (avoidance of confusion), Harm's scotoma, and

b. Suppression of the double image at the extra-foveal area of the deviating eye (diplopia point scotoma). Such scotomata can be charted with perimetry under binocular conditions. (Polaroid Scotometer, Synoptophore, Lees' screen, etc.).

Suppression may be **facultative** (operative under certain conditions only and disappears when the dominant eye is occluded, or **obligatory** (operative under all conditions, persisting even when the dominant eye is occluded — responsible for amblyopia).

Synergist, agonists muscles that work together for a particular action.

Sursum version: Straight upwards movement.

Sursum-adduction or surso-adduction: Upwards in adduction.

Sursum-abduction: Upwards in abduction: An operation in which the tendon is cut and a part excised. It may be **partial** (partial width) or **total** (full width).

Tenotomy (Greek, *teno* = tendon, *temnein* = to cut): An operation in which the tendon is cut.

Times Roman Test Types: A standard type of Near vision test types numbered N-3 to N-48 based on "point" (one point = 1/72 part of inch) size of the printing fonts.

Torsion: *See* cyclodeviation.

Triplopia: Appreciation of three images of an object seen binocularly or monocularly.

Vergences: *See* disjugate movements.

Vernier Acuity: A type of hyperacuity in which the **minimum separable,** or the ability to defect minimal differences in the horizontal alignment of two vertical lines is estimated. It is observed to be 2–10 seconds of arc in normal subjects. It is affected in amblyopia and appears to be a better test to screen amblyopia in infants, compared to **grating acuity** (vision charted by using gratings as optotypes). It can be tested on oscilloscope or in the preferential looking, Acuity card, format.

Versions: *See* conjugate movements.

Vision, visual acuity: The ability to test the minimum resolvable **(grating acuity)** the minimum recognisable **(recognition acuity** on Snellen's charts) and the minimum detectable (Catford's test) by using suitable optotypes. Optotypes may be in rows, line or with surround **(Line acuity)** or single **(single optotype acuity)** to detect crowding phenomenon.

Visual acuity may be charted at 6 m **(Snellen's),** 4 m (ETDRS, **Bailie-Lovie charts)** or for near at 33, 35 or 40 cm (Jaeger, Times Roman, M. Charts)

"V" phenomenon, V pattern: A type of horizontal squint in which the divergence is more in upgaze relative to the downgaze or primary position.

"X" phenomenon, "X" pattern: A type of horizontal squint in which the relative divergence is more, both for up- and downgazes compared to primary position.

"Y"-pattern: A type of horizontal squint in which the relative divergence is increased in upgaze whereas it is the same for downgaze and primary position.

Zero retinomotor value: Each point of the retina other than the fovea has a retino-motor value, indicating its urge to switch fixation to the fovea. The fovea itself has zero-retinomotor value and thus has central fixation. In case of eccentric fixation the eccentric point has the zero retinomotor value.

Index